ADVANCE PRAISE FOR KETOGENIC BODYBUILDING

"Sikes cuts through all the bro science and urban myths surrounding the keto diet to give you the real talk. He knows of which he speaks and walks the walk, having used his keto knowledge to earn his pro card and coach countless clients on the subject. This book covers everything from mindset to any nutritional question you could have about ketogenic bodybuilding. This is the Bible of ketogenic bodybuilding."

-Marcus Aurelius Anderson, mindset coach to elite CEOs, leaders and entrepreneurs, author of *The Gift of Adversity*, TEDx and international keynote speaker and host of *Acta Non Verba* podcast

"*Ketogenic Bodybuilding* is truly the only comprehensive guide you will ever need to optimize the keto diet to transform your body, especially for those competing in the sport of bodybuilding. Robert's passion for natural bodybuilding and the keto diet really comes through in this book and his personal story resonated with me on many levels. He used bodybuilding and ketogenic nutrition to not only transform his body, but to overcome personal struggles, disordered eating, and to instill a growth mindset to excel in business. The ketogenic diet has sharpened his mind to educate others on these topics. This book is a beacon of light to those that are confused about how to implement a keto diet for bodybuilding and gives readers a step-by-step plan. If you are a competitive bodybuilder, fitness model, fitness coach or just someone seeking to optimize body composition and overall metabolic health, this book is for you!"

> -Dominic D'Agostino, PhD, associate professor in the department of molecular pharmacology and physiology at USF Morsani College of Medicine

"When it comes to the nuances of cutting on the ketogenic diet, especially getting to stage-level leanness, Sikes is the one coach everyone thinks about."

> -Nsima Inyang, bodybuilder and co-host of *Mark Bell's Power Project* podcast

"Finally, a keto resource for bodybuilders! Sikes is an expert when it comes to prepping bodybuilders and physique athletes using a ketogenic diet. *Ketogenic Bodybuilding* provides you with insights into Sikes's own nutrition, training and mindset so that you can achieve your goal physique using a ketogenic diet."

> -Chris Irvin, MS, CMO of BioCoach

"When it comes to ketogenic bodybuilding, Sikes is the world's number one expert on the topic. He's got years of experience under his belt and has proven the effectiveness of his methods with results. Being an outlier and a contrarian in the field of bodybuilding, he doesn't shy away from challenging the status quo and is expanding the collective consciousness of what we know about muscle growth.

The book is an absolute gem for anyone interested in living the keto lifestyle while simultaneously getting after their dream physique."

-Siim Land, bestselling author, speaker and consultant

"Robert Sikes is a force to be reckoned with in the world of ketogenic bodybuilding and competition prep! His tried-and-true ketogenic approach has proven itself very effective for countless competitors, myself among them. Utilizing his program, I was able to win my 'pro card' and several other top three placings at natural bodybuilding competitions in 2021! His attention to detail is like no other. I highly recommend this book!"

-Greg Mahler, natural pro men's physique athlete

"Sikes has truly mastered the art and science of preserving muscle while burning fat on a ketogenic diet. If you follow the seven phases in *Ketogenic Bodybuilding*, you'll get stage-ready without experiencing the drastic post-contest weight gain that's common when adhering to mainstream cutting regimes."

-Mike Mutzel, MS, founder/CEO of Myoxscience

"Robert Sikes, the Keto Savage, is a fat melting wizard! I have worked with Robert to prep for two shows now and as much as I initially sought out his coaching for his expertise and knowledge around bodybuilding and the ketogenic diet, I have been absolutely blown away by his ability to perfectly adjust macros to melt away fat while maintaining muscle and hormonal health! I trust him implicitly and would more than recommend his book to anyone looking to use a ketogenic diet to prep for a show. I look forward to having him coach me again in the future!"

-Jen Pittaro, natural pro figure athlete

"*Ketogenic Bodybuilding* leaves no stone unturned. Robert Sikes has brilliantly broken down every step of the process for proven results. No detail was left out and you can feel his passion, warmth and humor along the way. As a doctor, it is important to me that athletes don't sacrifice long-term health for short-term gains. This book will change the world of natural bodybuilding for so many competitors."

-Dr. Jaime Seeman, Doctor Fit and Fabulous

"*Ketogenic Bodybuilding* is by far the most comprehensive book that exists on ketogenic nutrition and building muscle intelligently and sustainably. It is unapologetic and innovative. I recommend putting this book in the hands of athletes and coaches as quickly as possible so they can avoid many of the pitfalls I see people experience when trying to mix and match traditional methods with a ketogenic diet."

-Danny Vega, MS, CEO at Fat Fueled Family

"Never before has there existed an exhaustive and authoritative ketogenic bodybuilding guide like this. Finally, there is a clear cut, how-to manual that will show you how to get leaner with more muscle and avoid the pitfalls in the process. My highest recommendation."

-Shawn Wells, MPH, RD, LDN, CISSN, FISSN, author of the bestselling *The ENERGY Formula*, biochemist, dietitian, formulator and ketogenic lifestyle proponent

"Robert Sikes is the godfather of bodybuilding on a ketogenic diet, and this book is a goldmine of information. If you want to take your physique to the next level and do it the healthiest way possible, you need to read this book front to back."

-Jason Wittrock, fitness coach

"I always believed that if you wanted to get stage-ready, you had to suffer through low libido and other hormonal issues following a traditional bodybuilding diet of chicken, broccoli and rice. Robert Sikes broke that mold. He has the knowledge, track record and physique to prove that a keto diet works for bodybuilders."

-Andrew Zaragoza, co-host and producer of *Mark Bell's Power Project* podcast

A NATURAL ATHLETE'S GUIDE TO COMPETITIVE SAVAGERY

KETOGENIC BODYBUILDING

ROBERT SIKES

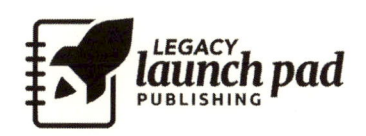

LEGACY
launch pad
PUBLISHING

Copyright © 2022 Robert Orion Sikes.

All rights reserved.

No part of this book may be reproduced in any form or by any electronic or mechanical means, including information storage and retrieval systems, without written permission from the author, except for the use of brief quotations in a book review:

ISBN: 978-1-956955-10-1 (ebook)

ISBN: 978-1-956955-07-1 (paperback)

ISBN: 978-1-956955-09-5 (hardback)

DISCLAIMER

I don't have any acronyms after my name—no MDs or PhDs. For some of you, that may entirely discredit everything that follows. Without a formal credential, how could I possibly speak on nutrition and body recomposition?

To that point, one of my biggest frustrations has been the utter division and malice within the nutritional and fitness communities lately. It has amplified considerably since the introduction of the internet and social media where everyone has a voice.

It happens on all sides. Everyone with a decent physique feels qualified to contribute their two cents. Every doctor or physician turns their nose up at anyone without a formal educational background. Studies get published left and right, but they seem to create more confusion than clarity. People cherry-pick studies to support their claims and back their arguments. I know people on both sides of the spectrum and everywhere in between.

This war doesn't just rage between those with formal schooling and those without. It exists within many of the same peer groups—doctors against doctors, influencers against influencers, athletes against athletes. You've got the vegans against the carnivores and the flexible dieters against the keto groups. Where does it end?

I don't know. I don't know where, when or how all this division will disappear. I don't like dealing in absolutes, and I'm not naive enough to suggest that the ketogenic diet is the best for everyone. In short, the best diet is the one most sustainable for you. That might seem like a cop-out, but it's true. Ideally, you should follow a nutritional protocol that you can adhere to long-term and create a lifestyle around. It should also improve your health and optimize your performance as well.

It just so happens that for me and so many others that optimal diet is the ketogenic diet.

Some come to keto because they can't control their binging tendencies with processed carbohydrates and sugars. Some come as a way of controlling their blood sugar and regulating their insulin. Some come with a focus on single-ingredient, wholesome foods they procure themselves through hunting or gardening, and others come because it's relatively easy, and they like the taste of bacon more than rice. Whatever the reason, it's impossible to ignore the ever-growing demographic of people discovering tremendous success following a ketogenic diet and lifestyle.

My motivation for writing this book stems from my love for the sport of bodybuilding and my passion for this diet. This diet liberated me from disordered eating tendencies and allowed me to discover true health. Leveraging the keto diet to excel in a sport traditionally viewed as requiring carbohydrates has been my major focus.

The principles I've outlined in this book aren't based on epidemiological studies, rat models or randomized controlled experiments. That's not to say that those experiments haven't been done; they just aren't my area of expertise. I'm a practitioner of what I preach—a "boots on the ground" kind of guy. This book is based on the very protocol that has worked incredibly well for me and the clients I've coached over the years.

As of this writing, my client list comprises well over 500 individuals—actual people living their day-to-day lives. They are people like you and me, not patients in a metabolic ward study or mice in a control group. These principles have worked exceedingly well for them, and they have the potential to work incredibly well for you.

Whether you find success with the principles outlined herein or move on to something completely different, I ask of you one simple favor:

Don't contribute to the negativity that runs rampant out there. Be a light in the sea of darkness. Be brave enough to speak your mind and share your thoughts but rational enough to know that there are many different ways of doing anything in life, especially nutrition! Be receptive to others views and keep an open mind. With that said, I hope this book helps you find the success you're looking for.

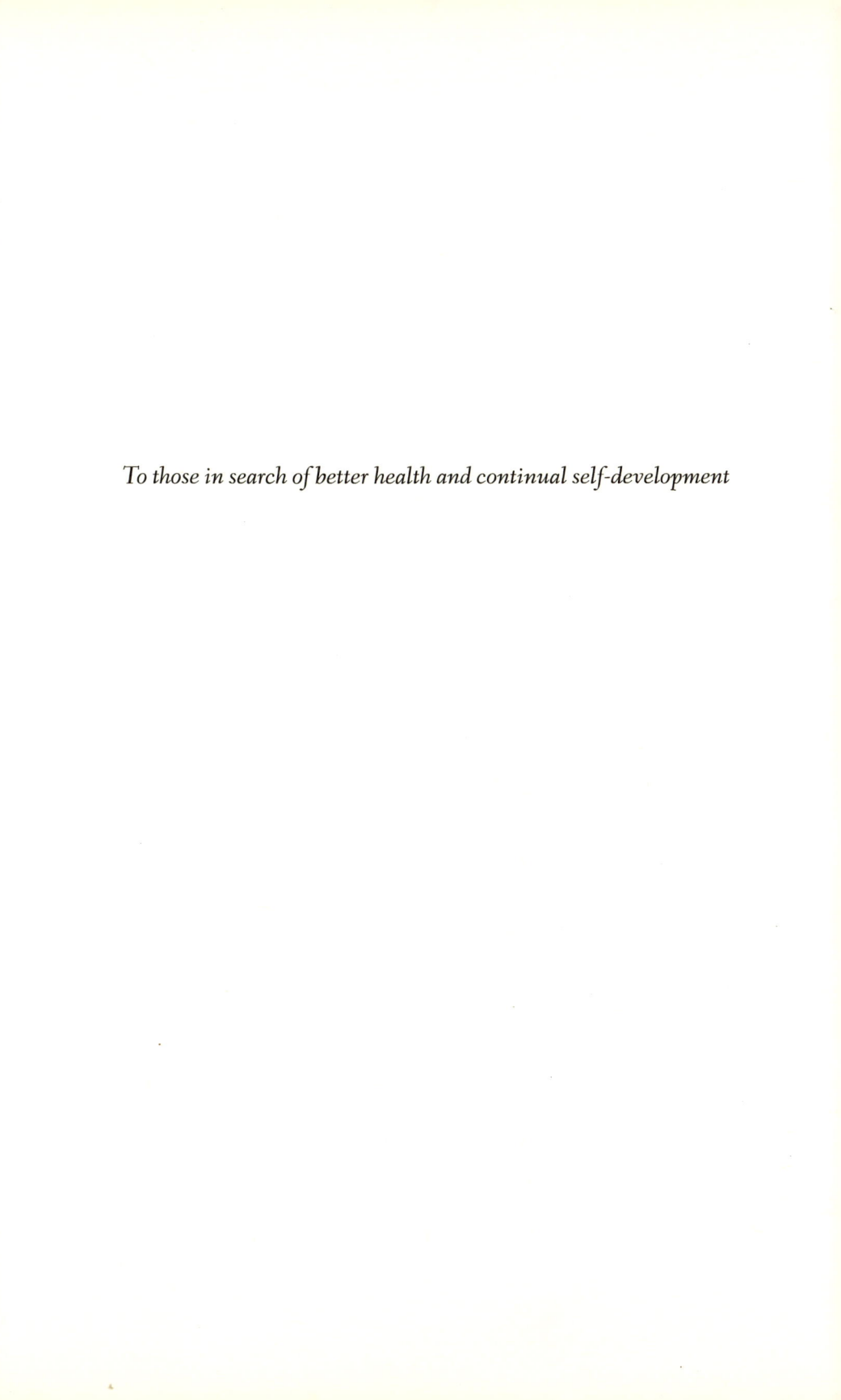

To those in search of better health and continual self-development

DOWNLOAD MY FREE COMPANION GUIDE

CONTENTS

ADVANCE PRAISE FOR KETOGENIC BODYBUILDING	1
Disclaimer	9
Download My Free Companion Guide	15
Introduction: Why Bodybuilding?	27

PART 1
PRELIMINARY GROUNDWORK

PREP FOR PREP	37
Psychological Prep for Prep	37
Technical Prep for Prep	42
Choosing a Show	50
Time Frame	50
Location	51
Choosing a Federation	52
Relationship With Food	53
Hormones	55
Overview	56
Guidelines and Keto-Specific Guidelines	58
Meal Frequency	58
Pre and Post Workout	60
Extended Fasting	62
Intermittent Fasting (IF)	62
Meal Preparation	64
Managing Willpower	66
Nutrient Density	66
Total Carbs vs. Net Carbs	69
Grass-Fed vs. Grain-Fed Meat	70
Fats and Sweeteners	71
Alcohol	73
Refeeds and Diet Breaks	74
The Keto Brick	76

PART 2
THE PREP

1. **PHASE ONE: ESTABLISH YOUR BASELINE** — 81
   - Weighing In — 83
   - Body Fat Percentage — 84
   - Ideal Body Fat Percentage — 86
   - Energy Balance and Starting Calories — 88
   - Calculations — 90
   - Activity Multiplier Guide — 95
   - How Long Should You Prep? — 103
   - Starting Caloric Intake — 106
   - Starting Macronutrients — 108
   - Standardize Before You Optimize — 112
   - Meal Examples — 115
   - Macro Ratios — 120
   - Fat — 121
   - Protein — 123
   - Carbohydrates — 124
   - Training Baseline — 125
   - Why Less Is More with Cardio — 126
   - Bloodwork — 128
   - Basic Lipid Panel — 129
   - C-Reactive Protein — 130
   - Thyroid Panel — 131
   - Hormone Panel — 131
   - Mindset — 133

2. **PHASE TWO: ESTABLISH YOUR PROTEIN THRESHOLD** — 136
   - Phase Two Objectives — 138
   - Phase Two Guidelines — 140
   - Increase Protein — 141
   - Decrease Fat — 142
   - Week By Week — 142
   - Tracking Metrics — 143
   - Protein Threshold Indicators — 146
   - Pattern Recognition — 147
   - Phase Two Mindset — 148

3. **PHASE THREE: TAPERING MACROS**   151
   Phase Three Objectives   152
   Phase Three Guidelines   154
   Decrease Protein   155
   Decreasing Dietary Fat   156
   Decreasing Dietary Carbohydrates   156
   Hold Macros Constant   157
   Meal Prep and Nutrient Density   157
   Meal Frequency   158
   Increase Cardio   160
   Resistance Training   163
   Tracking Metrics   165
   Concluding Phase Three   166
   Phase Three Mindset   168

4. **PHASE FOUR: INTRODUCING KETOGENIC REFEEDS**   170
   Phase Four Guidelines   172
   Dialing In Electrolytes   174
   Tracking Sodium, Potassium and Fluid Levels   177
   Minimize Veggies   178
   Calculate Refeed   178
   Best Practices   181
   Proper Electrolyte Manipulation   182
   Notes on Equilibriums   183
   Sodium Loading   185
   Potassium Loading   186
   Analyze Refeed Impact   187
   Further Manipulations   189
   Changes to Training   192
   Phase Four Mindset   193

5. **PHASE FIVE: PEAK WEEK AND SHOW DAY**   196
   Setting Expectations   197
   Phase Five Guidelines   200
   Traditional Peak Week   201
   Peak Week (Carbs, Water and Electrolytes)   201
   Peak Week Refeed Meal   205
   Peak Week Training Manipulations   208

Peak Week Cardio Manipulations	211
Peak Week Posing	213
Peak Week Stress	215
Travel Stress	218
Fear of the Unknown During Peak Week	220
Putting It All Together	221
Show Day	227
Morning of the Show	227
Show Day Nutrition	229
Show Day Routine and Training	232
Posing Onstage	235
Show Day Stress	236
Show Day Placings and Awards	238
After the Awards	239
The Day After	242
Phase Five Mindset	243
6. PHASE SIX: REVERSE DIET REFEEDS	**246**
Phase Six Objectives	247
Why Is Reverse Dieting Necessary in the First Place?	249
Have a Plan or Plan to Fail—There Is No "Finish Line"	251
Phase Six Guidelines	254
Raise Protein	255
Reverse Protein Threshold	256
Continuation of Refeeds	257
Rate of Increase	259
Metabolic Set Point	260
Reverse Diet Training	262
Phase Six Mindset	264
7. PHASE SEVEN: REVERSE DIET BASELINE AND BEYOND	**267**
Phase Seven Guidelines	269
Phase Out Refeeds	270
Increase Total Caloric Intake	270
Monitor Body Composition and Strength Progression	272

Training Adjustments	274
Cardio Adjustments	276
Don't Jump Right into Another Prep	277
Phase Seven Mindset	280
Afterword	285

PART 3
APPENDICES

Overview	289
1. NUTRITIONAL OVERVIEW AND OBJECTIVES APPENDIX	291
Meal Prep Basics	291
Grocery List	294
Fat Sources:	294
Protein Sources:	295
Vegetables:	295
Recipes	296
Zero Carb Meat Pancake	298
"Fathead" Pizza	300
Frittata	302
Organ Meat Burger	304
Baked Salmon	306
Buffalo Bacon Burger-Bites	308
Sweet and Simple Chaffle	310
Chicken Piccata	312
Drink Recipes	313
Keto Coffee	314
Keto Tea	314
Broth Drinks	314
Electrolyte Drinks	314
Carbonated Drinks	315
Hunger Hacks	315
Shirataki Noodles and Rice	316
Kelp Noodles	317
Eggs	317
Zero Calorie "Snow Cones"	318

Ready-to-Eat Foods	318
Keto Brick	319
Canned Sardines/Oysters	319
Parm Crisps	319
Meat Sticks	320
Pili Nuts	320
Pork Rinds	320
Post-Show Celebratory Meal	321
2. POSING AND JUDGING APPENDIX	323
Posing and Judging Criteria Overview	323
Women's Bikini	324
Competition Attire	324
Rounds Scored	324
Round 1: Fitness and Balance	324
Round 2: Physical Appearance	325
Face Front	326
Quarter Turn to the Right	328
Face Back of the Stage	330
Quarter Turn to the Tight	331
Front and Back Stage Walk	331
Scoring Each Round	332
Women's Figure	332
Competition Attire	332
Rounds Scored	333
Round 1: Symmetry	333
Round 2: Muscle Tone	333
Posing Execution	333
Face Front	334
Side Pose	336
Rear Pose	338
Presentation and Stage Walk	339
Overall Stage Presence	339
Prejudging Walk	339
Scoring Each Round	340
Men's Physique	340
Competition Attire	341
Rounds Scored	341
Round 1: Symmetry and Muscle Tone	341

Round 2: Presentation	341
Posing Execution	341
Front Pose	342
Side Poses	344
Back Pose	346
Individual Stage Walk	347
Scoring Each Round	347
Men's Bodybuilding	348
Competition Attire	348
Rounds Judged	348
Round 1: Symmetry	348
Round 2: Muscularity and Conditioning	348
Posing Execution	349
Symmetry Poses	350
Front Relaxed	350
Side Relaxed	351
Rear Relaxed	352
Side Relaxed, Opposite Side	353
Mandatory Muscular Poses	354
Front Double Biceps	354
Side Triceps	355
Abdominal and Thighs	356
Front Lat Spread	357
Rear Double Biceps	358
Hands-On Hips Most Muscular	359
Side Chest	360
Rear Lat Spread	361
Crab Most Muscular	362
Scoring Each Round	362
Men's Classic Physique	363
Competition Attire	364
Mandatory Poses	364
Front Double Biceps	365
Side Chest	366
Back Double Biceps	367
Abdominal and Thighs	368
Favorite Classic Pose (not Most Muscular, Vacuum Pose pictured below)	369

3. EXERCISE APPENDIX — 370
- Exercise Appendix Overview — 370
- Resistance Training — 370
- Cardio — 371
- Progressive Overload — 372
- Intensity — 372
- Volume — 372
- Frequency — 373
- How to Manipulate These Variables — 373
- Training for Keto — 375
- Advanced Training Techniques — 376
- Muscle Failure — 376
- Supersets — 376
- Giant Sets — 377
- Pyramid Sets — 377
- Drop Sets — 378
- Negatives — 378
- Forced Reps — 379
- Time Under Tension — 379
- Partial Reps — 380
- Yeah, Yeah—But What Should *I Do*? — 381
- Tracking Your Training — 382
- Deload Weeks — 385
- Adaptations to Training Over Time — 386
- Changes to Resistance Training Throughout Prep — 387
- Changes to Cardio Throughout Prep — 388
- My Training and Cardio Routine — 389
- Day 1: Squat Day — 390
- Day 2: Heavy Delts | Hypertrophy Back — 390
- Day 3: Heavy Triceps | Hypertrophy Chest — 391
- Day 4: Rest Day — 391
- Day 5: Heavy Back | Hypertrophy Biceps — 391
- Day 6: High Volume Legs — 392
- Day 7: Heavy Chest | Hypertrophy Delts — 392
- Day 8: Rest Day — 392
- Additional Work — 392
- Sample Cardio Progression Plan — 393

4. SUPPLEMENTS APPENDIX — 395

- Overview — 395
- Electrolytes — 396
- Sodium — 396
- Potassium — 397
- Magnesium — 398
- Calcium — 398
- Electrolyte Blends — 398
- Iodine — 399
- Vitamin D and K2 — 399
- Fish Oil and Omega-3 Fatty Acids — 400
- Creatine — 400
- Caffeine — 402
- Keto Bricks — 402
- Pre-Workout Drinks — 403
- Whey Protein, BCAAS and EAAS — 404
- Exogenous Ketones — 405
- Fat Burners and Diuretics — 407
- Steroids and Other Super Supplements — 407
- Banned Substances — 409
- INBF/WNBF Banned Substance List (as of Writing) — 409
- Testosterone — 411
- Growth Hormones and Peptides — 411
- Anabolic Agents, Pro-Hormones, Precursors and Metabolites, Derivatives and Related Compounds — 412
- Designer and Pro Steroids — 412
- Hormonal Precursors and Their Metabolites and Isomers — 413
- Pro-Hormonal Fat Burning Supplements — 413
- Fat Burning Pro-Hormone Derivatives — 414
- Prescription Thyroid Hormone Medication — 414
- Prescription Diuretics and Masking Agents — 414
- Clenbuterol — 415
- GHB — 416
- Miscellaneous — 416
- Other Anabolic Agents, Hormones and Metabolic Modulators — 416

    Ephedrine, Ephedra and Stimulants 418
    DMAA and Related Compounds 418
    WADA Banned Stimulant List 419
    Psychomotor Stimulants 419
    Cannabinoids & CBDs 419

5. MISCELLANEOUS APPENDIX 421
    Posing Suits and Trunks 421
    Hair Removal 422
    Hair Removal Techniques 423
    Tanning 424
    Tanning Beds and Sun Exposure 425
    Spray Tan 426
    Dream Tan 428
    ProTan and Jan Tana 429
    Hair and Makeup 429
    Travel 430
    Competition Music 432
    Competitor Check-In 432
    Competitor Weigh-In 433
    Weight Classes (5) – Men's Amateur Bodybuilding 433
    Bantamweight 433
    Lightweight 434
    Middleweight 434
    Light Heavyweight 434
    Heavyweight 434
    Weight Classes (3) – Men's Amateur Bodybuilding 434
    Lightweight 434
    Middleweight 434
    Heavyweight 434
    Drug Testing 435
    Running Format 437
    Stage Presence 438
    Back-to-Back Shows 439

Acknowledgments 443
About the Author 447

INTRODUCTION: WHY BODYBUILDING?

Why bodybuilding? That is a good question. Why would anybody be drawn to a sport where the payoff comes in the form of scantily clad individuals flexing their muscles in front of a panel of judges? It sounds more like the prelude to an R-rated movie than a test of physical and mental fortitude. Truth be told, the sport of bodybuilding is widely misunderstood. Contrary to popular belief, it is not simply an outlet for steroid-abusing freaks to hype themselves up and galivant around in tight-fitting posing trunks. Quite the opposite, really.

I may be a bit biased, but I would argue that the sport of bodybuilding is one of the most physically and mentally demanding sports one could pursue. You can't fake your way to success with bodybuilding. You must put in the work. There is also no "off" switch. You can't expect to compete at the elite level if you train hard during the day but then hit up the bars with your buddies when the sun goes down. You can't kill it in the gym and then half-ass your nutrition. It's an all-inclusive, never-ending ritual that you must live and breathe day in and day out.

You'll have to sacrifice much of what you love to be a successful bodybuilder. You'll have to say goodbye to the all-night keg stands, the tantalizing buffets, the care-free outlook towards exercise and your demoralizing circle of friends. You'll have to push yourself harder than you've ever pushed before, physically, mentally and even emotionally. Why would anyone agree to such madness? It's simple: the rewards and satisfaction at the end of it all are unparalleled.

To do this properly, you'll have to go to a place where you've never been before. You'll have to sacrifice more than you ever have and gnaw and tear your way to the top—but it will be the most incredible thing that's ever happened to you. I can guarantee this sport will change your life for the better *if* you commit to it fully. If you give it everything you've got and take zero shortcuts.

We live in a peaceful, plush era. Sure, we all have our hardships, but when was the last time you really woke up questioning if you would still be alive at the end of the day? We no longer need to hunt for our food or march into battle, sword in hand, to rage against our enemies. Our food is conveniently prepackaged for us at the nearest convenience store. Usually, the closest we get to being in a raging battlefield is at our office when we're disagreeing with a co-worker. We live in times that make it incredibly easy to become "soft." We are no longer warriors. We are peaceable couch potatoes perusing Netflix.

The sport of bodybuilding can be our cure. It can be our own manufactured hardship that forces us to toughen up and rise to meet our challenges. It can teach discipline and dedication. It can sharpen not only our bodies but also our minds.

The lessons learned in bodybuilding transcend the sport itself and bleed into all aspects of your life. With total confidence, I can say that being a bodybuilder is what gave me the foundation to become a successful businessman, husband and contributing member of society. It gave me purpose and became the backbone of my values. It did it for me, and it has done the same for so many others. It can do it for you, too.

WHY KETOGENIC?

So, on top of bodybuilding, why be ketogenic? The ketogenic diet has not always been popular, but it has certainly gained popularity in recent years. If you rewind the clock to the 1920s, you'll see that the ketogenic diet was used primarily as a method of treating children with epileptic seizures. Rewind a bit further to, say, the dawn of human existence, and you'll realize that ketosis is simply an evolutionary adaptation for survival in the absence of carbohydrates and glucose.

In the earliest days of humanity, before the advent of grocery stores and fast food, we had to hunt and gather our food to survive. Depending on location and seasonality, our furry forefathers often had a tough time finding sweet potatoes and juicy fruits. When the megafauna were plentiful, they would likely have consumed predominantly meat and animal fats. In times of extreme scarcity, they would consume nothing at all for extended periods. Carbohydrates provide fuel for a relatively short period, and we can only absorb so much to store for later. If we hadn't adapted to burning fat and ketones for fuel, we would have become extinct long ago. In its purest sense, being ketogenic or keto-adapted is a survival mechanism that keeps us alive and well when food is scarce.

Since about 2017, the keto diet has started to pick up speed. "Keto" has now become a household name, and many people have either tried it at some point or know someone who has. Companies are coming out of the woodwork to ride the hype train and now, seemingly every product is marketed as "keto-friendly." In the eye of the whirlwind of hype are the claims that keto is a miracle weight loss diet, guaranteed to trim inches off your waist (and in some cases, even cure brain cancer!).

Does it sound too good to be true? Yeah, probably so—but even if some of the claims get slightly overstated, there is a glimmer of truth in them when the diet is implemented correctly. In short, is there truly a benefit to following a ketogenic diet and lifestyle? Hell yes, there is!

While it's true that the ketogenic diet is commonly discussed in weight loss circles, it has proven effective in many other arenas as well. It has become popular among endurance athletes, ultrarunners, cyclists and swimmers. It even has momentum in certain CrossFit circles and more explosive sports.

Is it possible that the ketogenic diet can be leveraged in the sport of bodybuilding? Keto has historically gotten a bad rap in the bodybuilding industry, and I'm not entirely sure why that's the case. Bodybuilding's "bro diet" dogma is just so ingrained in the sport that it has been hard for athletes to look outside their nutritional norms for a potentially superior alternative.

Traditionally, a "good" bodybuilding diet consisted of whole grains, fiber and boatloads of protein for muscle building and recovery. Additionally, these diets included minimal dietary fat, theoretically because fat would clog your arteries and make it impossible to get lean. These diets typically consist of chicken and rice consumed every two or three hours to "boost metabolism." The outcome of it all is that bodybuilders become slaves to a meal plan of extremely bland food.

The "If It Fits Your Macros" (IIFYM) diet or "flexible dieting" is the current reigning champ in bodybuilding circles, which allows more flexibility and variety than eating plain chicken and rice all the time. My issue with this philosophy is that it often places minimal attention on nutrient quality and puts all the emphasis on calories alone. However, there is more to the equation than just calories; for instance, our hormones are often compromised when following a stereotypical IIFYM approach because of lower-quality foods and minimal dietary fat.

There is a strong argument to be made for implementing a well-formulated ketogenic diet when you look at the science and consider the long-term effects of your nutritional protocol, but the emphasis there is on "well-formulated." I would never recommend a "lazy keto" approach in which the bulk of your calories come from butter, cheese and bunless burger patties. There is no perfect diet that works for all seven billion-plus people on the planet; however, I *would* argue that a well-formulated keto diet comprised of whole, nutrient-dense foods gives human beings the most bang for their proverbial buck.

Contrary to what you may think, we didn't evolve to perform on a mainline diet of Hot Pockets and veggie burgers. We ate meat—a lot of it! Industrial agriculture is relatively new in the timeline of human existence, so it only makes sense that our biology is better positioned to function on diets that mainly consist of the foods we've been consuming for the last three million years—but I digress.

Much has been written on this topic, and the point of this book is not to give you a history lesson. Instead, I'd like to turn our attention to how you can leverage the ketogenic diet to excel in your transformative bodybuilding endeavors. While your peers and competitors are sucking down rice cakes and bland sweet potatoes, I'm going to teach you to eat juicy ribeye steaks and kick all their asses onstage!

WHY ME?

What makes me qualified to write this book in the first place? That's a fair question. After all, since the ketogenic diet has become popular, keto coaches are now a dime a dozen. Everyone seems to know how to coach you on your keto journey and what meals and macros will help you reach the goal! Still, optimizing your nutrition, especially in the context of preparing for a bodybuilding competition, shouldn't be taken lightly.

So, what makes the principles laid out in the following pages more qualified than any of the other keto resources that turn up in a simple Google search? Well, for starters, I'm an actual bodybuilder. I am a natural athlete and have decided never to introduce illegal, performance-enhancing drugs into my protocol. I'm also keto-adapted and have been for the past seven years—no "falling off the wagon," no carb-laden uncontrolled binge fests and no compromises! I practice what I preach, and I do so every damn day!

Before finding keto, I had followed a traditional, "bro-dieting" approach to my nutrition. I would eat every two or three hours, and I would count my calories and macros to the gram. I followed this protocol for the first five years of my bodybuilding career. I experienced "success" in the sport in the sense of building muscle and being able to get incredibly lean for a competition, but that success was short lived, and it was far from sustainable. I developed severe eating disorders and had a terrible relationship with food. My hormones would take a nosedive with every prep I went through. I all but lost my mental clarity. I was the poster boy example of a stereotypical bodybuilder: chicken and rice at every meal, disordered eating and zombie mode toward the latter half of my prep. I experienced massive drops in strength and stamina, I had zero sex drive and I went through harmful surges of body fat after shows, followed by the negative cycle repeating all over again. I was not the perfect picture of health, and I had no idea where to turn.

In 2014, I started dabbling with "carb-backloading," a dieting approach in which you remove all carbs during the day and only consume meats and veggies. At night, you are supposed to ingest a large bolus of high glycemic carbohydrates to intentionally spike insulin and provide fuel for the following day's workout. This was all fine and dandy, but I noticed that I had GI distress on the days following the massive carb-ups. I decided to avoid them entirely and see what happened. Lo and behold, I felt better in the absence of carbohydrates. I didn't know it at the time, but this was my first foray into the keto diet.

In 2014, there was zero hype about the ketogenic diet. There were no food products, no podcasts, no books, no nothing. I was in uncharted territory, but I was experiencing benefits and decided to run with it. I noticed an almost immediate improvement in my relationship with food, and my battle with disordered eating started to subside—that alone was reason enough for me to stick with it, but that wasn't all that changed. I experienced a drastic improvement in my gym performance.

My inflammation disappeared, and I cut my recovery time in half. My energy, both physically and mentally, shot through the roof! My strength steadily improved, and it was much easier to maintain a lean physique without all the chronic calorie counting. I didn't know exactly what I was doing, but I knew I was on to something!

In 2017, I decided it was about time to step onstage again. By that point, I had been following the keto diet for a few years, and I felt pretty confident about its effects on my overall health. I was unsure how competitive I would be on a bodybuilding stage with keto, but I figured it was worth a shot and that I'd blaze my trail or die trying.

There were no keto coaches at that time and certainly none that were competitive bodybuilders, so I was flying blind and learning as I went. I tracked every morsel of every macro that went into my mouth. I tested blood ketones, glucose, hormones, *everything*! I took detailed progress pics and measurements, tracking my training and assessing how I felt. I left no stone unturned and documented everything to the best of my ability. I wanted to learn as much as humanly possible and pave the way to a healthier protocol for competition prep dieting.

When the show day finally arrived, I was at peace with myself. I knew I had put in the work, and I was prepared to let the judges take it from there. I meditated until it was my turn to step onstage. Fortunately, the judges liked what they saw.

I brought a level of conditioning that I had never achieved before. My skin was paper-thin, showcasing every artery, vein and capillary that could possibly be seen. I filled out and had a crazy pump that took all the other competitors by surprise. As I waltzed onto center stage, I knew I had just brought a level of conditioning to the table that was going to redefine what was possible in the world of natural bodybuilding.

And what's more, I did it following a strict ketogenic protocol that I developed myself through rigorous trial and error and self-experimentation. I earned my bodybuilding pro-card that day. From then on, I proudly wore the title of professional, natural, ketogenic bodybuilder—one I still hold very dear and carry with pride.

I've since dedicated my life to refining my methods and teaching others these techniques. I genuinely believe it to be significantly healthier than traditional dieting methods. It's incredibly sustainable, as I've followed it flawlessly for the past seven years. My performance has only improved, and my lifestyle is optimized. Unfortunately, the industry is still filled with doubters clinging to their dogmatic beliefs about carbohydrates being required in the sport of performance bodybuilding. Their ignorant interpretations of the diet can sway you—or, you can listen to me.

I've coached hundreds to success with my methods, many of whom have earned their pro status and since become coaches themselves. I don't have all the answers, but I am confident I know one thing pretty damn well: how to optimize your health and performance by leveraging the ketogenic diet. I've quite literally made this my life's purpose. After battling with disordered eating for years and being lost in a sea of endless information regarding human performance, I set out to discover the solution. Ketogenic natural bodybuilding is that solution. So, if the possibility of taking control of your nutrition, removing the guesswork from the sport of bodybuilding and becoming an overall badass excites you, please continue to the next page.

[PART 1]
PRELIMINARY GROUNDWORK

PREP FOR PREP

PSYCHOLOGICAL PREP FOR PREP

As I mentioned earlier, bodybuilding is a mental sport, not a physical one. That said, I feel I would be remiss if I started this manual by talking about macros, protein and body fat. No, we must start this off in the actual beginning and lay the proper foundation to see success. We must start with the mind. So, let us begin this contest prep with a psychological prep!

Why? Why do you want to compete in a bodybuilding show? Maybe it's to look good naked? Perhaps it's to prove somebody wrong? Maybe you don't have a clue and the concept just sounds cool. I highly encourage you to sit with yourself and explore your thoughts on this topic. Bodybuilding is not a trivial thing and cannot be taken as such. What you are about to embark on will change your life; there is no doubt about it. It's essential to have a strong enough "why" to sustain you through the ups and downs, the trials and tribulations. If your "why" is not rock solid, you will fail. You'll crumble at the first sign of resistance.

My "why" is simple: I want to create a self-imposed hardship I can chip away at every damn day for the purpose of self-discovery. I genuinely believe bodybuilding to be the ideal vehicle for learning your capabilities and understanding your limits. Nothing embodies the core values of patience, discipline, persistence and work ethic quite like this sport. If you master this sport, by definition, you master those character traits. Those traits then bleed into every area of your life, and everything begins to flourish. Bodybuilding has become my "life hack" for being a better person.

It's also the best thing you can do for your health and physical well-being. I've always said that resistance training paired with the ketogenic diet is the closest thing we've found to the fountain of youth. Consistent training coupled with a well-formulated ketogenic diet adhered to daily will compound over time and manifest into true health that lasts well into your golden years. I'm confident that I'll have many more quality years with my loved ones due to the health and lifestyle decisions I've made since adopting this protocol of ketogenic natural bodybuilding.

The point is simple: establish your "why" and keep it top of mind. Know what drives you and hold it close. It will keep you moving in the right direction.

Secondly, you should recognize and accept the fact that you can't half-ass a competition prep. It must consume you and become your main priority. The absolute worst outcome that could happen is to walk off that stage when it's all said and done and be filled with regret, the regret of knowing that you cut corners. Regret that you didn't go the extra mile when you should have.

That kind of regret is a cancer that can spread into other areas of your life as well. Don't let it. Give this prep your everything and confidently know within your heart of hearts that you didn't hold back. Do that, and I promise you'll be able to hold your head high, regardless of how you place.

Giving something your everything requires sacrifice. Competitive bodybuilding requires a significant amount of sacrifice. You'll have to sacrifice many aspects of your social life. Meal flexibility will become a distant memory. Skipping a workout because it doesn't jibe with your day is not an option. Boozing it up with your buddies is forbidden. Life, as you know it, is about to change drastically.

Do I say this to scare you? Not at all! Many outliers are blessed with fantastic genetics and can play a bit more loosely with their meals. Some competitors skip many training sessions and still look amazing on show day; however, this book and my overall philosophy toward bodybuilding are not geared toward seeing what you can get away with. Instead, the essence of my message and my prep protocol is to truly pull out all the stops and optimize your prep and performance as much as humanly possible. To truly optimize, you must not only accept but embrace a certain degree of sacrifice. Let that fact excite you! So many people desire an easy life. I encourage you to smile in the face of adversity.

I want to lay down some groundwork in terms of expectations. What are your expectations? Be honest with yourself. Are you expecting to have six-pack abs and negative two percent body fat in 45 days? If so, come to grips with the fact that you're in for a rude awakening. Do you expect to do your first show, go pro, and then be on the Olympia stage within a matter of a few years? If so, go ahead and pinch yourself, because you need to wake up from your dream.

Having the right expectations at the onset of this journey is paramount. I've known many a competitor who started their prep with delusions of grandeur only to hit a wall one month in and become discouraged and depressed. I can't promise you that this book will guarantee you your pro status. I can't promise that you'll be the next Arnold Schwarzenegger making your living as a competitive bodybuilder. But, I can promise you this:

You'll be given the tools to push your body further than it has ever been tested before. You'll have the guidance necessary to optimize your competition prep while following a ketogenic diet and lifestyle. You'll be equipped to continue improving your body long after your prep is over, and you'll be capable of bringing your absolute best package to the stage with the time and resources you have at your disposal.

I'll even take it one step further. If you follow my protocol to the absolute best of your ability and push yourself beyond what you thought possible, you'll have something to show for it. You'll be proud of what you've accomplished. With those expectations, you cannot fail.

One more piece of psychological prep before we commence:

We are all individuals. The macros that work well for me may not be appropriate for you whatsoever. The same is true with our mindset and our outlook on life. My approach to something may be different than what you respond to. Still, with each prep I've gone through, I've made massive advancements in my mindset. I want to share some with you and set you up for success. As I mentioned in the beginning, bodybuilding is a mental sport, not a physical one. Wrap your mind around these concepts, and you'll be primed for the adversities that arise.

Play the long game. What does that mean exactly? It means to be patient. Never make a rushed decision that sacrifices your integrity, health or moral code of ethics. Be excited about how you look, feel and perform when you're 80 years old, not just this summer. Don't opt for a "quick win" only to sell yourself short down the road.

As I said before, natural bodybuilding paired with the ketogenic diet is the closest thing I've found to the fountain of youth, and you shouldn't throw that away—especially when you don't have to! Eat right, train hard and repeat, repeat, repeat. If you do that, you cannot fail. This is a lifestyle in which the victors are the most disciplined and the most consistent. You don't have to be blessed with the best genetics or be born with exceptional natural skills. You just have to embrace the daily habits and routines that move you in the right direction. If you commit to daily habits and routines in line with your nutritional and training guidelines, you will succeed.

The old adage that you can't rush greatness is nowhere truer than in natural bodybuilding and the ketogenic lifestyle. Building quality muscle takes time; there are no quick fixes. Becoming deeply keto-adapted is an ever-improving physiological phenomenon. Being strictly keto-adapted for six years is significantly different than six months. It just keeps getting better and better. Know and accept this fact and be excited for the journey. If you want instant gratification, you should put this book down now.

For best results with this guide, be a stoic. What is stoicism? It is a philosophy of personal ethics informed by its system of logic and its views on the natural world. I would describe a stoic individual as someone who doesn't let circumstances outside their control negatively impact their emotions and actions. It is the ability to analyze your current situation, make the most of it based on reason and then be at peace with that decision.

My introduction to stoic thinking came from *The Obstacle is the Way* by Ryan Holiday. The book had a profound impact on how I view the world and my place in it. It has guided me in times of adversity, and I listen to it in audio format every single time I go through a competition prep. As I've experienced firsthand, there are hardships during prep just as there are hardships in life. Knowing how to interpret them and make reasonable judgments on how to move forward is crucial, and a stoic mindset is your key.

The final suggestion I'd like to make is this: find your stillness. We live in a world in which everyone and everything seems to be in a perpetual state of chaos. We are constantly jumping between tasks, and this trend has only been amplified by the rise of social media. We are constantly tethered to our devices, and we are never able to be alone with our thoughts.

A competition prep has a funny way of forcing silence upon us. Embrace it with open arms. Perhaps it's because calories get so low that we have little energy for anything else, or perhaps it's the laser focus on a goal. Whatever it is, take full advantage of it.

I fully tapped into this "stillness" during the last month of my competition prep. After every training session, I would go to the park and run for a mile or two as a means of light cardio and meditation time. After the run, I would sit against a tree and just be present, totally and completely. It was beautiful. While I was in that state, the rat race of the world had no hold on me. Instead, I began to see things more clearly. By doing the same, you will be able to pick out the meaningful from the superficial. Rather than skating from one mindless objective to the next, you can take the time to pause and reflect. Everything you do has a purpose.

This stillness is powerful, and you'll know when you feel it. Please take full advantage of it and don't squander the moment. Breathe it in and let it awaken you. Leverage its power long after the prep is over. Life is too short not to be present in the moment. Fashion your day-to-day so that it contributes to the future, but don't live mindlessly. Soak up every second of the journey and learn from every lesson it teaches you. Tap into your stillness and let it transcend the prep. Let it into your entire life. Let it become your voice of clarity.

TECHNICAL PREP FOR PREP

Let's switch directions slightly and talk about the physical aspect of prep. Having the right mindset is crucial, but it's all for naught if your body isn't on the same page. So, let's roll up our sleeves and dive into the technical prep work next. Once we establish this framework, you'll be golden.

Be honest with yourself: what is your experience in the sport of bodybuilding? How a seasoned veteran goes about a contest prep will differ significantly from a first-time rookie who has just gone through their first season of "newbie gains." Building solid muscle takes time, just as shape, proportion and symmetry do. Muscle maturity is a legitimate thing, so accept this fact and have the self-awareness to know where you are on the spectrum.

If you've just started your fitness journey, great! That is a massive step in the right direction. Still, I don't necessarily suggest you jump straight into a competition prep. If you've just started training, your body is experiencing many new stimuli, and each training session is an opportunity for further growth. You're primed to build size and strength at a rate faster than you'll ever experience again! The absolute worst thing you can do is stunt your growth period by diving deep into a caloric deficit and focusing on the stage. Keep that desire burning, but I recommend you keep it in your back pocket and save it for later.

I see so many young athletes shoot themselves in the foot by pursuing a show too soon. Instead, I recommend building a rock-solid foundation first. Learn about the different exercises. Establish a true mind-muscle connection. Gain some perspective on how your body responds to certain foods and caloric intakes. Manipulate your cardio, and be in tune with your body before you ever commit to stepping onstage. If you do that, you'll be much more competitive when you do!

The same principles hold for your level of keto-adaptation. Becoming deeply adapted doesn't happen overnight. Just as you can't step onstage after six months of training, you can't truly optimize your keto prep if you've only been following this nutritional protocol for a matter of months. Give your body the time it needs to learn how to metabolize fat and ketones for fuel. Being keto-adapted and being in ketosis are two entirely different things. Deciding to ditch the carbs for a week and then registering 0.5 mM on a ketone meter does *not* mean your body is prepared for ketogenic competition prep. Tap the brakes and lay the foundation. I followed a strict ketogenic diet for two solid years before I ever *attempted* to go through a competition prep.

Again, the keyword there is "strict"—not "keto-ish," not "lazy keto," not "mostly keto." None of that crap. When you decide to change your body's primary fuel source completely, your level of discipline matters. Like most things in life, you get out of it what you put in. If you half-ass your keto nutrition, you'll never truly adapt to your full potential, and you'll likely stay in a state of nutritional purgatory, never fully benefiting from carbs and glucose and never fully optimizing with fat and ketones. Pick the option that is most sustainable for you and commit to it fully.

Our bodies are pretty damn smart. They are capable of truly making the most of what we put in them. If you only consume quality ketogenic foods, you'll become more and more keto-adapted and your body's ability to function on fat and protein will become increasingly effective. This begs the question of metabolic flexibility: should we introduce high glycemic index carbs on occasion and take advantage of a "dual fuel" energy system? *No!* Not if your primary goal is proper human optimization from a fat metabolism approach.

Think of metabolic flexibility as having the ability to be a jack-of-all-trades. You'll have more options, but you'll be a master of none. This isn't necessarily a bad thing; it's just a matter of preference. Personally, I gravitate to going "deep" on a given concept rather than going wide.

You won't lose your ability to metabolize carbohydrates and glucose if you keep it strict keto; our biology doesn't work like that. Introduce carbs again and, rest assured, your body will know what to do with them. You may feel like crap for 48 hours and retain a ton of fluids, but your body will reacclimatize pretty quickly.

My question is: why would you want to? Is the momentary bliss of binging on a chocolate cake worth it? I accept that I'm a bit of an extremist. Still, I continue to stand by my philosophy that staying strict and disciplined with your nutrition is far superior to operating in the "gray zone" and constantly flirting the edge. That doesn't necessarily mean you have to continually track your macros and weigh everything out to the gram; I actually *don't* recommend that.

It's essential to take a mental and physical break from the rigors of strict macro tracking. It's what having a more relaxed building phase is all about (though I'll dive into the concept of sustainability and making your keto "relaxed" later in this book). The main point I want to make here is this: if you're genuinely trying to optimize for a ketogenic diet and lifestyle, you're better off avoiding unnecessary carbohydrates. If you want to have more flexibility and "fit in" at social gatherings and enjoy more carbs, that is fine. Just accept the fact that your ability to reach your ketogenic potential will be hindered. One is not right or wrong; it's all a matter of what you value and place as your priority.

Speaking from personal experience, maintaining a ketogenic diet indefinitely without reintroducing carbohydrates is sustainable! I become more efficient at using fat and ketones for fuel with each day that passes, and I'm excited to see how my body continues to adapt as I maintain my consistency.

There are ketogenic alternatives to every single carbohydrate-based meal that exists. For that reason, I never feel like I'm missing out or sacrificing anything. Many argue that life is too short not to enjoy certain foods. People even go as far as to suggest that I'm missing out on my closest relationships by not indulging in certain foods with loved ones. I would argue that if my relationship with loved ones is dependent on the types of foods I choose to consume, it's not much of a relationship in the first place.

Life is more than the food you stuff in your mouth, so don't place so much importance on what you eat. Food can absolutely be enjoyed, and it should be enjoyed! Even so, recognize that food is fuel, first and foremost, and don't put it on a pedestal. For me, it's more rewarding to know that everything I consume contributes to my overall betterment. That realization is far more exciting than the short-term high I would feel from a carb-laden sugar rush. If you can't say the same, then what's truly in control—you or your food?

All right, enough of my soapbox. Let's talk about some of the physical benefits of staying strict with keto by turning our attention to glycogen.

Glycogen is the substance deposited in muscle tissue and the liver as storage of carbohydrates. It's basically what provides our energy while training during highly glycolytic exercises. When you first cut out carbs, your body burns through its glycogen stores and you may experience a period in which you look a little "flat" and depleted. Many of the gym bros will tell you this is why you can't build muscle and look your best while following a ketogenic diet, but this is far from the truth.

As you become more deeply adapted, your body becomes increasingly efficient at replenishing stored muscle glycogen. The FASTER (Fat Adapted Substrate use in Trained Elite Runners) study illustrated that long-term keto-adaptation resulted in rates of glycogen replenishment that were similar to the carb-based control group. That same study also indicated that peak fat oxidation was 2.3 times higher in the keto group. So, burn more body fat and have the same efficiency at restoring glycogen—that sounds like a win for the keto group!

One key point to observe here is that your ability to replenish glycogen is directly correlated to your level of fat adaptation. The more fat-adapted you are, the better you are at restoring glycogen. In other words, the more strictly you adhere to a well-formulated ketogenic diet, the more efficient you become at replenishing glycogen and the better your ability to "fill out" and obtain a great pump while training.

Speaking of "pumps," following the ketogenic diet typically results in a loss of excess water weight. This reduction in extracellular water weight causes your skin to appear thinner, resulting in more noticeable vascularity. Thinner skin, more vascularity and muscle glycogen replenishment is all a recipe for freakish pumps! The best pumps I've ever gotten were achieved while following a ketogenic diet. If the gym bros tell you that you can't get a solid pump on keto, they've never been legitimately keto-adapted.

Do you ever train to failure in a set? Where you push yourself so far and so hard that you experience an incredible burning sensation deep within your muscle tissue? A temporary build-up of lactic acid causes that sensation. Lactate is a byproduct of glucose breaking down in a process called glycolysis. This process occurs during intense strength training. It isn't a bad thing, just an everyday physiological phenomenon; however, it does tend to put a damper on the number of reps you can hit in a set. You can push through it for a while but eventually, it becomes intolerable, and you have to rest. I used to experience these moments all the time when I first started weight training.

Interestingly enough, I never experience them anymore. Why is that? Deeper levels of keto-adaptation have been shown to improve the lactate threshold. One possible reason for this is the increase in monocarboxylate transporters. When you become more deeply keto-adapted, your body produces significantly more ketone bodies, and it needs to find a way to handle that increase in supply. It adapts by building more monocarboxylate transporters (MCTs). These MCTs are membrane proteins that act as carriers for ketone bodies. They don't just move ketones, though. They are also capable of shuttling lactate and pyruvate, another byproduct of glycolysis. This increased shuttling ability enables you to clear lactate in a much more efficient manner. More effective lactate clearing results in, you guessed it, more intense training sets in which you can perform additional reps without running into a lactate burn. In layman's terms, being keto-adapted allows you to push through a workout with minimal burn and recover from the training session much more efficiently!

I am just barely scratching the surface of the physiological effects long-term keto-adaptation has on the body. Honestly, the effects it has on the brain are even more exciting! However, I do not intend this book to be a deep dive into our biology or the impact ketones have on us at a cellular level. I just wanted to briefly touch on these points because they are very misunderstood topics within the bodybuilding community. Mainstream bodybuilding is under the impression that you cannot get a good pump or train hard with keto. Both assumptions are inaccurate, and more and more ketogenic athletes are popping up daily proving otherwise!

I will stress this point, though: your ability to truly thrive as a ketogenic athlete improves with the length of time you are deeply keto-adapted. The longer you are adapted, the more efficient your body becomes at replenishing glycogen. The more ketone bodies you produce, the more MCTs your body creates and the better you become at shuttling ketones and lactate throughout your system.

What other factors are worth considering? We've established that it's best to go into a contest prep after at least a few years of resistance training. We just illustrated the benefit of being deeply keto-adapted before jumping straight into a competition. What else needs to be dialed in and optimized? Your caloric and metabolic baseline! Resistance training and the ketogenic diet can help set this baseline at a higher level; still, I want to look at this variable independent of both activities and the type of diet you're following.

Sadly, we live in a world in which chronic dieting and caloric depletion are the norms. This constant down-regulation of calories results in a corresponding down-regulation of your metabolic rate. Your body is competent; it has evolved to survive. If you don't consume enough fuel, your body throttles back on its rate of caloric expenditure and your metabolism dives. Multiply this trend over years and years of chronic under-eating and you're setting yourself up for a world of hurt.

I'll dive into this in greater detail later, but I'd like to set the stage for a particular train of thought. Think of bodybuilding—and sustainable body recomposition, for that matter—as existing in two different phases. You have a building phase and a cutting phase. The building phase prioritizes adding lean muscle tissue. You won't be your leanest during this phase, and that is okay. On the opposite end of the spectrum is the cutting phase. This phase consists of lower calories, more detailed tracking and much more visible abdominals. You won't be hitting any crazy PRs in the weight room during this phase, and that is okay.

Knowing and embracing these two different phases is critical. You can't half-ass one and expect to excel in the other. The two phases are a perfect illustration of yin and yang. They are both dependent on each other, and both are necessary to truly improve.

Having a legitimate building phase does *not* give you an excuse to eat like an ass and stuff your face with copious amounts of low-quality foods. It does, however, allow you to eat at a slight surplus and prime your body for building more lean muscle tissue. The increase in lean mass helps improve your metabolism, and so does the additional caloric intake. Therefore, you can effectively increase your basal metabolic rate and caloric maintenance intake if you implement a proper building phase. In addition, this building phase puts you in a much better position to have an effective cutting phase.

I've seen numerous athletes start a competition prep at far too low a caloric intake. What happens to them? They are forced to drop their calories even further and they begin to lose hard-earned muscle at an alarming rate. Their hormones take a massive hit, and they become incredibly depressed and discouraged. The incredible sport of bodybuilding becomes a negative in their lives, and they often give it up entirely. This happens much more than it should, and this downward spiral can easily be avoided.

Be honest with yourself: have you eaten far too little for far too long? Have you allowed yourself to become trapped in the vicious "summer shred cycles" and never really given yourself ample time at a caloric surplus to build any additional muscle? Are you hungry all the time and eating far below your metabolic baseline now? If so, jumping into a contest prep may not be in the cards right now.

First and foremost, focus on your metabolic health and caloric intake. Ensure that you are eating enough to start prep. Think of it like this: the higher your starting calories and the higher your metabolic baseline, the longer your caloric "runway" is at the onset. Leverage that longer runway, have more room to taper macros, manipulate certain variables, fine-tune things and dial in to peak conditioning. If you try to start prep with zero runway, then there will be nowhere left to go, no room to taper macros and no chance of making it through without seriously screwing up your metabolism. No runway is no good. You'll surely crash and burn!

CHOOSING A SHOW

Next, I want to turn our attention to the details of the show itself. Bodybuilding as a sport has steadily grown in popularity over the years, and as a result, there are many different ways to pursue it. What federation do you want to compete in? What does your prep timeline look like? Do you want to compete in a natural federation or a non-tested show? Since there are lots of different options to choose from, let's roll up our sleeves and see what makes the most sense.

TIME FRAME

First, I highly encourage you to give yourself enough time to prep for a show and do it right; there's no sense in trying to rush this process. The faster you have to diet down, the more susceptible you'll be to losing hard-earned lean muscle tissue. Personally, I like to budget four to six months for competition prep. As a natural athlete, I feel that provides ample time to gradually diet down without risking any severe damage to hormones, metabolism or lean mass.

Be honest with yourself and your current conditioning. If you have more than 50 lb to lose, you're likely going to need to diet for much longer, and you may be better off breaking your prep into multiple phases and postponing stepping onstage.

I recommend staying within 15-25 lb of stage weight in the off-season. There is no inherent benefit to letting yourself get any heavier than that, and it just makes competition prep more gruesome if you do. I've gone through incredibly intense preps in which I've lost 70 lb in 12 weeks to diet down for a show, and I certainly don't recommend it. It was miserable, and I sacrificed a ton of muscle in the process. Now, I stay within about 15-22 lb of my stage weight, giving myself a solid five months to diet down. This enables me to enjoy the process. It's not miserable; it's just calculated. It's much better to slowly chip away at the fat and sculpt yourself into a figure of art than to hack away haphazardly and hope that you don't miss your mark.

Look at your calendar. Do you have any massive events planned in the coming months? If so, can you move them around? What is the priority? Bodybuilding is a lifestyle, and it's meant to be enjoyed in tandem with the other aspects of your life. That said, recognize that you can't be the best version of yourself on the bodybuilding stage if the previous week was spent at a family vacation in Hawaii sipping margaritas.

I like to block out my calendar and avoid committing myself to any demanding events that could conflict with my ability to train and track my nutrition. That's not to say that everything else gets put on absolute hold; you can still be a world-class bodybuilder while being a fantastic parent, spouse, employee, employer, contributing member to society and everything in between.

The stars will never align perfectly, and your environment will never be perfect for bodybuilding; that's life. Accept that, embrace it and make the most of it. Be stoic when obstacles arise and charge forward anyway. I'm simply suggesting that you be as proactive as possible with your planning and scheduling. If you know you're going to start prep, try and dedicate the next several months to your primary focus. Make sure your family, friends and loved ones are on board. Having their support and respect is going to make the entire journey much more enjoyable!

LOCATION

Next, consider the location of the show. Are you okay with traveling to the venue? Are you lucky enough to have a great show local to you? Factor these considerations into your planning. If you have to travel for a show, set it up so you can minimize stress. Plan on getting there a day or two early and letting your body acclimate. The more stressed you are, the more extracellular water you'll retain, which is not a good look on show day. Consider the budget you have for this prep and the competition itself. You'll need funds for the venue, travel, tickets, fees, tanning, hair and makeup, a posing suit and photography. All these factors help dictate your location, federation and timeframe.

CHOOSING A FEDERATION

Initially, there were only a handful of federations and options were limited. Now, new federations seem to be popping up every day. Not all federations are created equal, though, and each has its own rules and regulations regarding posing, suit style, division and so on.

Consider the prestige of the federation. Do you want to compete to make a name for yourself in the bodybuilding industry? If so, you'll want to associate yourself with well-respected federations and compete accordingly. If you're doing this more for your personal development, then the federation itself doesn't matter as much. All the same, more popular federations tend to attract more competitive athletes, and I always encourage you to push for a challenge. Knowing that you'll be stepping onstage with elite athletes is a very motivating factor.

As a natural athlete, I tend to categorize federations as being either untested or natural. On average, untested federations tend to garner more attention and popularity. The main federation in this category is the National Physique Committee (NPC) and their pro counterpart, the International Federation of Bodybuilding (IFBB). The pro IFBB competitions get the bulk of the media coverage. They are the federation that hosts the Arnold Classic and the Olympia. They are also the federation that has the most significant payouts and prize winnings. This is where the majority of money resides in the sport of bodybuilding.

With so much money, fame and potential on the line, this has become an incredibly competitive federation. Athletes are always trying to push the envelope beyond what is naturally possible. Unfortunately, this has led to an abuse of performance-enhancing drugs such as steroids. Not all athletes that compete in the NPC and IFBB abuse drugs, but many of them do.

Due to the increase in drug use, it became apparent that there needed to be a separate federation catering to natural athletes. As a result, new federations such as International Natural Bodybuilding and Fitness (INBF) and North American Natural Bodybuilding Federation (NANBF) were formed. Each natural federation does things a bit differently, but all usually require some form of drug test. Typically, this takes the form of a polygraph and a urinalysis test. Federations are often broken into two sectors: an amateur division and a pro division. Rules and regulations will differ, but generally speaking, you'll need to win in an amateur, pro-qualifying show to earn your pro card and compete as a professional athlete.

I don't want to dive too deeply into the hierarchy of different federations and divisions. Instead, I'll link to a few references in the appendix that you can use to do some research and see what best fits your competitive aspirations. There are pros and cons to each federation, so I highly encourage you to explore your options. One word of caution, though: many federations "don't play well with others." You could potentially earn your pro card in one federation and then be banned from competing in another. Unfortunately, there are politics in the sport of bodybuilding as well. Be mindful of this, and do your homework on the federations you compete in.

RELATIONSHIP WITH FOOD

One topic that often gets overlooked in bodybuilding but is of utmost importance is your relationship with food. Have you ever or are you currently dealing with any form of disordered eating? Binging, purging, bulimia, obsessive-compulsive consumption or anything of that nature? If so, I highly encourage you to be honest with yourself about it and prioritize improving that relationship before diving into a prep. Trust me on this one. My first competition prep was effective in the sense that I was able to get incredibly lean, but it was an utter disaster as it related to my relationship with food.

After months of stringent dieting, I went off the rails and started eating everything in sight. I gained over 20 lb in 48 hours. Unfortunately, I continued to struggle with disordered eating for more than two years after that first competition. I would binge on copious amounts of food and then feel incredibly guilty for my actions. I'd cuss myself for not having more self-discipline and willpower. This behavior would inevitably lead to a vicious cycle of purging and self-inflicted starvation. I'd then become so hungry that I'd binge again, and the terrible process would start all over. Sadly, this happens within the bodybuilding community all the time.

I would argue that there are more athletes who struggle with their relationship with food than those who don't. In all honesty, the ketogenic diet and this lifestyle was the most significant contributing factor to me beating this downward spiral. It is the main reason I'm so passionate about pairing natural bodybuilding and the ketogenic diet together. I believe it can help so many people, just as it helped me! Regardless of where you're at in your bodybuilding and ketogenic journey, take a moment and ask yourself where you're at in your relationship with food.

This contest prep will require some incredibly detailed macronutrient tracking. It's sustainable, but it is very restrictive for a finite period. There will be times when you're downright hungry. You'll never be starving, but you'll be hungry. Are you prepared for that? Are you prepared to say no to the foods you desire and crave? Are you prepared to stay on track when all your friends indulge in the foods you love? Can you step back and look at the brevity of what you're doing?

Know that this is a moment in your life, not your entire life. You can do anything for four to six months. Do it right and embrace the sacrifice. Know that you'll be a much better person for the experience; however, acknowledge that it will be a massive test of your discipline and willpower. The desire for more food will gnaw at you in the evening hours. Will you be strong enough to resist when that time comes?

In the context of contest prep, try and view food as fuel and fuel alone. Food can be enjoyed, but it's not meant to be the highlight of your day. Instead, it is serving the purpose of powering your body and mind for something great. That great thing is the highlight; the food is just a means to an end. Don't put it on a pedestal. I know this shift in thinking is much easier said than done, especially in our society. Still, if you're truly able to master this outlook, you'll be empowered throughout the entirety of this contest prep. You'll overcome any cravings and urges you have to eat outside of the plan, and you'll have something transformative to show for it!

HORMONES

There is another topic worth mentioning, namely a quick discussion of hormones. Whether you are male or female, I highly encourage you to get a baseline hormone panel checked before commencing this prep; it's honestly just good information to have. Knowing that your testosterone, estrogen, progesterone and thyroid levels are all functioning as they are supposed to will give you peace of mind. In addition, a competition prep, with its intense training and caloric restriction, will likely impact those metrics.

I like to get baseline checks at the onset, halfway through and after the prep. It's normal to see a drop in hormonal functions, but it's crucial to quantify that drop and know that you are staying within a healthy window. If you don't get these numbers checked initially, you'll have no metrics to measure against.

If you are a female, know that your monthly cycle could potentially change throughout this prep. Being fertile and having the ability to grow another human being is no small feat. Your body demands a certain degree of health and safety for that to be possible. If you're training like crazy and in a steep caloric deficit, your body will likely shift its priorities from making babies to simply surviving. As a result, you may lose your period during the tail end of this prep.

It is not "natural" in the biological sense of the word for females to lose a ton of body fat and perform at a level that is not conducive to growing a child—but who said bodybuilding is normal? If you lose your cycle, know that this is only temporary and is very common among female athletes. Recognize that this is not ideal and prioritize returning to a healthy baseline and regaining your menstrual cycle when you're done.

Now, for one last technicality before we begin this journey.

This is the "cover my ass" clause. I'm not a doctor, and I don't want to play one on the internet. Consult with your physician prior to beginning any intense training and dieting protocol. If you are taking any medication, know the symptoms and implications that your medications may have on any of the changes you make during this prep. Some types of drugs and antibiotics can cause varying degrees of water retention, some may impact your hormonal levels and some may negatively impact sleep and recovery. Do the legwork and understand the implications that may result, and consider that before beginning this prep.

Now, let us begin!

OVERVIEW

Ahh, you feel that? That feeling of anticipation. That feeling of angst. That feeling of excitement. It is the feeling of something looming—something significant. Buckle your seat belts, ladies and gents, and prepare for takeoff. This journey is about to commence!

I've broken the bulk of this book into seven primary phases. These phases comprise the entirety of what I define as my ketogenic contest prep protocol. If you adhere to the recommendations in these seven phases, you'll be set up for success. What's more, you'll learn about your body and how it responds to various nutritional manipulations. You'll be able to take the lessons learned forward in life and put them to use long after this contest prep. With no further ado, let me introduce these seven phases, so you know what you're getting yourself into.

Phase One is all about establishing your baseline. Initially, I didn't intend for this to even be a phase. In the past, I'd brush over this part of the journey, assuming that the athletes I was working with would already have a solid idea of their baseline. Unfortunately, that was an inaccurate assumption. If you don't know where you're starting, you can't possibly know where you're going to end up. Being honest with yourself is of utmost importance. We determine body composition and initial starting macros in this phase.

Phase Two involves the manipulation of our macronutrient allocation and percentages to determine your protein threshold. Everyone has their own protein threshold; it depends on a host of factors such as your level of fat adaptation, your training intensity, lean mass, fat percentage and, to a degree, your body's personal preferences. Manipulating macros to define this threshold is critical as it allows us to set the stage for tapering our macronutrient intake in Phase Three.

Phase Three is all about the slow, steady and consistent tapering of your food intake. We'll gradually drop your macronutrients throughout this phase, and we'll manipulate the rate of that drop based on feedback from your body and how you feel. This is where discipline really comes into play. There is nothing sexy about this phase, but it's absolutely crucial.

Phase Four introduces ketogenic caloric refeeds. By this point in the prep, your calories are getting low, and you'll likely start to experience a slight down-regulation in your metabolic rate. By strategically implementing keto caloric refeeds, we can mitigate that metabolic slowdown and push your body through any potential plateaus.

Phase Five is the part you're looking forward to: peak week and show day itself. Peak week is all about adding the finishing touches and the last little bit of polish. We'll manipulate your training and nutrition slightly to allow for proper show day peaking.

Phase Six will begin the reverse diet. There is no "finish line" during this contest prep. If you go off the rails post-show, you'll pay for it—so this phase ensures that doesn't happen! We'll leverage the refeeds we implemented in Phase Four and start ramping your caloric intake back up.

Phase Seven is all about reestablishing your new baseline. This will get us through the entire reverse diet and prepare you for what lies beyond the contest prep. By the end of this phase, you'll know what your caloric and metabolic thresholds are and how to set yourself up for success going into a building phase.

GUIDELINES AND KETO-SPECIFIC GUIDELINES

There are a few guidelines and keto-specific differences I'd like to take the time to point out. While some standard practices implemented in contest prep are shared between all dieting protocols, there are many differences when you decide to go through a contest prep in a state of strict nutritional ketosis. This section isn't intended to compare a keto prep with other methods such as flexible dieting, IIFYM, the vertical diet or any other plan. Instead, this is my attempt at throwing some wisdom your way that hopefully allows you to avoid common pitfalls.

Not only does much of the traditional prep dogma not apply to ketogenic contest prep, but it can also actually have an adverse effect and negatively impact your ability to peak on show day. I've made many of these mistakes myself, and I'd love to save you the trouble. So, throw whatever you think you know about contest prep nutrition out of the window and adopt the following guidelines as your new standard.

MEAL FREQUENCY

How often you should eat is a massive point of contention between different dieting philosophies. Conventional "bro dieting" suggests that you consume six to seven meals a day, eating every two to three hours. This supposedly boosts your metabolism and ensures that you are never in a catabolic state, allowing your muscles to constantly brim with nutrients so you can add slabs of muscle to your frame.

I followed this train of thought for years. My first five years of weight training consisted of Tupperware piled with chicken and rice. I would carry these with me everywhere I went. If I was ever caught without my Tupperware and the clock hit three hours since my last meal, I would quite literally go into a panic attack. I assumed all my hard-earned muscles were melting away. This is just no way to live. Under this philosophy, you become a slave to your meal timing. You can't afford to be spontaneous without the fear of being caught without your next meal. Luckily, this is not necessary (and certainly not recommended).

The beauty of the ketogenic diet is that you are not forced into incredibly rigid time constraints around your feeding windows. I can go all day without eating if I so choose. When you become fat-adapted, your body can harness a much larger fuel reserve: all your stored adipose tissue. By tapping into this larger reserve, you can effectively fast for days on end without a noticeable decline in lean mass.

Since this is a book on bodybuilding, I'm not going to spend much time on fasting. It's a great tool and can be used strategically when needed. I mention it here to simply illustrate the fact that, contrary to popular belief, you will not wither away to nothing if you happen to miss your meal. In the context of bodybuilding and preserving lean mass, I've found that consuming two to three meals a day is optimal. As calories get lower during prep, I'll often switch to one meal a day (also known as OMAD). I've found that having fewer, larger meals is more enjoyable than smaller meals spread throughout the day. The timing isn't nearly as critical, and I can be much more flexible. This flexibility is genuinely liberating. Rather than being a slave to the Tupperware and eating on the hour, you're able to simply live your life and eat when it's convenient.

The benefits go beyond convenience alone. By eating fewer meals throughout the day, you allow your digestive system to take a breather and your nutrient absorption of the food you are consuming improves. You're also much more likely to keep your blood glucose and insulin more stable with decreased feeding frequency. As a result, you're faced with significantly fewer cravings and a stabler mood.

PRE AND POST WORKOUT

On the subject of meal frequency and timing, it is also worth discussing pre- and post-training nutrition. Conventional wisdom instructs us to "carb-up" before a training session to fuel the workout. Since carbs are out of the equation on a strict ketogenic diet, "carbing up" is clearly not an option. Pre-training nutrition depends heavily on training time. Ideally, you won't have a ton of undigested food sitting in your stomach prior to an intense workout. That would not only weigh you down and impede your performance (a situation I'd prefer to avoid); it's also likely to come back up if your training is particularly intense.

Long-chain fatty acids typically take longer to absorb and be used readily by the body as fuel. Your daily nutrition will likely contain a large percentage of these fatty acids if you're following a ketogenic approach, and this is not a bad thing at all. This slower rate of absorption is one reason we can perform quite effectively after prolonged periods of fasting; the food that we do consume is still fueling us long after we actually ingest it.

This is also why it makes no sense to mainline a large ketogenic meal filled with proteins and slow-digesting fats immediately before a training session. Your body won't assimilate the nutrients in time, and it will only hinder your training. I recommend a solid three to four hours between your meal and your workout. If you train in the morning hours, and you don't want to wake up super early just to get a meal in, no worries. Just consider the last meal of the previous day your "pre-workout" nutrition. After a whole night's sleep, your body will have had the time to break down the nutrients in the food you consumed at dinner, and you'll be ready to rumble when the morning's workout rolls around.

What if you train in the afternoon or evening hours? Simple: try to time things so your lunch meal is several hours before your intended training time.

I don't want you overthinking this piece of the equation. If you're consuming adequate protein and enough dietary fat, your body will be totally fueled within a revolving 24-hour period. You should have no problem killing a workout and pushing through from a fuel standpoint. Time your meals around your daily schedule in a manner that is convenient for you. Don't sweat the small stuff, and don't be a slave to the clock. This is one of the main benefits of the ketogenic diet, so take full advantage of it!

So, what about post-workout nutrition? Do you need to slam a protein shake within 30 minutes of your training session? Nope.

I used to think this was the case. If I didn't consume a protein shake with at least 25 g of whey protein concentrate, I felt that the brutally intense training I had just endured would be a waste. Fortunately, this just isn't true. The "anabolic window" is the time following a training session in which the body willingly and readily absorbs nutrients to fuel muscle repair and recovery. Traditionally, this was thought only to be about 30 minutes. Modern science illustrates that the crucial factor isn't the immediate ingestion of protein post-workout but rather adequate total protein intake for the day.

What does this mean exactly? If you're consuming enough total protein throughout the course of a day, your body will have the fuel and nutrients necessary to rebuild, repair and grow more lean mass. However, in the context of contest prep, you'll most certainly be in a caloric deficit and, at times, may not be consuming enough protein to optimize for recovery. In this scenario, I advise consuming a meal with a large percentage of your daily protein intake within a few hours of training. This doesn't mean you need to rush to a protein shake or start the timer; simply eat a meal with a solid portion of protein sometime within a few hours of training.

I would consume a meal within two to three hours of training if you're in a deep caloric deficit and opt for an OMAD approach to your meal frequency. It's not critical, but it's a great way to hedge your bets and ensure that you're not any more catabolic than absolutely necessary while deep in prep.

EXTENDED FASTING

Fasting is very popular within the low carb and ketogenic communities, and for good reason, too! Fasting offers a host of benefits that go far beyond losing body fat and shedding a few pounds. Fasting is excellent for jumpstarting cell autophagy, our body's way of cleaning out damaged cells and clearing the way for the regeneration of new, healthy cells.

There is a ton of scientific debate on the best extended fasting protocol. Some experts recommend a monthly 48-hour fast. Many implement a quarterly three-day fast. Others suggest an annual weeklong fast. Personally, I like to do a quarterly fast and time it such that it falls within a de-load week because the less intense training works out perfectly with my non-existent caloric intake during an extended fast.

While extended fasting is great, I do *not* recommend incorporating an extended fast into your competition prep or during the initial phases of your reverse diet. Fasting is a strategic stressor on the body but a stressor nonetheless, and competition prep also puts significant stress on the body. Doing both simultaneously is more likely to backfire on you than offer any significant benefit. Rather than overloading your body, focus on one thing at a time and give yourself the necessary time to recover in between prep and an extended fast.

INTERMITTENT FASTING (IF)

IF is excellent, and it goes hand in hand with following a ketogenic lifestyle. Since the fats you eat while on keto digest more slowly than carbohydrates, your hunger throughout the day is likely going to plummet. This is true even as calories start to taper. As a result of this decreased hunger, implementing an intermittent fast can happen almost by default.

There are a million different protocols for IF, though the standard 16:8 is one of the most popular. You fast for 16 hours and have an eight-hour feeding window. Depending on how many meals you consume throughout the day, this can easily be achieved. For instance, say you finish your final meal for the day at 6 pm. You wake up the following morning, drink a black coffee, head to work and eat your first meal when you get hungry, probably around noon. Congrats, you just implemented a 16:8 IF! It's that easy.

Intermittent fasting works well with most people's schedules, and it pairs perfectly with the keto diet. IF helps regulate your hunger hormones and you won't constantly be spiking your blood glucose and insulin as you would be if you were ingesting calories every few hours. Also, as we discussed earlier, your lean mass will not waste away if you go several hours between meals assuming you're consuming enough nutrients.

IF also offers significant psychological benefits. By decreasing your meal frequency and consuming one or two substantial meals a day, you'll appreciate these larger meals more, especially as you near the end of the prep and your hunger starts to ramp up. For whatever reason, one large meal that actually offers some satiety is much more preferable than multiple smaller meals that always leave you wanting more.

How you structure your daily IF and meal frequency is totally up to you but, for illustrative purposes, I'll share how I set mine up below:

> 3:00 am: Wake up.
> 3:30 am: Keto coffee with a fat source (usually heavy cream or coconut creamer),"fat fasting" protocol.
> 6:00 am: Train.
> 8:30 am: Cardio.
> 10:00 am: OMAD meal (at the very beginning of my prep when calories were too high to fit comfortably in one meal, I ate two meals).
> 8:00 pm: Sleep.

Following this model, I implemented a 17:7 Intermittent Fasting protocol with no issue whatsoever.

MEAL PREPARATION

If you only need to eat once or twice a day, does it make much sense to prepare your meals in advance? Bodybuilding often evokes the image of piles of prepared meals and long, drawn-out meal prep days. Is any of that necessary with a ketogenic prep?

It's not required, and you certainly don't have to prepare your meals in advance. In general, it's relatively painless to prepare one or two consistent meals fresh every single day; however, I personally prep every meal in advance, and I advise you to do the same.

One of the main benefits of strategic meal prep is the reduction in decision fatigue. If your allocated macros for the day are already prepared and ready to go, you're significantly less likely to stray away from the plan. That consistent discipline and devotion to the program separates the pros from the amateurs in this sport.

As you follow this ketogenic prep protocol, your macros will change every week. I recommend keeping your meals for a given week the same every single day. Feel free to change them the following week as you adjust your macros. By maintaining this consistency at a given macro goal, you'll effectively be removing numerous unnecessary variables. The more variables you can control throughout a prep, the more effective your manipulations will become.

Imagine trying to dial in macros based on your body's response while also changing the source of those macros every single meal. It would be nearly impossible! Instead, try and eat the same thing every day for a week and then adjust the following week accordingly. I recognize that this removes a ton of variety from your plate and your palate, so you don't *have* to heed this advice. All the same, I'm confident the package you bring to the stage on show day will be infinitely better if you do. In my mind, sacrificing a little bit of food variety seems like a worthwhile trade for that payoff.

How can you put this into practice? Once you know your macros for the week, simply plan your meals accordingly. Using your macro tracking app, calculate what combination of foods can be prepared to hit those macros accurately. Then, simply prepare those meals for the week in advance and keep them in marked Tupperware containers stored in the fridge. Since you are likely only eating once or twice a day, this won't take up a ton of space in the refrigerator.

Personally, I like making the foundation of my meal prep around ground beef and eggs. Both are incredibly nutrient-dense and easy to manipulate. If my fat ratio is higher, I can opt for a fattier ratio in ground beef, like a 75/25; as my protein goal increases, I can swap out the fattier ratio for a leaner one such as 90/10. Eggs come in very handy because they are almost a perfect 1:1 ratio of protein to fat, each coming in at about 5 g. Since I typically adjust macros by 5 g each week, manipulating my egg consumption is a simple adjustment.

MANAGING WILLPOWER

As you go deeper and deeper into this prep, your willpower will likely diminish. It's hard to stay incredibly disciplined and consistent for months on end. On top of that, you'll also still have your typical day-to-day responsibilities. Staying the course and not wavering from your planned macros gets harder and harder, even for seasoned veteran competitors. With that in mind, the fewer decisions and choices you'll have to make, the better.

Remove the variables and decision fatigue from your meal planning. Become a machine and optimize for your body's fuel and nutrient demands. This rigidity may sound tedious and unenjoyable, but it's actually liberating. You'll be amazed at how much more productive you are when you don't spend so much time planning your next meal and trying to make it fit your macros. Prep your food in advance and free up that mental bandwidth for other things that need your attention.

By now, we've covered the concepts of meal timing and frequency in enough detail. Let's dive deeper into the nuts and bolts of what your meals should consist of. First and foremost, I want to focus on the importance of nutrient density.

NUTRIENT DENSITY

Nutrient density trumps all else, especially in the context of a caloric deficit. If you're dieting down for competition prep, every single calorie you consume matters. Everything you consume is taken in by your body and put to use; therefore, it only makes sense to prioritize the most nutrient-dense options you have at your disposal.

Honestly, this is one of my most prominent issues with the IIFYM community. I don't want to stereotype that entire community but, in large part, the IIFYM dieters place most of their focus on macros rather than the nutrient density of the foods that make up those macros. That is a big mistake!

Consider the macronutrient and ingredient make up of margarine vs. butter. They both have virtually the same macro profile of about 11 g of dietary fat, but look a bit deeper into the ingredients. The primary ingredient in margarine is a highly inflammatory, hydrogenated soybean oil; after that is a laundry list of highly processed ingredients. A high-quality butter is made from cream—that's it! The ingredient list is much simpler, but the natural butter also contains MCT's and is high in vitamins A, E, D and K2. They have the same macros, but the ingredients tell a very different story.

As I mentioned earlier, this quest for the most nutrient-dense foods becomes increasingly important as your calories get lower and lower. For this reason, I'm a huge advocate for incorporating organ meats while in competition prep.

Organ meats are often given a bad rap because people don't like the taste. I get it; a plate full of liver and onions may not be for everyone. Still, don't let your taste buds sway you from incorporating one of the world's most incredible superfoods! Several companies have started creating desiccated organ meat pills that contain various animal parts such as heart, liver and kidney. These pills are easy to swallow and are virtually tasteless. I'd recommend something like this over a typical daily multivitamin any day of the week.

The nutrient density in organ meats is unrivaled by anything the plant kingdom has to offer. Kale is often hailed as a superfood within nutritional circles, but if you compare kale and beef liver side by side, you'll see that there is no competition between the two. Rather than sucking down green smoothies to optimize your prep, consider implementing the benefits of high-quality organ meat.

Personally, I'm a sucker for liverwurst sausage. It contains a mixture of beef, beef heart, beef liver and beef kidneys and is typically mixed with a variety of spices. The sausage has an incredibly mild flavor, and I usually mix it in with scrambled eggs in my meal prep. The taste is incredible!

As far as nutrient density is concerned, prioritize single ingredient, whole foods that are sourced from reputable farmers and ranchers and aren't heavily processed. I've included a list of quality food options in the appendix of this book to simplify your selection. What about the things you should avoid?

I caution against incorporating a ton of high-volume filler ingredients for two reasons. For one, any filler ingredients you ingest are taking away from potential nutrient-dense calories you could consume in their place. Secondly, filler foods may inhibit the complete absorption of the high-quality foods you're trying to prioritize.

I don't want to villainize fiber, but it may not have much place in the context of competition prep. First of all, fiber isn't nearly as necessary as conventional health wisdom indicates. The main benefits of fiber are to blunt the spike in blood glucose resulting from eating a diet high in carbohydrates and help move unabsorbed food through your digestive tract. Both are non-issues if you're following a well-formulated ketogenic diet and in a caloric deficit.

If you're truly keto, you shouldn't be experiencing any massive spikes in blood sugar. If you're prioritizing nutrient-dense foods and eating in a deficit as you will be on this prep, you're highly unlikely to have much food waste to push through your system. I'm continually amazed at how so many people fear not eating enough fiber, yet when they do minimize their fiber intake and prioritize nutrient-dense foods, they notice incredible benefits! Bloating almost always decreases, they still stay regular and they have zero gas or indigestion. Fiber isn't the secret; eating quality food is!

Now, does this mean you can't eat a salad or a plate full of greens? Not at all. I'm not a hardcore carnivore by any means. I'm simply suggesting that you prioritize hitting your macronutrient goals with high quality, nutrient-dense fats and proteins rather than green smoothies. If you're craving a salad, by all means figure it into your macros for the day. Just don't expect that salad to offer as much of a performance boost as a more nutrient-dense option would.

TOTAL CARBS VS. NET CARBS

All this talk of fiber begs one question: should you count total carbs or net carbs? I'd like to cut to the chase on this one. I advise you to remove the term "net carbs" from your vocabulary. Be honest with yourself and count the total carbohydrates in the food you consume.

There is no "free lunch" when it comes to nutrition. Net carbs is defined as total carbs minus the dietary fiber in a given food. Counting only the net carbs suggests that dietary fiber doesn't impact your caloric load for the day, that the fiber just passes through you and is a wash. This is absolutely ridiculous!

Everything counts when it comes to your nutrition. Accept this fact and be honest with yourself in how you calculate your daily intake. Count total carbs, and you'll get total results!

By now, you can probably tell that I'm not putting plants and dietary fiber on a pedestal. Does that mean you should just cut them out entirely and do this prep following a carnivorous protocol? You certainly can if you like!

I keep my total carbs very low throughout competition prep. The highest my carbs get is around 20 g, and I'll go as low as 0 g. If you're following a strict ketogenic protocol, you're not getting your fuel from dietary carbs, so you are totally fine to eliminate them entirely.

I genuinely have found no performance gain from incorporating the carbs, and a well-adapted athlete is safe to remove them from the equation. However, veggies do offer the benefit of some dietary variety. Every once in a while, I'll find myself craving a salad or a handful of Brussels sprouts. On those rare occasions, I figure them into my macro goals and indulge. If you want to go through this prep as a carnivore with zero greens, that is fine. If you're going to implement some daily greens, that is fine, too.

Some people experience adverse reactions to vegetables and others don't. This variability is where the protocol becomes a bit more individualized and customizable to fit your personal preferences. If you do decide to go carnivore, I suggest that you diversify your food sources. Don't just eat 80/20 ground beef straight for the next six months—mix it up so that you're covering all of your micronutrient needs.

You'll be consuming quite a lot of meat throughout this prep, so it's worth noting that not all meat is created equal. Sourcing is essential—not only across different animal species but also within the same species. For instance, red meat from beef will contain a more favorable amino acid and micronutrient profile than the white meat in a chicken breast.

I encourage you to diversify where you're getting your proteins. Try and make the foundation beef-based but mix in fish, pork and some poultry as well. Opt for fattier cuts whenever possible, since it will make hitting your overall macro goals much more straightforward.

GRASS-FED VS. GRAIN-FED MEAT

A constant debate rages within meat-based dieting circles about grass-fed vs. grain-fed meat. Which should you choose? Honestly, it all depends on the source.

There are very high-quality cuts of beef that are finished on grain and still have a superior fatty acid profile to their grass-finished counterparts. However, the reverse can also be true. Generally speaking, grass-fed beef is a bit leaner than grain-finished, and the omega-3 to omega-6 ratios are more favorable. Even so, it's hard to know for sure which is the better option unless you know exactly where your meat is coming from—and that is a nearly impossible task if you purchase from a grocery chain that sources all its beef from one or two large suppliers.

Ideally, you can find a local butcher or rancher who knows precisely where their livestock came from and what it was raised on. These cuts will typically be a bit pricier than what you'll pay at your local grocer, but that is to be expected. As with most things in life, you get what you pay for, and quality trumps quantity when it comes to sourcing your groceries.

Throughout my entire prep, I incorporated ground venison that I personally shot and butchered the year prior. Venison is much leaner than most meats, so I had to pair it with a quality fat source, but wild game is incredibly nutrient-dense, so I figured it was a worthwhile trade-off.

The micronutrient profile of wild game is incredible, and I was proud to put my own food on the table, but I don't mean for this to turn into a rant about how everyone should hunt and support their local farmers. It is something I'm passionate about and want to touch on, but I recognize that higher-quality foods are generally much more expensive, and the financial burden may be a barrier for some. Don't let that be a limiting factor for you. I did my first competition prep when I was a sophomore in college and could barely afford Ramen noodles. Simply consume the best quality food you can afford.

I certainly don't expect you to head into the wilderness to hunt all your own food before beginning your contest prep. Suffice it to say that I do place significant importance on the quality of the foods you consume. Take care of your body, give it the highest quality fuel you can, and you'll benefit for years to come.

I've also included an appendix at the end of this book that lists recommended foods and ingredients to make things easy.

FATS AND SWEETENERS

Just as all food and meat aren't created equal, all fat isn't created equal either. When choosing your dietary fats, I highly encourage you to prioritize quality saturated fats and monounsaturated fats. Most polyunsaturated fats come from heavily processed sources and can contribute to unnecessary inflammation. Contrary to popular belief, saturated fats are not evil, and they will not independently clog your arteries and give you a heart attack (though I'm assuming that if you're keto and have been adapted long enough to be interested in this book, you already know that). As is true with everything we've discussed thus far, focus on the quality of the source. If you're getting quality cuts of meat that are high in saturated fats, you are good to go.

As far as unsaturated fats are concerned, keep it simple. Prioritize natural monounsaturated fats such as those found in avocado and olive oil. When it comes to polyunsaturated fats, try to consume an omega fatty acid profile that is not heavily weighted with omega-6 relative to omega-3. Quality fish and supplemental fish oil that contain both DHA and EPA are a good bet. Avoid processed polyunsaturated fats such as vegetable oil, canola oil and soybean oil.

A discussion on natural and artificial sweeteners could quickly become a book on its own. At the time of this writing, there are 56 different names for sugar alone in common food products. That is crazy! This confusing nomenclature can easily mislead the average consumer. Of course, what's worse is that most companies are not interested in educating the consumer. Instead, they are interested in driving sales. This results in marketing tactics that lead people down the wrong path. Sadly, this has become a reality within the ketogenic space as well.

Riding the hype, many companies are simply slapping "keto" on their packaging to drive revenue. Because of that, it's not enough to merely look at the list of macronutrients. You must dive into the ingredient list and know on a deeper level what you're buying.

When it comes to sweeteners, I recommend keeping things simple: go natural and choose options that have a minimal impact on blood glucose. **Stevia** is my preferred sweetener, with **monk fruit** coming in second. These two seem to have a negligible effect on my blood glucose levels and they typically do not trigger any cravings.

Erythritol and **Xylitol** are both chemical compound sugar substitutes. They also have a minimal impact on blood glucose compared to sugar. **Allulose** has become a popular sweetener within the low-carb space, but I do not recommend it due to its adverse effects on most people's digestion. Everything else is pretty much out of the question. An occasional treat sweetened with Sucralose or Ace-K won't kill you, but I certainly don't recommend them.

The sweetener debate goes beyond just the impact on blood glucose and requires a deeper dive into the biological details. The cephalic phase of insulin secretion occurs soon after you anticipate something sweet or ingest something that triggers a sweet response in the brain. This phenomenon elicits an insulin response regardless of what is happening with your blood glucose. This secretion often triggers increased cravings and temporarily disrupts the natural sensation of true satiety. Basically, eating sweet foods can increase cravings and temporarily blunt satiety—not a desirable combination when you're deep in contest prep.

ALCOHOL

Is there any place for alcohol within a contest prep, especially within a ketogenic one? Well, to be honest, no. You can probably drink some alcohol without being totally derailed, but I prefer elimination rather than moderation when it comes to alcohol consumption. For one, alcohol has caloric load. One shot of vodka contains about 100 calories. When you're in a caloric deficit trying to prioritize nutrient density, do you really want alcohol eating away at your allotment for the day? Probably not. That reason alone is compelling enough for me to steer clear of alcohol during prep.

Will alcohol kick you out of ketosis? It depends. Alcohol is going to be burned preferentially by the body before carbs, fats and ketones. Suppose your body is well adapted and tapping into your stored body fat and dietary fat for fuel. In that case, you can expect the oxidative process to temporarily slow down after a significant consumption of alcohol. This doesn't mean you can't drink at all while following a ketogenic diet, but try and consume alcoholic beverages that are relatively "clean" and don't contain a ton of added sugars. Gravitating to something like a dry red wine that has been tested for residual sugars, plain vodka or whiskey is going to be your best bet. Still, as I mentioned earlier, ideally you don't want to sacrifice your daily calorie allotment for something as nutritionally void as alcohol.

If you absolutely cannot make it through the day without your glass of red wine, figure it into your macros and optimize for the variables you can control. If you want to optimize everything from the ground up, I highly advise avoiding alcohol during prep altogether.

REFEEDS AND DIET BREAKS

Refeeds and diet breaks are also terms that get thrown around quite a bit within the context of dieting. Put simply, refeeds are a temporary surge in calories. They are not an all-out binge but rather a calculated manipulation of macronutrient intake for the day.

Refeeds can be leveraged to help give your metabolic rate a little boost and as a psychological break. Looking forward to a temporary increase in calories after months of dieting is a helpful way to disconnect. It makes the dieting process much more sustainable. Refeeds are also implemented during peak week to add a bit of "polish" to your physique and help your muscles fill out for the show. A properly implemented refeed can significantly improve your muscle definition and vascularity. In some cases, it can be the deciding factor between first and second place.

Traditionally, refeeds include a significant increase in dietary carbohydrates (surely, you've heard the term "carb loading"). The primary objective for loading up on carbs is replenishing glycogen stores and bringing out a fuller look, but there is some risk associated with carbing up before stepping on a stage.

If you miscalculate your carbs, water or sodium intake, you could "spillover" and wash out all of your hard-earned definition. This is when water spills out of your muscle tissue and gets held within the subcutaneous layer of skin. This is the last thing you want to happen after months of dedicated training and meal prepping!

If you're reading this book, I'll assume you're keto-adapted and want to follow a proper ketogenic contest prep. Luckily for you, there is no need to implement any carbohydrates in your refeeds. If your body is accustomed to deriving all its energy from fat, why would you want to switch it up right before the show? Let's bypass that risk altogether and stick with an actual ketogenic diet! We'll still implement refeeds, but they won't include any carbohydrates. They'll be ketogenic caloric refeeds with a strategic increase in dietary fat and protein (I'll be doing a deep dive into keto refeeds in a later chapter, but I wanted to introduce them here so that you'll have an idea of what is to come).

Diet breaks are, as they sound, legitimate breaks from the diet. If you're following a ketogenic diet and lifestyle, a diet break doesn't necessarily mean breaking out of ketosis and eating a ton of carbs. Diet breaks are more of a complete break from caloric deficit, and they are often used bi-weekly.

For example, imagine you are dieting for four months straight in a caloric deficit. If you wanted to implement diet breaks and make the process a bit more sustainable, you could implement a diet break every other week and return to maintenance. This is not a bad idea if you have a ton of weight to lose as it could make the process of losing weight much more enjoyable, and you wouldn't have to spend every waking day of your life for four months in a deficit.

However, there is a drawback to diet breaks. Since you'll be in a deficit for half the time, it will likely take you twice as long to reach your desired composition. What would have taken four months to accomplish will now be closer to eight months. At the end of it all, you're not really spending any less time in a caloric deficit, you're just drawing it out over a much longer window.

Personally, I would recommend this as more of a lifestyle tool and not use it for actual competition prep because it adds far too many variables to the equation. It's better to optimize everything for prep to maximize your efficiency and effectiveness. In the grand scheme of things, prep isn't that long—only four to six months. It's better to give that period your all and devote yourself entirely to it than go back and forth between dieting and living everyday life.

THE KETO BRICK

There is one more thing I'd like to touch on before diving into Phase One: the Keto Brick. I may sound a bit biased (being the company owner and all), but I formulated the Keto Brick to optimize my competition prep nutrition long before it was ever a product available for sale. In the beginning, I never even intended to turn it into a business. It was, and continues to be, a tool to leverage for increased performance and optimized ketogenic nutrition. You certainly don't have to use Keto Bricks, but I would be remiss if I didn't explain what they are and how you can incorporate them.

The Keto Brick is a 1,000-calorie, shelf-stable meal replacement brick that delivers the perfect ketogenic macro ratio with zero filler ingredients. I formulated it back in 2017 when I was prepping for my first ketogenic competition and needed to simplify my meal prep without compromising my nutrition.

There was nothing available in the marketplace at the time, so I set out to create something for my consumption needs. Thus, the Brick was born. Unlike most keto "fat bombs," the Brick doesn't melt at room temperature, making transporting it significantly more convenient. Depending on the flavor, the average Keto Brick has about 82% of its calories from fat, and the total carb count for each 1,000-calorie brick is around 12 g. Unlike the vast majority of the keto bars on the market, the Brick contains zero filler ingredients and no artificial sweeteners. Every single ingredient has a purpose and contributes to your nutritional demands and performance needs.

I'll always advocate quality wholesome foods over pre-packaged foods and supplements, but the Brick is an excellent addition to your other food sources. Since it has such a high-fat ratio, you can pair it with leaner or fattier meat cuts depending on your macronutrient goals—and it doesn't result in any bloating or digestive distress, so you don't have to worry there. Each Brick contains a solid dose of sodium, which makes getting in your electrolytes a bit easier.

I've eaten a Keto Brick every single day since I started making them. I consumed a whole Brick every day during my contest prep, and many of my clients have as well. It's not a "snack bar" or a guilty treat; it's also not a magical weightless supplement. It's a performance Brick that helps optimize your nutrition.

I totally believe in and vouch for the Bricks, and I'm confident they will help you dial in your macronutrient goals more efficiently and effectively. Because I make them in-house with my team, I oversee the entire production process and ensure that zero compromises are made. The Brick is a tool that I highly encourage you to leverage if you so choose. If not, that's totally fine, too—more for me!

[PART 2]
THE PREP

[1]
PHASE ONE: ESTABLISH YOUR BASELINE

Alrighty, ladies and gents, the time has come. Enough of the preliminary prep talk; let's get this show on the road!

Welcome to the very beginning of the prep itself, Phase One, which we're going to use to:

- Determine your current caloric and metabolic baseline
- Establish your initial starting macronutrients
- Develop your initial training and cardio outline

The primary objective of this phase is to look under the hood and see what we're working with. After all, you can't possibly know the best route to your desired destination if you don't even know where you're starting.

If you're a data nerd and already track all your nutritional and training metrics, this phase will fly by. If you're coming in with a solid understanding of your current caloric and macronutrient intake, then you've already done a lot of the heavy lifting. If you have no idea how to track your macros, we've got some serious work ahead.

If you want to jump into a competition prep, I'll assume that you have some baseline knowledge of macronutrients and how to track them using one of the many popular applications such as MyFitness Pal or My Macros+. If you don't know what I'm talking about, I highly encourage you to download one of these apps and spend some time familiarizing yourself with it. As I pointed out in the introduction, a competition prep requires some serious fine-tuning and goes beyond the scope of intuitive eating. Know how to track your intake using one of the apps mentioned above or something similar.

If you have no clue what your current nutritional intake is, I highly recommend eating intuitively as you have been for a few weeks and tracking all the numbers. See what kind of intake your body naturally gravitates to and establish a baseline. Remember, the priority of calculating your initial starting macros is ensuring that you're eating enough at the onset of the prep to begin with. If you're already in a deep caloric deficit, then you should rethink your competition prep plans. Ideally, you want to start Phase One at your caloric and metabolic baseline—not too far above it and not too far below it. If you've been tracking religiously for quite some time before beginning the journey, you likely have a solid grasp of your baseline.

Many macro calculators and formulas are used to establish these baseline numbers, but please realize that they are only estimations. When working with a new client and setting their starting macros, I always prefer to base it on their current macros and unique history. This is much more accurate than simply plugging their stats into a generic macro calculator or formula. In a perfect scenario, you'll have an excellent grasp of your individual caloric baseline at the onset. Ideally, that baseline is within a healthy range and gives a ton of runway to taper calories. If your caloric baseline is at an unhealthy level and far too low to safely begin a prep, refer to the technical prep for prep at the beginning of this book.

If you have some knowledge of what your caloric baseline is (i.e., the caloric intake your body can handle without experiencing a weight gain or loss), then write that number down. We'll calculate the macronutrient ratio you should start at to hit that caloric intake later.

If you don't know your current caloric baseline, get ready to do some math. The formulas and calculations that follow will be employed to determine your initial caloric intake.

Note: I encourage anyone reading this to go through these mathematical calculations—even those of you that do feel confident in your current baseline estimations. The more data you have, the better, and all of these calculations will be combined as a safeguard to ensure you are set for success as efficiently and healthily as possible.

* * *

WEIGHING IN

Bodyweight is a tricky subject; many people don't like stepping on the scale every morning. It can become an obsessive habit that has a negative connotation associated with it. Some people can step on the scale and not think twice about the number reflected to them. Others step on the scale, don't like the number, step on the scale four more times and then let it ruin the start of their day.

Let's start by changing our relationship with the scale entirely. That data it shows is not good or bad; it's simply data. It's a measurable statistic that we can use to control for certain variables in the future. It's not going to magically or drastically change overnight, and you shouldn't expect it to. It's much better to weigh in daily than only to weigh once a week while in competition prep. Why is that? We are trying to see what direction you're trending over time. That is best accomplished by measuring your average gain or loss over a week, one week after another.

If you only weigh in once a week, you won't see nearly as accurate a depiction of your weekly average. You won't truly dial in electrolytes and see how subtle changes like sleep quality can impact your scale weight. Something as trivial as eating a few extra pickles can significantly impact your level of water retention, and that will result in a measurable increase in scale weight.

A temporary inflammatory response from an intense leg training day almost always increases scale weight; these things are normal and to be expected. We can't accurately account for them if we only see a momentary blip in time on the scale. My suggestion is to weigh in daily, first thing in the morning after urination—no need to jump on the scale multiple times throughout the day. Weigh yourself once, record that weight and be done with it.

Weight loss and weight gain are not linear processes. There will be days when your weight goes up and others it goes down. There will even be times when it seems like you're stuck and your weight seems immovable. Keep tracking and stick with the process.

I used to weigh myself every morning and then write that number on a calendar, which I pinned above the bathroom scale. I then graduated to an Excel spreadsheet that made plotting the numbers much more visual. Now, I use Heads Up Health.

Heads Up is a software application that syncs with my smart devices such as my macro tracker, bathroom scale, Oura Ring and blood glucose/ketone monitor. The nice thing about using Heads Up is that I can chart multiple different data points against one another and find correlation. For instance, I can graphically see how a gradual decrease in my caloric intake is correlated to my corresponding drop in bodyweight. Leveraging Heads Up Health is certainly not required, but it does make the process of tracking these various data points much more convenient and informative.

BODY FAT PERCENTAGE

Total bodyweight is excellent, but what is that weight composed of? How much of that is lean muscle tissue relative to body fat we need to lose? The figure we're looking for here is body fat percentage, and there are many ways to measure it.

The medical standard is the **DEXA scan**. A DEXA machine

measures bone density and is widely used to assess skeletal strength for patients with osteoporosis. Besides measuring bone density, DEXA machines can also determine your percentage breakdown of fat tissue and lean muscle mass.

To do so, you lie on the machine and let it scan your entire body (a process that takes about 10 minutes). Pricing is usually between $50-$150 depending on your location. Most hospitals have a DEXA machine they make available to the public. The best way to find one is through a simple Google search looking for DEXA scans in your area. I like to get a DEXA scan at the very beginning of my prep, about halfway through and at the very end.

A **bio-electric impedance analysis (BIA)** is also another great way to measure your body composition. In a BIA, a weak current flows through the body and measures the voltage on the other side to calculate impedance or resistance. Most of our body's water is stored in the muscle tissue. More muscle equals more body water, which equates to a lower impedance score.

The **InBody scan**, which uses a non-invasive scale you step on to measure impedance, is a very popular method for testing your BIA. The only downside to this method is that your level of hydration can profoundly impact your level of bio-electrical impedance. I would try and stay as consistent with your water consumption and activity level as possible before each scan. Many supplement shops have an InBody scan they offer to customers for free or for a small fee of $10-$15. If you have a BIA scale available nearby, try and jump on it biweekly.

The **skinfold caliper test** is another popular method that tests the thickness of your skin and the underlying fat at specific points on the body. These points are plugged into a formula to determine overall body fat percentage. This method is also non-invasive and is reasonably convenient if you have a volunteer who can test it for you in the comfort of your own home.

I use the **Jackson-Pollock seven point test** method for my caliper tests; to do the same, google this method and plug in the millimeter measures from each skinfold site to determine your estimated body fat percentage. The nice thing about this testing method is that it's free after purchasing a simple skin caliper and is also incredibly convenient and non-invasive. Because everyone tests a bit differently, having the same person test you is the best way to control for any variability. I have my wife perform this test on me every two weeks.

Many bathroom scales can also test for body fat; however, these are the least accurate of all the different testing methods. Some scales use BIA technology while others use a generic formula calculated from your age and weight. Often, these scales calculate the BIA of your lower body and then use a rough estimation to calculate your upper body composition. This is far from accurate, which is why I recommend one of the other methods to determine your initial body composition.

Calculating your initial body fat percentage is crucial for knowing where you're starting and how far you have to go. Don't measure once and be done with it, though—test your body composition on a bi-weekly basis. There are many times throughout a contest prep where your weight may not be changing but your body composition is changing drastically. If you only track scale weight, it can be easy to get discouraged and veer off-plan; however, if you can see a measurable change in your body composition independent of the scale weight, maintaining the motivation to stay the course becomes easier.

IDEAL BODY FAT PERCENTAGE

What body fat percentage should you shoot for to be competitive onstage? The sport of competitive bodybuilding demands a lot more than simply getting lean; you have to be freakishly shredded. Getting shredded entails detailed tracking, manipulations and tweaks to showcase your full potential, and different divisions within the physique sport require different "looks."

Judges of an open bodybuilding division, for example, will be looking for a leaner, grainier physique than judges for a men's physique class. The same is true for female divisions: women's physique is going to demand a leaner look than women's bikini. Know what division you're preparing for and strive for a look that fits best. Typically, I recommend erring on the leaner side; leaner tends to be more impressive and can help you stand out from competitors.

The open bodybuilding division demands the leanest competitors and requires the lowest body fat percentage. On the amateur level, it's rare to see competitors come in with striated glutes and insane vascularity, so strive to be one of the athletes who does! If your glutes are popping while everyone else is looking soft, the judges' eyes will immediately be drawn to you and you'll stand out from the pack.

I've included a table below to illustrate what a rough estimation of goal body fat on show day could be depending on the division and method of testing. These are not hard numbers but rather a reliable estimation with tangible numbers to shoot for.

*Notice the larger range with the BIA method as a result of fluctuations in fluid levels.

Body Fat Analysis

Division	Caliper	DXA	BIA/Inbody
Men's Bodybuilding	2-4%	4-6%	3-10%
Men's Classic Physique	3-5%	5-7%	4-11%
Men's Physique	4-6%	6-8%	5-12%
Women's Physique	7-9%	9-12%	9-16%
Women's Figure	8-10%	10-13%	11-17%
Women's Bikini	9-12%	11-14%	12-18%

ENERGY BALANCE AND STARTING CALORIES

Okay, now that you know your starting weight and body composition, where should you start with caloric intake? As I mentioned previously, it's best to already have hard evidence of what your approximate metabolic and caloric baseline is. If you don't know, use the following equations to establish a starting point. Still, I want to preface this discussion of calories and the energy balance with a straightforward statement: it's not *all* about calories.

There is a constant debate among different dieting communities about the significance of calories. Some traditional bro and IIFYM dieters think calories are the end-all be-all; on the opposite end of the spectrum are ignorant low-carb and keto enthusiasts who genuinely believe calories don't count and it's all about hormones, specifically insulin.

As is true with most things in life, the answer lies somewhere in the middle. All these details are important and have an impact, but calories and energy balance are crucial parts of this equation and are some of the more controllable variables. I can control the number of calories I consume more effectively than I can manage my hormonal fluctuations. I'm not suggesting that one matters more than the other; I'm just choosing to focus on the one I have the most control over.

As a side note, know that it is relatively impossible to know your actual caloric intake and expenditure with utmost certainty. The food industry grants nutritional labels 20% amnesty in both directions. Food labels aren't 100% accurate, and you can't possibly know how many calories your body is burning. As a result of this inaccuracy, many argue that it's pointless to count calories in the first place.

Here's the thing: if you consistently track your caloric intake the same way every time, these inaccuracies average out over time, and you can make reasonable assumptions based on these averages. Competition prep is all about controlling for variables and holding as many things constant as possible. If you're living a very structured, routine life as is recommended throughout your prep, you'll be able to dial in despite any inaccuracies.

Let's start this discussion with a few simple definitions:

Metabolism: Metabolism is the set of life-sustaining chemical reactions present in all living organisms. There are three primary purposes of metabolism:

1. The conversion of food to energy to run cellular processes.
2. The conversion of food to building blocks for proteins, lipids, nucleic acids and some carbohydrates.
3. The elimination of nitrogenous waste.

Calories: A calorie is a measured unit of energy. Technically speaking, a "small calorie" or "gram calorie" is the amount of heat energy required to raise one gram of water temperature one degree Celsius; most of us are more familiar with the "large calorie" or "food calorie," which comprises 1,000 small calories and is known as a "kilocalorie" or "kcal." Of course, nutritional labels illustrate these kilocalories simply as "calories." If you're eating a 1,000-calorie ribeye steak, you're technically eating a 1,000,000 small calorie meal. Since this is incredibly confusing, from now on, whenever I mention "calories," I mean the ones we're most familiar with: the larger "food calories."

Maintenance Calories: This is the caloric intake you must regularly consume to maintain your current body weight and composition.

Calorie Deficit: This involves consuming *less* than your maintenance intake. Consuming at a deficit for a long enough period will yield a drop in body weight. This drop is often comprised of both lean mass and body fat (though ideally, the majority is fat).

Calorie Surplus: This involves consuming *more* than your maintenance intake. Your ability to build lean mass is much more effective when consuming at a surplus and providing your body with the fuel necessary to build more tissue; however, this can also increase body fat.

Metabolic Adaptation: This is the adaptation that occurs when your caloric intake shifts, and your body is forced to compensate. This is a natural evolutionary survival mechanism. For instance, if you were stuck in Paleolithic times and suddenly found yourself short on food, your body's metabolism would down-regulate to conserve energy and adapt to this shortage. This also occurs when you hit a dieting plateau.

Energy Balance or **Energy Homeostasis** is a biological process that involves the coordinated homeostatic regulation of food intake (energy inflow) and energy expenditure. This balance is often referred to as "calories in, calories out" or CICO, but it goes much deeper than just calories. For whatever reason, this concept of energy balance became a red flag to many people in the low-carb dieting communities. This is likely because keto and low-carb enthusiasts hold hormones and insulin in such high regard as it relates to losing body fat and being healthy. Hormones and insulin secretion play a massive role in our body's storage and loss of adipose tissue; however, it makes no sense to disregard the fact that the amount of calories you consume has a profound impact on your ability to gain or lose weight. This holds regardless of the type of diet you are following. As such, we will give it the attention it deserves when establishing maintenance calories and determining the caloric deficit necessary to lose body fat for a competition optimally.

CALCULATIONS

Let us start by determining our initial caloric intake for maintenance. Remember, our maintenance calories are the calories we need to consume to maintain our current weight and composition. If this were illustrated as an equation, it would simply be:

Maintenance Calories = Total Daily Energy Expenditure (TDEE)

So, how do we go about establishing our TDEE? Let me preface this entire discussion by saying that these are all estimations at best. There will be outliers for which these numbers will not apply. The most effective method for determining your true TDEE is through trial and error and a lot of self-experimentation, even if these calculations will get us in the general ballpark for most of the population.

The human body is incredibly complex and does not operate in a closed system. There are many other factors and variables that are not accounted for in these equations; instead, these estimations are a perfect illustration of the 80/20 principle. Basically, of all the different factors that impact our metabolic needs, these energy balance calculations get us close enough to make a measurable difference. Rather than spending 100% of our time trying to manipulate every little detail, a better strategy is to spend far less time on factors we can't control or know and focus on those we can (i.e., caloric intake, energy balance, macronutrient make-up, micronutrient density and so on).

TDEE = BMR + NEAT + Exercise + TEF

Basal Metabolic Rate (BMR) is the energy intake necessary to stay alive—in other words, the energy you would burn if you were in a coma. It doesn't account for activity outside of normal bodily functions.

Non-Exercise Activity Thermogenesis (NEAT) accounts for all the movement you do throughout the day outside of planned exercise. This activity includes fidgeting, walking around, taking a shower, cooking a meal, doing your laundry and whistling while you work. NEAT takes a massive hit when your calories are in a steep deficit. On the other end of the spectrum, NEAT activity intensifies when calories are consumed at a significant surplus.

Exercise is exactly what it sounds like: these are the calories burned while training and are dependent on the intensity and duration of the session. There are many different apps and wearables that calculate total energy expenditure while training, but keep in mind that all of them are just estimations.

Thermic Effect of Food (TEF) is the energy you burn to process the energy you consume. If you eat a steak, the bodily functions that metabolize that steak and break it down into energy also require energy from calories. Of the three macronutrients—proteins, carbs and fat—protein has the highest TEF. As it relates to metabolism and total caloric expenditure, the thermic effect of food has a fairly minimal impact. A significant increase in dietary protein does not translate to a significant increase in total calories burned.

There are many different mathematical calculations for determining BMR, but we'll use the Muller Method for simplicity's sake as it accounts for lean body mass (LBM), fat mass (FM), age and sex. The Muller method for calculating BMR looks like this:

BMR = (13.587 x LBM) + (9.613 x FM) + (198 x Sex) - (3.351 x Age) + 674

Sex is notated as "1" for males and "0" for females in this equation. **Age** is notated as the number of years you've been alive.

We'll need to know our **Lean Body Mass (LBM)** for this equation, so let's start by defining that.

LBM is everything in our body that isn't body fat. This includes skin, bones, muscle tissue, water, hair, nails and everything else that is *not* adipose. Your LBM will fluctuate throughout prep. For instance, your body's total water retention will dip when you start tweaking electrolytes. That will result in a drop in your lean body mass but by no means indicates that you've lost a ton of muscle. Recognize that your LBM is simply everything that does not include fat mass. We'll use our body fat percentage that we calculated earlier to find LBM using the following equation:

LBM = Body Weight - (Body Fat Percentage x Body Weight)

With all these calculations, body weight is represented in kilograms rather than pounds. To convert to kilograms, simply multiply pounds by 0.45359237.

To illustrate, I'll make all these calculations using myself as an example.

At the time of this writing, I am 28 years old and weigh about 180 lb. I am coming in at about 12% body fat via the caliper tests.

Based on my numbers, my LBM would be calculated as follows:

180 lb x 0.45359237 = 81.65 kg
LBM = 81.65 - (0.12 x 81.65)
LBM = 71.85 kg

Since my LBM equals 71.85 kg, my fat mass (FM) would be 9.8 kg.

Body Weight - LBM = FM
81.65 - 71.85 = 9.8

Taking this one step further and plugging these numbers into the Muller equation to find my BMR would look like this:

BMR = (13.587 x 71.85) + (9.613 x 9.8) + (198 x 1) - (3.351 x 28) + 674
BMR = 1,848.61

This estimation would indicate that my individual Basal Metabolic Rate is 1,848.61 calories. I need to eat 1,848 calories simply to keep the lights on.

For the sake of being thorough, let's also include an example for females. Let's say our female is 140 lb, 25% body fat and also 28 years old. The calculations would look like this:

140 lb x 0.45359237 = 63.50 kg
LBM = 63.50 - (0.25 x 63.50)
LBM = 47.63

After establishing the LBM, we can then find the fat mass:

Body Weight - LBM = FM
63.50 - 47.63 = 15.87 kg

Please note that if you want to convert kilograms back into pounds, simply multiply the kilogram measurement by 2.20462262.

In this case, our female is carrying about 34.99 lb of body fat:

1 kg = 2.20462262 lb
15.87 x 2.20462262 = 34.99 lb

Now, let's calculate our female's estimated BMR. Females are denoted as a 0 in the equation for their sex rather than males, who are expressed as a 1.

BMR = (13.587 x 47.63) + (9.613 x 15.87) + (198 x 0) - (3.351 x 28) + 674
BMR = 1,379.88

Our female has a basal metabolic rate of about 1,379.88 calories.

* * *

Now that we've established our basal metabolic rate, our next calculation is to determine our total daily energy expenditure as mentioned above. Remember, this figure is calculated as follows:

TDEE = BMR + NEAT + Exercise + TEF

The Thermic Effect of Food is a noteworthy variable, but due to its low overall impact, we will let its effect average out over time rather than figuring it into our initial calculation here.

Following this ketogenic contest prep protocol means that protein intake will fluctuate quite a bit over the course of months. Many traditional "bro" dieting methods leave protein intake as a fixed variable that doesn't fluctuate. Since we'll be manipulating protein, it makes more sense to let its impact average out rather than factoring it into our initial TDEE calculation.

That said, we do want to account for our NEAT and exercise caloric expenditures. The best way to factor these variables in is to assign them via an "activity multiplier." This activity multiplier exists in a range from 1.2-1.9 and is designed to be a rough estimation for the types of activities you do throughout the day. A simple guide is illustrated below:

ACTIVITY MULTIPLIER GUIDE

1.2: Sedentary

You work a 9-to-5 desk job and do not train at all. You come home after work and watch Netflix with your feet propped up. You definitely aren't hitting a 10,000-count step goal. If this is you, you're probably not reading this competition prep manual.

1.375: Light activity

This category would encompass those of you that work a desk job but also train on occasion—possibly at-home workouts with calisthenics and resistance bands when the mood strikes. On the other hand, perhaps you don't train at all but work at a slightly more active job that keeps you on your feet all day.

1.55: Moderate Activity

This is where the vast majority of people reading this manual will likely fall. You may work a desk job but then absolutely kill it in the gym; or, you may not train at all but instead have a demanding job doing something like construction where you are constantly moving and lifting heavy objects.

1.725: Very Active

If you are very active, you're moving throughout the entire day. You train consistently throughout the week with quite a bit of intensity, but you also have a physically demanding job that requires you to move constantly.

1.9: Extra Active

If you're operating out of this category, you're burning some serious calories throughout the day. You likely train like an animal five or six days a week and have a highly demanding job pouring concrete or something similar.

***

Using this activity multiplier guide, determine which multiplier fits you best and multiply that by your BMR, which we calculated earlier. Keep in mind that there is no point in having an ego here; it won't do you any good. A little bit of self-awareness goes a long way.

If you think of yourself as a Trojan warrior who trains intensely non-stop and would be a 1.9, but you actually just watched the movie

Troy and think you look like Brad Pitt, you're probably closer to a 1.375 multiplier. Don't try and overestimate your activity as it will only slow you down later.

In the case of our male example (me), I would say that I'm about a 1.55 on the activity multiplier. I resistance train six days a week very intensely, and I go for a run every single day. I often hike on the weekends, but my career involves a ton of computer work for which I sit at a desk. I doubt I'm burning a significant number of calories while podcasting or writing this book.

Using that 1.55 multiplier, I can determine my estimated total daily energy expenditure. The TDEE will be a close approximation of what our maintenance calories should be.

TDEE = Maintenance Calories*
***(Remember, we decided to negate the Thermic Effect of Food (TEF))**

TDEE/Maintenance Calories = BMR x Activity Multiplier

In my case:

TDEE/Maintenance Calories = 1,848.61 x 1.55
TDEE/Maintenance Calories = 2,865.35

Now, through trial and error and years of self-experimentation, I know my actual maintenance caloric intake to be around 3,100, but 2,865 isn't too far off in the grand scheme of things, and it certainly didn't take me years to calculate it.

As far as our female is concerned, let's assume she is a 1.725 on the activity multiplier. She resistance trains six days a week and takes her dogs for a brisk walk every day. Unlike me, her career path is a bit more physically demanding. She is a registered nurse and spends 98% of her day walking the floor and treating patients rather than sitting at a computer. Her maintenance calories would be calculated as follows:

TDEE/Maintenance Calories = BMR x Activity Multiplier

TDEE/Maintenance Calories = 1,379.88 x 1.725
TDEE/Maintenance Calories = 2,380.30

Again, this is just an estimation, but it's a good starting point. There are many other factors at play such as hormones, muscle maturity and stress, but in theory, consuming less than 2,380 calories would yield a drop in weight for our female.

One other important thing to realize is this: it's better to start high and give yourself more time than to start too low. As far as overall caloric consumption is concerned, I highly advise starting on the higher end to ensure that you have enough time to diet down. This will result in far less muscle loss over time and ensure that you take advantage of your actual caloric threshold. If you start much lower than necessary, you may lose weight faster at the onset, but you'll be more likely to plateau later on. The more "caloric runway" you have to taper from, the better.

Okay, now that we know our current body fat percentage and our estimated maintenance calories, we can begin to determine how long we need to prep. Once again, this is also just an estimation—some people are much more responsive to the prep than others, and it's always better to peak early and manipulate variables to stay dialed in than it is to peak too late and overshoot the show day entirely.

I'll also say this: while getting in peak condition, you can lose a lot more weight than you might anticipate. Not all the weight we lose is adipose tissue; some is LBM. This LBM loss is normal and to be expected, and the percentage of LBM lost will likely be higher in natural athletes than those using performance-enhancing drugs. Remember, this drop in LBM isn't all coming from muscle tissue;

most of it is water weight. It's essential to account for it, though, to have a clearer picture of our expected total weight loss.

The first time I prepped for a competition, my starting weight was 230 lb. This was long before I ever started the ketogenic diet and I had just finished an incredibly "dirty" bulk. I assumed that I would lose 30 lb and step onstage as a shredded, 200 lb natural bodybuilder. I was wrong. Eighty pounds later, I jumped onstage as a lean and wiry 150 lb bodybuilder.

My perception of what I had to lose was skewed, and it cost me. I didn't give myself nearly enough time to prep, and I lost a ton of lean muscle tissue in the process because I dieted down far too aggressively. This is where self-awareness comes into play. Be honest about your actual body fat and how you look in the mirror. Give yourself enough time and do it right.

Also, keep in mind that the judges don't care about your body fat percentage. There won't be any DEXA scans on show day. It's all about how you look, and that is going to be highly individualized. I've seen athletes at 6% body fat who look significantly leaner than competitors at 4% body fat. It's not all about the number; it's about the total package you bring on show day.

That said, having some actual numbers to strive for provides some helpful context. Referencing the chart below, we can begin to put together some hard numbers and create a rough timeline.

Body Fat Analysis

Division	Caliper	DXA	BIA/Inbody
Men's Bodybuilding	2-4%	4-6%	3-10%
Men's Classic Physique	3-5%	5-7%	4-11%
Men's Physique	4-6%	6-8%	5-12%
Women's Physique	7-9%	9-12%	9-16%
Women's Figure	8-10%	10-13%	11-17%
Women's Bikini	9-12%	11-14%	12-18%

Using myself as the male example, let's say I'm starting at 12% body fat via the caliper test. I know from personal experience that my glute striations start popping and I'm show-ready when the caliper puts me at 3% body fat. For the sake of calculation, let's say that means I'll shoot for a body fat goal of 3% via the caliper test on show day.

If I currently weigh 180 lb (81.65 kg) and my body fat is 12%, I'm carrying 9.8 kg of body fat, as we calculated earlier. If I need to get down to 3% body fat to be competitive on show day, I need to lose about 9% body fat between now and peak week. Nine divided by 12 yields 0.75; this means I need to lose 75% of my current body fat to be competitive.

9.8 kg x 75% = 7.35 kg of fat to lose during prep

7.35kg x 2.20462262 = 16.20 lb of fat

Does this mean my total expected weight loss is about 16 lb, and I can plan on stepping onstage at around 164 lb (180 lb minus 16)? Nope, not even close.

Inevitably, you will lose some lean body mass as you go through this process. As I mentioned earlier, most of that will likely be attributed to water and other fluids, but some could very well be muscle mass. I do think one of the main benefits of following a ketogenic protocol throughout your contest prep is that you are significantly less catabolic than those guzzling carbohydrates and minimal dietary fat.

I lost a significant amount of strength and muscle tissue during contest prep when I leveraged "bro" dieting and IIFYM principles. I'd keep protein intake very high to minimize this loss in muscle, but I'd always experience a noticeable dip. Once I switched over to keto, I experienced minimal, if any, drop in actual muscle tissue during the prep, and I've been able to replicate this same response in all my prep athletes since.

I honestly believe this is a result of the highly anti-catabolic effects of ketones combined with the stabilized hormone levels that result from higher dietary fat consumption prescribed in this protocol. Traditional bro dieters hail protein and carbohydrates as being anti-catabolic, and they are correct. I've just observed a greater muscle sparing effect from leveraging the increased circulating blood ketones and higher levels of dietary fat relative to other macros within the context of an extreme caloric deficit.

When you are keto-adapted, you tend to hold less unnecessary fluid. Since you're not constantly over-saturating your glycogen stores, you're not continually retaining excess water weight. As we discussed earlier, water is a significant contributor to LBM. At first glance, it may seem like you have less LBM while following a ketogenic diet than you would if you were consuming large quantities of carbohydrates.

As it relates to your water storage, this is probably true. Make no mistake though: having less LBM due to less fluid retention isn't necessarily a bad thing at all. I'd much prefer having slightly less LBM and have it come from a drop in unnecessary fluid. Your ability to retain actual lean muscle tissue is improved when following a strict ketogenic protocol. Maintaining more lean muscle tissue is significantly more appealing than maintaining more water weight.

Keto or not, you can expect to lose some LBM during a prep. You can minimize this with proper training and nutrition, but some loss is still inevitable. For the sake of simplicity, I would estimate that about 75% of the weight you lose will be adipose tissue while the remaining 25% will be LBM. For this reason, we can expect to lose more total weight than is illustrated by just body fat alone. As we calculated earlier, I need to lose 7.35 kg of fat during this prep. Let's divide that by 75% to determine our total weight loss required.

Total weight loss = body fat loss required / percentage of weight from body fat lost

7.35 / 75% = 9.8

Thus, I need to lose 9.8 kg throughout this contest prep, which equates to 21.61 lb of total weight to lose. That would put me onstage at a total body weight of 158.4 lb.

How much does our female need to lose? Let's say she is competing in the figure division and is also testing her body fat using the calipers. Remember, she started this journey at 25% body fat, and her initial weight was 63.50 kg. Let's assume she needs to get down to 9% body fat to look optimal.

25% - 9% = 16%
16/25 = 0.64

She needs to lose 64% of her current body fat to be competitive on show day. Her initial fat mass (FM) was 15.87 kg.

15.87 kg X 64% = 10.16 kg of fat to lose during prep

10.16 kg X 2.20462262 = 22.40 lb of fat

Remember, about 25% of all the weight she loses will be LBM, so we have to figure that into the equation.

Total weight loss = body fat loss required / percentage of weight from body fat lost

10.16 / 75% = 13.55 kg of total weight to lose
13.55 kg x 2.20462262 = 29.87 lb of total weight to lose

Thus, our female would be stepping onstage at around 110 lb (140 lb - 29.88 lb equals about 110 lb).

HOW LONG SHOULD YOU PREP?

Now that we know how much total body weight we should aim to lose during contest prep, we can also estimate how long prep should be. Of course, there are many different trains of thought around this question.

My very first competition prep was a whopping 12 weeks long. I allotted 12 weeks to lean out simply because that's what I read all the pro bodybuilders did in *Muscle & Fitness* and *Flex*. That was a huge mistake. I went from a sloppy 230 lb to a lean 150 lb in 12 weeks, but I lost a ton of muscle in the process. I had to diet far too aggressively, and the entire process was miserable. I wound up with eating disorders, and my relationship with food took years to recover fully.

I've learned a lot since that first prep, and I do things much differently now. It's better to take a slow and systematic approach. Give yourself all the time in the world because it's more sustainable. As a natural athlete, you'll retain more lean muscle mass if you don't diet down too quickly.

I like to keep it super simple and shoot for an average of one pound per week. In the example above, I need to lose 21.61 lb over the course of the prep, so I'd round that up to 22 lb and plan for a 22-week prep (our female example needs to lose 29.87 lb, so round up to 30 lb and prepare for a 30-week prep).

This plan doesn't necessarily mean that you will lose a pound every week. There may be weeks when your weight goes up a few pounds. There may be weeks when nothing changes, and you get frustrated every time you step on the scale. There may be weeks when you randomly drop five pounds. Weight loss is *not* a linear process. Take the fluctuations as they come and don't lose any sleep over it.

Now, let's be honest with ourselves: 30 weeks is no walk in the park. That is a long time to stay strict while tracking macros, consistently training, posing and sacrificing social events. There is a point of diminishing returns in which a longer prep starts to have a negative effect. Fifty-two weeks makes up an entire calendar year. If you're spending more than half of your year in a caloric deficit, are you genuinely going to be enjoying the process?

There is a fine line between prepping long enough to maximize muscle mass conservation and prepping so long that it becomes miserable. The longest prep I've personally endured is 22 weeks. I could have kept going, but I certainly wouldn't have wanted to go much beyond the 25-week mark. It's why I advise against going off the rails in the off-season and implementing a "dirty bulk."

The more sloppy weight you add, the more you will have to lose later. The more you have to lose, the longer your competition prep cycle. I've found that my "sweet spot" is to stay within about 15-20 lb of my ideal stage weight year-round. If I go much beyond that, I feel a bit sluggish and look softer than I like. Contrary to popular belief, you don't need to blow up like a balloon in the off-season to put on quality muscle. Stay healthy throughout the year and always be within reach of that 15-20 lb window.

One more caveat: recognize that your weekly caloric intake will gradually drop over the entirety of contest prep. If you're prepping for 20-30 weeks, make sure you're starting at a high enough intake to ensure you're not running on fumes by the end. You can expect to be consuming very little by the end, but it's essential to make sure that it's still a healthy intake. There is a significant difference between consuming very little and straight-up starvation.

Have a caloric floor and don't go below it because doing so will likely do more damage to your metabolism than it's worth. I've seen far too many competitors tank their metabolism by going too deep into a deficit for far too long. Caloric floors are highly individual, but have enough self-awareness to know where it is for you.

From experience, I don't take my female clients below 1,300 calories—maybe 1,200 at the *absolute* bottom if they are significantly shorter than average and carry much less total muscle. Similarly, I don't like taking my male clients below 1,500 total calories. Also worth noting is that these floors are finite and short-term. I recommend only staying that low for a week or two before the show. Context is also important.

When calories are at their lowest, it's good to incorporate ketogenic caloric refeeds once or twice a week. This helps bump up the overall caloric average for the week, which makes things more sustainable. Do *not* stay at an extreme deficit for weeks on end. If your coach recommends you go below 1,000 calories, fire your coach. They are not interested in your overall health and wellness.

I'll dive more into metabolism and reverse dieting to ramp metabolism back up post-show later in this book, but I mention it here to bring the fact that your calories will be dropping continuously throughout prep to the front of your mind. It's the reason why it's critical to start your prep at a healthy caloric intake to begin with. If your metabolism and caloric intake are not in a healthy range at the onset, you should probably rethink your competing plans and come back to them later. The last thing I would want your prep to result in is any form of long-term damage to your metabolism, hormones or overall health.

STARTING CALORIC INTAKE

We have now established our starting body fat percentage and have calculated our basal metabolic rate. We have a rough approximation of how many calories we need to consume daily to maintain our weight based on our total daily energy expenditure. We have a good idea of how many total pounds we need to lose, counting adipose tissue and lean body mass, to step onstage at our desired conditioning. We also know how many weeks we should budget for reaching that conditioning goal. Now what?

The next step is to determine starting calories: how much of a deficit do we need to torch away the body fat?

This is a fork in the road where my protocol differs substantially from other prep coaches. If you were following an IIFYM or bro dieting coach, this is when they would calculate required deficit based on the caloric load of body fat and lean mass. They would establish how many grams each would need to be cut based on a weekly weight loss goal, and then they would determine how many calories would result in that number and then slash maintenance calories accordingly. It's not uncommon to see coaches automatically start prep at 500-1000 calories below maintenance. This is *not* what we are going to do.

Why not? Well, first of all, athletes and bodybuilders work so hard to ramp up their metabolic rate and increase their caloric threshold coming into a prep. All the training over the years and all the healthy eating works overtime to improve their metabolism and allow them to function optimally at a higher caloric intake without risking unnecessary body fat gain. The last thing I want to do is slash that caloric threshold significantly.

If you make a massive manipulation such as cutting your calories by 500, it's relatively impossible to know where the tipping point truly is. As such, you run the risk of leaving a good deal of that caloric runway behind. Another disadvantage of this method is that it practically guarantees that you will hit a plateau. You may indeed see some initial weight loss, but your body is competent; it will adapt and correct course. Your metabolism will acclimate to this drop, and your progress will come to a grinding halt. You'll be forced to slash calories again to regain your momentum, which becomes a vicious cycle that inevitably leads to consuming far less than necessary. Rather than estimating our deficit based on how many calories are in a pound of body fat and then cutting accordingly, I prefer to let our bodies show us precisely what we need to know.

Use your maintenance calories as your starting point. Rather than hacking away at that number, gradually taper that intake throughout the entire prep. I like to manipulate macros every week, slowly chipping away at total caloric intake and tweaking the macronutrient ratios to get things dialed in. This protocol is slow and methodical, but it's incredibly effective and leaves the guesswork out of the equation. By slowly tapering caloric intake, we apply just a slight amount of pressure continually throughout the entirety of prep. Our body responds to this pressure by burning through body fat with a minimal drop in lean tissue.

True, you may not lose as much scale weight right off the bat using this method. That can be discouraging at first, but make no mistake: that doesn't mean nothing is happening internally. We are priming the pump to ensure sustained fat loss for this entire prep, not just the first quarter.

I like to think of it like a sculptor chipping away at a massive rock wall. Chisel and hammer in hand, he chips away daily, hitting the same spot on the wall. It seems like nothing is happening for weeks but he continues to chip away, constantly applying that pressure. One day, he carefully places his chisel in the same spot, rears the hammer back and drives it forward. He hits his mark, and a massive piece of rock breaks off and falls to the ground below.

It wasn't that single blow that resulted in the shattered rock; it was the constant application of pressure over several weeks. The same concept holds to what we are doing with this prep. We're not using dynamite on that rock wall. We're applying gradual pressure and keeping it steady over several weeks. There's no one single manipulation that makes a ton of difference; instead, it's the compounded effect of all of the seemingly insignificant changes we make. So grab your chisel, and prepare to create a masterpiece.

STARTING MACRONUTRIENTS

Remember that fork in the road we talked about earlier? The one that separates this ketogenic protocol from that of other prep coaches? That fork starts going the opposite direction at this point, so get ready. Take everything you think you know about carbs, fats and proteins and how much you need to consume daily and throw it all out the window. What follows are my recommendations for determining your initial macronutrient intake and macro ratio profile.

Typically, prep coaches will calculate your protein requirements based on the LBM you're carrying. Protein will stay constant throughout the prep and carbohydrates will fuel your energy demands. They'll typically leave enough fat in the diet to keep the body functioning, but dietary fat is often stripped to a bare minimum. We obviously aren't going to go that route since we are keto-adapted athletes; we leverage dietary fat and stored body fat as our primary fuel source.

A standard ketogenic diet is often viewed as 75% dietary fat, 20% protein and 5% carbohydrates, so should we start there? No. We are going to err on the extreme side of things. We'll begin this journey with 80% of our caloric intake coming from dietary fat.

As far as protein and carbs are concerned, we'll base them on a ratio of our total caloric intake rather than LBM. I know that sounds crazy, but trust me. Let's cap total dietary carbohydrates at 20 g to begin with, and the remaining caloric load will be allocated to protein.

Using our male and female examples, let's establish our starting macronutrient intake and ratios:

Male: TDEE/Maintenance Calories = 2,865.35

Fat Macros = 80% of total calories
Fat Macros = .80 x 2,865.35
Fat Macros = 2,292.28 total calories

Since there are nine calories in a gram of fat, divide 2,292.28 by nine to determine fat grams.

Fat Grams = 2,292.28 / 9
Fat Grams = 254.70 g

I like manipulating macros in 5 g increments, so let's round this up to 255 to keep things convenient.

We'll cap total dietary carbohydrates at 20 g. There are four calories per gram of carbohydrates, so that would be 80 calories used up by carbs.

20 x 4 = 80 calories from carbs

Let's now calculate our initial protein intake by subtracting our dietary fat and carbs from the equation.

Protein Calories = Total Calories - Fat Calories - Carb Calories
Protein Calories = 2865.35 - 2,292.28 - 80
Protein Calories = 493.07

Like carbs, there are four calories per gram of protein. To determine our protein grams, simply divide our protein calories by four.

Protein Grams = 493.07 / 4
Protein Grams = 123.27

Again, to keep things simple, let's round this up to the nearest 5 g increment. Our starting protein intake will be 125 g.

Thus, our starting macro/caloric intake for our male example will be as follows:

Calories: 2,875

Fat: 255 g
Protein: 125 g
Total Carbs: 20 g

Note: Our calorie count is slightly higher than our calculated TDEE/Maintenance intake because we rounded our macro goals to the nearest 5 g increment.

Now before you get yourself all worked up about that low starting protein intake, relax. I'll explain the higher fat and low protein macro goals in just a minute.

Before that, let's also calculate our starting macros for our female example:

Female: TDEE/Maintenance Calories = 2,380.30

Fat Macros = 80% of total calories
Fat Macros = .80 x 2,380.30
Fat Macros = 1,904.24 total calories

Fat Grams = 1,904.24 / 9
Fat Grams = 211.58 g (round to 210 g)

Carb Grams = 20 g total

Protein Calories = Total Calories - Fat Calories - Carb Calories

Protein Calories = 2,380.30 - 1,904.24 - 80
Protein Calories = 396.06

Protein Grams = 396.06 / 4
Protein Grams = 99.02 (round to 100 g)

Thus, our starting macro/caloric intake for our female example will be as follows:

Calories: 2,370
Fat: 210 g
Protein: 100 g
Total Carbs: 20 g

Note: Again, calorie count is slightly different than our calculated TDEE/Maintenance because we rounded.

I want to re-emphasize a significant point now that we have our starting macros: these are estimates! It's not the end of the world if you start a few grams higher or lower than what we've just calculated. These macronutrient targets will change every single week of this prep. For that reason alone, it's not critical that you nail your body's exact TDEE with the starting macro goals, so be a little flexible.

It's essential to have enough self-awareness to use an activity multiplier that accurately defines you and gets you in the range you want, but nothing here is set in stone. The main goal of this prep up to this stage is to establish a solid foundation.

Everybody's body will respond differently to the manipulations I'll suggest here, which is why adjusting macros weekly gives us so much wiggle room. We can react on the fly and be very agile with our tweaks, so there's no need to feel locked in on any specific macronutrient set. Establish your initial starting macros and then *start!* Don't be a perfectionist in Phase One. Analysis paralysis is the biggest killer of would-be prep athletes!

STANDARDIZE BEFORE YOU OPTIMIZE

So, now that we have our starting macros, what's next? Well, if you were following an IIFYM approach, you would simply throw together a random combination of foods that fit your desired intake—but is that the optimal approach?

Generally speaking, there are two schools of thought on what to do next. The first suggests that you eat whatever you desire as long as the daily total falls within your desired macronutrient and caloric range. This offers a ton of variety, and you likely won't get bored of the meals you are consuming.

The other suggests that you prep your meals in advance and structure your meal plan around specific foods that hit your target macros. This option provides much less variety, but it takes out all the guesswork.

The direction you take depends a lot on your personality. Do you get stressed out and frustrated with the monotony of doing the same thing day after day? Do you think of meal prepping as a shackle that keeps you confined to a rigid way of eating? Will this likely result in you abandoning the plan altogether and binging on other food, sabotaging your macronutrient targets? If so, then feel free to grant yourself some variety and flexibility. Eat quality foods that let you to hit your targets and make the process as sustainable as possible.

I'm just the opposite. Too much variety is what stresses me out, whereas having a structured plan is liberating. Macros will likely change week to week, so meal prepping for each week at a given macro count makes a lot more sense in my mind. I can eat the same meals day after day for a week and not get bored with them. Then, as my cravings change, I can change my meal prep with my macros the following week.

This strategy takes the guesswork out of daily planning. I don't have to stress about finding foods to hit my target macros because the food is already prepared and ready to go. I don't have to constantly stare at my macro tracker, swapping foods in and out to make the numbers work. Rather than wasting time being flexible, I save time by being consistent.

I recognize that we are all different, and what works well for one athlete may be a total dead-end for another. Have enough self-awareness on this topic to know where you stand and structure your meal planning accordingly. You could easily implement a hybrid model that looks something like this:

Meal prep on Sunday for the following week. Only meal prep for six days, Monday through Saturday. Sunday is a flexible day where you can mix up your foods and have something outside the norm—still within the target macros but outside the foods you typically consume. This will still yield a quality result and may be more sustainable for you.

There is no hard rule on this subject; the main thing is to implement a strategy that's both effective and sustainable. Sticking to a strategy consistently is what makes the magic happen, so recognize that too much flexibility can make standardizing this process much more difficult. It's important to standardize before you can optimize.

Consider this scenario: you hit your target macros every single day but you're mixing and matching your foods daily, so no two days are ever the same. One day you are down a pound and feeling great; the next day, you're up two pounds and feel like you're holding unnecessary water weight. The ending macros were the same for both days, so what gives?

Well, let's say one day you ate a container of coconut yogurt, and for some reason, your body didn't respond well to it. You would have a hard time noticing that if you ate something different every day. There is often a lag in response time between what you consume and how your weight and composition are affected. If you consistently eat the same thing every day for a week, it is straightforward enough to eliminate any outside variables and pinpoint whatever causes an adverse reaction.

Think of this contest prep as a scientific experiment and your body as the test subject. You want to control for as many variables as possible and manipulate one variable at a time. That way, you know with a substantial degree of certainty how your body responds to each manipulation. If you're changing 15 things at once, it's impossible to know how your body responds to each one. This is why I recommend standardizing your meals rather than giving yourself free rein to eat whatever you want within your target numbers. Standardize the foods you consume and you'll be able to optimize your fuel intake to reach your desired goal of getting shredded as hell!

MEAL EXAMPLES

Assuming many of you are visual learners, I want to include an example of what these starting macros could potentially look like. By no means do you need to feel trapped within these specific food items; you have a ton of flexibility in that regard. I just like to keep my food simple and easy to manipulate. Since we make minor adjustments to the macros each week (usually in 5 g increments), I like to incorporate foods that can easily be measured out and adjusted by 5 g of protein or fat.

Putting this "ease of manipulation" concept into practice, a starting meal plan for our male example may look something like this:

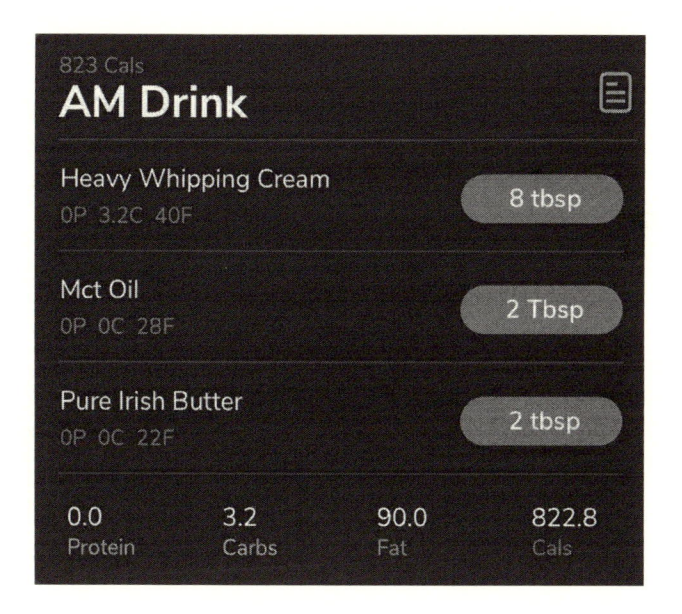

823 Cals
AM Drink

Food	Macros	Amount
Heavy Whipping Cream	0P 3.2C 40F	8 tbsp
Mct Oil	0P 0C 28F	2 Tbsp
Pure Irish Butter	0P 0C 22F	2 tbsp

0.0	3.2	90.0	822.8
Protein	Carbs	Fat	Cals

Meal 1
914 Cals

Liverwurst — 150 Grams
26.79P 0C 10.71F

Olive Oil — 1 Tbsp
0P 0C 14F

Egg Whole — 4 Large Egg
25.2P 1.56C 20F

Sardines, Wild, in Extra Virgin O... — 3 oz
15P 0C 12F

Pure Irish Butter — 1 tbsp
0P 0C 11F

| 67.0 Protein | 1.6 Carbs | 67.7 Fat | 914.1 Cals |

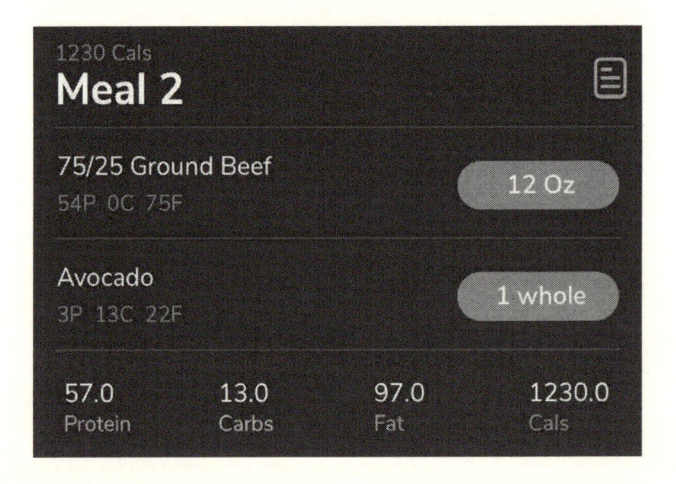

Meal 2
1230 Cals

75/25 Ground Beef — 12 Oz
54P 0C 75F

Avocado — 1 whole
3P 13C 22F

| 57.0 Protein | 13.0 Carbs | 97.0 Fat | 1230.0 Cals |

Daily Totals	
Calories	2966.9 / 2875
Total Fat	254.7 / 255
Saturated Fat	90.25
Monounsaturated Fat	7.60
Polyunsaturated Fat	2.72
Carbs	17.8 / 20
Fiber	9.00
Sugar	0.00
Protein	124.0 / 125

Calories: 2,875
Fat: 255 g
Protein: 125 g
Total Carbs: 20 g

Note: In this particular example, I would probably split the "AM Drink" into two separate cups of keto coffee to be consumed throughout the morning hours.

These screenshots were taken using my macro tracking app: MyMacros+. Notice that the calorie count isn't exact. For whatever reason, macro tracking apps are often slightly skewed in caloric measurements. Focus on the macronutrient gram goals. If you consistently get within 5 g of your macro goals, the calories will work themselves out over time.

An example starting a meal plan for our female client would look very similar, just scaled down a bit to compensate for the lower macros:

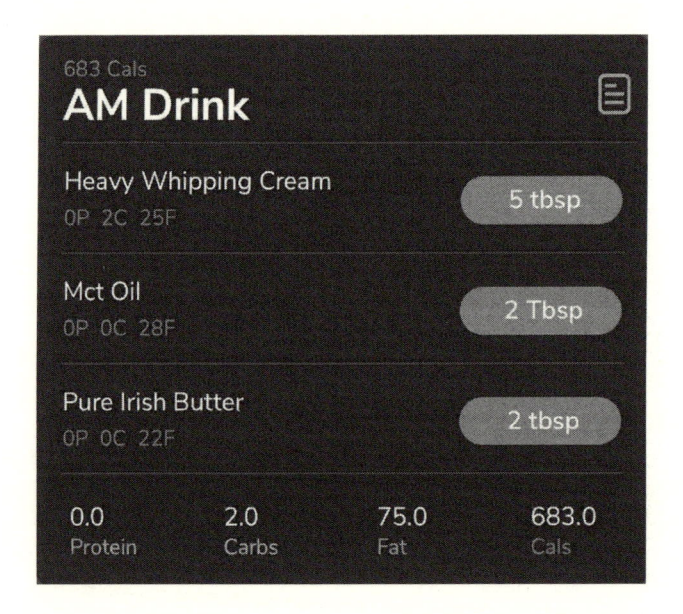

683 Cals
AM Drink

Heavy Whipping Cream 0P 2C 25F	5 tbsp
Mct Oil 0P 0C 28F	2 Tbsp
Pure Irish Butter 0P 0C 22F	2 tbsp

0.0	2.0	75.0	683.0
Protein	Carbs	Fat	Cals

858 Cals
Meal 1

Liverwurst — 150 Grams
26.79P 0C 10.71F

Olive Oil — 1 Tbsp
0P 0C 14F

Egg Whole — 4 Large Egg
25.2P 1.56C 20F

Sardines, Wild, in Extra Virgin O... — 2 oz
10P 0C 8F

Pure Irish Butter — 1 tbsp
0P 0C 11F

62.0	1.6	63.7	858.1
Protein	Carbs	Fat	Cals

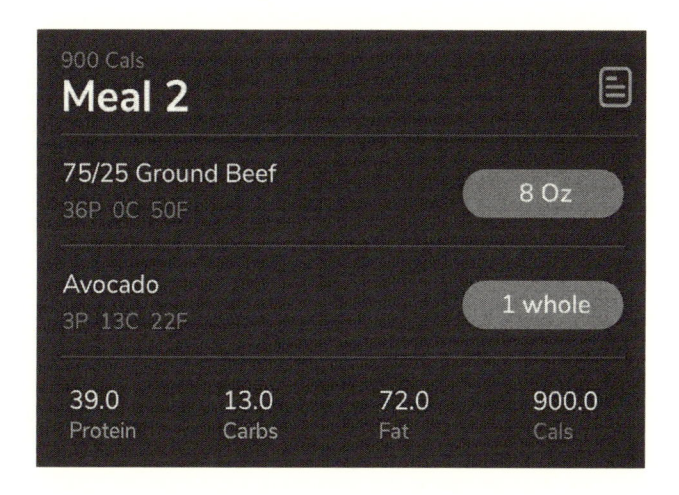

---

900 Cals
Meal 2

75/25 Ground Beef — 8 Oz
36P 0C 50F

Avocado — 1 whole
3P 13C 22F

39.0	13.0	72.0	900.0
Protein	Carbs	Fat	Cals

Daily Totals	
Calories	2441.1 / 2370
Total Fat	210.7 / 210
Saturated Fat	68.00
Monounsaturated Fat	7.60
Polyunsaturated Fat	2.72
Carbs	16.6 / 20
Fiber	9.00
Sugar	0.00
Protein	101.0 / 100

Calories: 2,370
Fat: 210 g
Protein: 100 g
Total Carbs: 20 g

MACRO RATIOS

You may be looking at these initial starting macros thinking to yourself, "Why is this fat ratio so high?" or "Why is my protein so low?" Those are valid, reasonable concerns. After all, if you want to lose body fat, it only makes sense to cut down on the dietary fat, right? If you're going to conserve lean muscle tissue, you need to be eating at least 1 g of protein per pound of lean mass, right? Not exactly.

The method behind the madness here is what separates this prep protocol from other dieting methods. You won't find these techniques in any other prep manual, they won't be listed in any encyclopedia of bodybuilding books and you certainly won't find them in a *Flex* article. The methods that follow result from years of self-experimentation on myself, refined and polished with each competition prep I've done.

Do you really want to put your faith in my n-of-1 experiment? Is my anecdotal evidence really enough to hang your hat on? It shouldn't be, so I've also incorporated these macro recommendations into all of my clients' contest preps over the years. Hundreds of clients have gotten the leanest they have ever been using these techniques, ones that go against the recommendations of every other contest prep coach. These techniques seem to conflict with common wisdom even within the keto and low-carb community.

Many of the keto coaches out there today were once my clients. They benefited from these techniques and then created their own platform with their own inherent style. That's fine with me; the more people that preach this practice, the better (because rest assured, it works)! Even so, get ready to throw away everything you think you know about macros and reach an entirely new level of keto-adaptation!

FAT

Let's start with the extremely high fat ratio. How in the world could it make sense to start this journey with 80% of your total caloric intake coming from dietary fat? The answer is quite simple: if you've been keto-adapted for any length of time, you are familiar with the fact that dietary fat and body fat have become your primary fuel source.

Stored body fat is burned and ketones are produced. These ketones and fatty acids are what replace carbohydrates and glucose as your primary source of energy. Many experts in the low-carb space suggest that minimizing dietary fat and forcing the body to tap into stored fat is the best way to lose weight. That may be true, but it comes at the expense of optimizing performance. If your primary energy supply comes from fat, the last thing you want to do is eliminate or significantly reduce it from your diet.

As a bodybuilder, your goal is not simply to lose weight. Your goal is to optimize performance while efficiently losing as much body fat as possible *while* retaining as much lean tissue as possible. If your performance sucks, your ability to train appropriately and preserve lean tissue is significantly reduced. Do you think you're going to be able to optimize your training if you're missing your main source of energy? Not likely.

By starting this journey with a very high intake of dietary fat relative to protein and carbs, you force the body to become incredibly efficient at leveraging fat, both dietary and stored. If your protein started out higher than fat, our body would function with much less efficiency. Dietary protein and lean muscle tissue would catabolize through a process called gluconeogenesis to provide energy. This glucose creation is a natural phenomenon and shouldn't be viewed as negative. It's just simply not optimal in the context of what we are trying to accomplish. The high intake of dietary fat prioritizes ketone production and utilization over gluconeogenesis. Our initial goal is not to torch body fat. Our initial goal is to improve our body's ability to metabolize fat and use it as the primary driver of energy.

This may sound oversimplified, but it makes complete sense.

Our body is an intelligent system designed to adapt and overcome any hardship. We've evolved over hundreds of thousands of years to survive in any environment. From an evolutionary, long-term perspective, our species survived by consuming animals high in fat and protein. Our Paleolithic ancestors were not chowing down on heavily processed, high glycemic Hot Pockets and Pop-Tarts, ladies and gents. It makes sense that we would function better after returning to a diet that more closely mirrors what we evolved from rather than a diet that only emerged as a result of large-scale industrial agriculture.

From an environmental and short-term perspective, our body will make the most of the materials it has at its disposal. If you primarily fuel it with protein, the body knows to convert that into energy through gluconeogenesis. Primarily fuel it with carbs and glucose metabolism takes effect. Consume a high ratio of dietary fat and a deeper level of keto-adaptation occurs. That deeper level of adaptation and fat metabolism is what we are after!

PROTEIN

But what about the relatively low protein intake—surely that can't be optimal, right? Let me put your mind at ease: your protein intake will increase significantly in the next phase, so there's no need to worry.

If you talk to bro dieters or IIFYM gurus, it's clear that they put protein on a pedestal. All their calculations are based on protein as a priority. In those diets, protein is kept high throughout the entirety of the prep. Protein is absolute.

Ask a hardcore low-carb athlete chasing high ketone numbers, and it's the exact opposite. It's almost like they fear protein and gluconeogenesis! Too much protein spikes blood glucose and hinders ketone production. There have even been arguments that too much protein can have the same effect as a chocolate cake when it enters your system (specious though they may be).

Again, there's a balance to strike here. You can most certainly manipulate protein to efficiently reach your goals. There are times when it's beneficial to have it low and times when it makes sense to have it high. Protein is incredibly important, but it shouldn't be held constant and shouldn't necessarily be put on a pedestal.

Over-consuming protein is counterproductive and unnecessary. Too much protein can lead to GI distress and a poor distribution of available calories. Still, under-consuming protein isn't optimal either. Consuming optimal protein is optimal. So, what is "optimal?" Protein requirements differ if you're trying to optimize for muscle gain or prioritize fat loss, but we'll focus on the fat loss objective here since this is a contest prep manual. During contest prep, we'll vary our protein intake to fit the different phases we go through.

The initial phase starts at a lower protein intake for a few primary reasons. The first is to support our primary objective of becoming more deeply keto-adapted. Having a lower protein intake at the onset of prep goes hand in hand with a higher dietary fat intake. As we discussed earlier, eating more fat forces our body to become increasingly efficient at using fat and ketones for fuel. By minimizing our initial protein intake, we also eliminate the risk of our body metabolizing a surplus of protein through gluconeogenesis. This ensures the prioritization of fat oxidation and ketone production.

Secondly, starting with a lower intake of dietary protein allows us to gradually increase those levels in Phase Two so we can establish an individual "protein threshold." If we were to start at a relatively high protein intake, we would have no way of finding the tipping point. At certain levels, excess protein results in bloating, brain fog and inflammation—and there's no sense in experiencing that if you don't have to.

By starting at a lower intake, we can gradually fine tune our protein intake and establish our individual protein threshold. Though we'll cover this in more detail later, rest assured that your hard-earned muscles will not wither away. Remember: in the beginning, our primary objective is to reach a deeper level of keto-adaptation and start with macros that yield a greater production of ketones and fat metabolism. Ketones are incredibly anti-catabolic. The more efficient you become at using fat and ketones for fuel, the less you have to concern yourself with muscle wasting.

CARBOHYDRATES

Let's also touch on total carbohydrate intake to round out this discussion on macro ratios. We are starting this prep with a 20 g total carb ceiling. Let me re-emphasize the *total* there—there's no sense in lying to yourself and only counting net carbs.

When you are indeed in a deep state of ketosis and have adapted so that all your body's fuel requirements are derived from fatty acids and some amino acids, there's no longer a need to consume more than

20 g of total carbohydrates. As a side note, I realize that the brain still requires a minuscule amount of glucose even after keto-adaptation; that trivial amount is easily provided through a slight level of gluconeogenesis that will naturally occur. No dietary carbohydrates are necessary. In fact, you could go through this prep following a zero-carb meal plan and be fine.

I've allotted the 20 g here simply as a buffer for the trace carbs that will be consumed through ketogenic foods (such as heavy cream, vegetables, eggs and other sources). We'll start this prep at the 20 g ceiling, but that will likely dwindle closer to 10 g as we get deeper into the cut. If you're coming from a traditional, carbohydrate-based prep, 10 g of total carbohydrates may sound entirely impossible.

On the contrary, it's entirely possible and quite manageable. You'll be amazed at how much tighter you'll become after simply dropping your carb intake to that low amount. You'll retain far fewer unnecessary fluids, and you'll be able to achieve a look that is nothing short of amazing.

Perhaps you're following a carnivore or zero-carb approach at the onset, and you don't want the 20 g of carbs to start. That is fine. Reallocate the 80 calories you would be getting from the carbs and partition them evenly between your dietary fat and protein intake. I'm writing this manual in the context of following a traditional ketogenic diet, but feel free to tweak it slightly if you want to take a carnivore approach. After all, carnivore is just another subset of keto, so all the same principles still apply.

TRAINING BASELINE

Just as we did with nutrition, we also need a baseline for resistance training and cardio. If you're considering stepping onstage as a competitive athlete, I'll assume that you're no stranger to the gym and that you have a respectable knowledge of exercise programming and technique. You've probably been following some structured training block and have some foundation already established.

If so, start with that. If you see success from your current training protocol, there is no sense reinventing the wheel. As is true with our nutritional goals, I would recommend some form of standardization in your training. Track your activity just as you would track your macros.

I used to train completely intuitively, and I'd never keep tabs on my exercises, weight lifted, reps or volume. That wasn't necessarily a bad thing, but it's not optimal during contest prep. When you're in prep and calories start to dip, your NEAT activity will begin to drop, without question. It's imperative to resist that dip when it comes to your structured resistance training. You likely won't be hitting any new PR's, but it's crucial to maintain your current level of intensity and volume if at all possible.

You can use an app, a spreadsheet or simply pen and paper, but try and keep tabs on your exercises, total volume, strength and intensity. Continually lifting hard throughout prep is one of the best things you can do to ensure maximum muscle retention. Suppose you drastically cut the physical demands of your body and start lifting much lighter in the context of a deep caloric deficit. In that case, your body will recognize that carrying all that lean tissue around is unnecessary and will start catabolizing your hard-earned muscle for fuel. You can fight this process by keeping that hard-earned muscle in high demand. In all reality, resistance training is one of the most muscle sparing activities you can implement during prep.

WHY LESS IS MORE WITH CARDIO

When it comes to cardio, I like to think of it as having an inverse relationship to calories. Use cardio as a "trick up your sleeve," so to speak. So many people decide to lose fat or begin prep and automatically ramp up their cardiovascular activity tenfold. Why is this?

Mainstream media and conventional wisdom suggest that hours on the treadmill are key to losing body fat, but this couldn't be further from the truth. Just as your body adapts to decreasing calories by downregulating metabolism, it adapts to cardio by establishing a "homeostatic norm." For instance, if you go for a five-mile run every single day, that becomes your new norm. Your body will acclimate to that cardiovascular demand and adapt accordingly.

You may lose a little bit of weight at the onset, but eventually, your body will maintain homeostasis and you won't see any additional fat loss. You'll be forced to ramp up the cardio and knock out six or seven miles to see any effect. This can lead to a massive downward spiral in which you're spending all your time and energy doing cardio to get your body composition to shift in the direction you want. Again, this can have a catabolic effect and result in a loss of lean tissue, which, in turn, has an overall negative impact on your metabolism and ability to lose body fat.

How does cardio have an inverse relationship with calories? At the beginning of this prep, calories are the highest; therefore, cardio should be at its least intense. Let's see how much of a change in body composition we can experience solely from manipulating our macronutrients. Then, if at any point our body starts to plateau and becomes unresponsive to the macro changes, we can introduce some cardio—nothing crazy, just a slight increase. That small increase will likely be enough to bump us past the plateau without pushing into a never-ending cardio spiral.

As calories get lower and lower throughout the prep, we'll gradually increase cardio more and more since we will have started with such a small amount to begin with. The less cardio you're doing at the onset, the more cardio runway you have to play with and the more room you have to make subtle changes and tweaks. Don't OD on cardio; instead, try and implement a minimum effective dose.

Just as with resistance training, try and find a way to standardize your cardio. It's much harder to get an accurate measure of your progress if you do hill sprints one day, battle ropes the next, follow that up with the Stairmaster and then top it off with a stationary bike. With a cardio split like that, how could you possibly pinpoint what your body best responds to?

Try and implement a form of cardio that is easily tracked and scaled. Personally, I tend to use the Stairmaster, and I begin my prep at an incredibly low intensity and duration. For instance, I may start with one day a week of cardio and accomplish that by spending eight minutes on the Stairmaster at level five. That isn't too crazy at all, but that may be all I need to get my scale and body composition moving in the right direction. Of course, I can also gradually bump up the intensity, duration and frequency as needed.

The actual nuts and bolts of training do not change drastically from one phase to the next; as such, rather than spending a lot of time on training within each different phase, I've dedicated an entire section of this book exclusively to training techniques and principles. In that section, I've also included some sample training templates and my personal training split that you're more than welcome to use if you don't have a structured plan of your own.

The main takeaway for Phase One correlates perfectly with the principles we discussed regarding our starting nutritional requirements: standardize before you optimize!

BLOODWORK

Getting bloodwork done at the onset of prep is certainly not required, but if you're anything like me, you like to gather as much data as humanly possible. Competition prep is no trivial endeavor. You'll likely be training harder than you ever have before, you'll most certainly be eating less and you'll assuredly be leaner than you ever have been. Even your sleep will be impacted.

Competition prep can be a physiological miracle and a nightmare all wrapped up into one. All of these "extremes" can have a profound impact on the body. It's wise to have a pulse on those changes, and getting preliminary bloodwork done is a great way to do so. What follows is a list of some of the labs I test for. Again, don't feel obligated to test for these; draw from it as you please or add your own tests as well.

BASIC LIPID PANEL

This test generally includes a measurement for total cholesterol, HDL cholesterol, LDL cholesterol and triglycerides. These markers are often the cause of a lot of concern for people on the ketogenic diet.

We've been told for so long that fatty cuts of red meat are guaranteed to clog our arteries and give us a heart attack, but this is simply not true. Cholesterol is essential and should not be demonized. Cholesterol is the precursor to testosterone, which is obviously a worthwhile hormone to have flowing through your body in abundance if you are trying to maximize performance, both in the gym and in the bedroom.

It's not uncommon to see cholesterol numbers above the "ideal range" when first starting a ketogenic diet. After all, you consume a significantly higher intake of lipids when you switch from a Standard American Diet to a ketogenic lifestyle. However, after you become keto-adapted, your body learns how to assimilate these lipids and use them for fuel. Since they are readily used, they aren't left floating around in the bloodstream to turn into plaque and cause a heart attack.

I'm certainly not a doctor, and I don't want to pretend to be an expert on cholesterol. However, I can confidently say that scientists have learned a ton about cholesterol over the past few years, and much of the conventional wisdom in circulation to this day is simply not true. Also, the "ideal range" for cholesterol is likely skewed because it's based on a sample size that predominately eats carbohydrates for fuel. Excess lipids combined with a diet based on carbohydrates is a recipe for disaster; however, this does not apply to those following a ketogenic lifestyle, since we don't consume excess carbohydrates.

As such, an essential lipid panel's "ideal range" may not be the best proxy to measure against. Generally speaking, if I see a high HDL and a relatively low triglyceride count, I'm pretty happy. I don't concern myself if LDL is slightly higher than what mainstream society deems to be "normal."

If you want to dive deeper into cholesterol, I highly encourage you to check out the work by Dr. Nadir Ali and many others in the low-carb space. Dave Feldman is also a great resource and offers an interesting hypothesis for cholesterol levels in athletes. According to his theory, it may be common for those described as "Lean Mass Hyper Responders" to have slightly elevated LDL levels. If you're an athlete following a ketogenic lifestyle, you likely fit within this LMHR definition.

Again, let me reemphasize that I am *not* a doctor, and I am not giving medical advice here. Take your health into your own hands. No one cares about it as much as you do, including your doctor. If you have a conventional doctor who is still preaching old-school methodologies and believes that carbs are great and fat is the devil, I encourage you to dive a bit deeper. They are likely stuck on what they learned in medical school back in the '70s during their limited training on nutrition. There are numerous excellent resources for you on this subject matter, so put in some work and learn something.

Finally, know that your lipid numbers are subject to change in the context of a caloric deficit. I like to test at the beginning of the prep and near the end to see how my body responds to my manipulations. Remember: what can be measured can be managed!

C-REACTIVE PROTEIN

Another practical test is C-reactive Protein or CRP. CRP is a homopentameric acute-phase inflammatory protein, which is basically a fancy way of saying that its level of expression is elevated in times of acute inflammation. It's been used as a marker for various inflammatory disorders, and I like to keep tabs on it to ensure that none of the nutritional or training manipulations I'm making are resulting in unexpectedly high levels of stress on the body.

THYROID PANEL

If you have the means, this is another test I strongly suggest. The thyroid's primary role in the endocrine system is to regulate metabolism. It is directly tied to our ability to break down food and convert it efficiently into energy. The thyroid works with our pituitary gland and hypothalamus to produce and excrete the appropriate amount of hormones to keep our metabolism functioning as it should.

Having very high levels of thyroid hormone (hyperthyroidism) or unusually low levels (hypothyroidism) can both have a profound impact on our appetite and energy levels. Getting a preliminary thyroid panel that tests for T_3, T_4 and Reverse T_3 at the beginning of prep is a wise move to ensure you start with a solid foundation.

HORMONE PANEL

Whether you decide to go the route of performance-enhancing drugs and anabolic steroids or keep it natural, rest assured that your hormone levels will most certainly change throughout prep. A complete hormone panel is a practical test regardless of sex; both males and females can benefit from it.

I test for total testosterone, free testosterone, sex-hormone-binding globulin (SHBG), estrogen and estradiol. Being in a caloric deficit, training intensely and reducing sleep can have a massive impact on your hormone levels, and it's imperative to try and keep these levels in a healthy window. Having healthy testosterone levels directly influences our ability to build muscle, decrease body fat, have proper mental focus and be confident. We want to be sure of and optimize these things while going through contest prep and life in general.

Honestly, this is where following a ketogenic prep protocol truly shows its superiority to traditional dieting methods. Conventional "bro" wisdom suggests a significant drop in dietary fat while dieting down for a competition, but this extreme drop in dietary fat directly impacts our ability to produce and maintain proper levels of testosterone and estrogen in our bodies.

If you drastically cut dietary fat, rest assured that you'll experience a severe dip in energy, mood, recovery and libido. It's no wonder traditional "bro-dieters" walk around like zombies in the latter stages of prep with no hustle, no energy and no sex drive. Keep yourself and your significant other happy and eat more dietary fat!

While going through this ketogenic prep, you'll be keeping your dietary fat intake relatively high by default. This is a great way to ensure your hormone levels remain balanced, even if you experience a significant dip as you drop deeper and deeper into a deficit.

To illustrate, I tested for hormone levels at the onset of my 2020 competition prep. I started with total testosterone of 718 ng/dl. At the time, I was 29 years old, so my numbers were well within the range of what one would expect from a natural athlete at that age. I tested again at the end of my prep six months later, and the results came in at 436 ng/dl. That is not a trivial drop.

A competition prep will have a severe impact on your hormone levels regardless of your age, sex, dieting protocol or level of experience. This is why it's so crucial to give yourself ample time to recover in between cutting phases. Take some preliminary bloodwork tests to ensure you have a solid foundation, give the prep everything you've got, experience a temporary dip in hormone levels and then go through a proper reverse diet and building phase to ensure your body can return to a solid baseline. This is how you turn bodybuilding into a sustainable lifestyle and not a recipe for disaster!

Again, starting a competition prep does not require a ton of preliminary bloodwork. There's nothing appealing about sitting in a hospital lobby for hours, waiting to get blood drawn; however, analyzing information from that data is a great way to ensure that you start the journey from a solid foundation. There's nothing worse than finding out four months into a six-month prep that you've got underlying hormonal issues and have to pull the plug. It's always better to simply gather the data at the onset and give yourself peace of mind.

If you have the means and the interest, try to get the same labs done after prep as well. This is a great way to quantify how much of an impact the journey had on your body, both metabolically and hormonally. So many competitors dive straight into another prep, which is one of the worst things you can do. I think this habit of transitioning right back into a cutting phase could easily be mitigated if more data were available.

Most competitors inherently know that prep is hard on their hormones, but since they don't see their numbers, they play the "ignorance is bliss" game. If you can see exactly how many points your hormone panel dropped, you'd likely put a little more thought into your future prep plans and give your body the time it needs to recover. Be smart and be strategic!

I do recognize that getting these basic labs drawn can be a hassle, and the more of a hassle something is, the less likely we are to do it; that's just human nature. As such, I've bypassed the hospital lobbies and insurance companies. I order all my bloodwork tests through an independent company and simply schedule an appointment with a Quest Diagnostics center to draw the blood. These independent lab companies are starting to pop up everywhere to meet increasing demand from people wanting to know their numbers. Directlabs.com is a site I've used several times in the past with great success.

MINDSET

Phase One of this journey is all about establishing our baseline. We measure our current stats, calculate our initial calories and macros, standardize our training, analyze our bloodwork and make sure we are primed to begin. But there is one more critically important factor that requires our attention: mindset.

Each of these phases will include a standalone section that focuses specifically on mindset. Why spend so much time on such an arbitrary metric? Because it is the most influential one of all! Each phase will require some changes in perspective. I will provide you with a perfect blueprint full of detailed instructions on optimizing your body for competition day, but I'd be remiss if I didn't properly equip your mind as well. You could start this prep with bulletproof bloodwork, amazing macros and a rock-solid training plan, but you will fail if you don't have the right mindset.

As it relates to Phase One, our mindset should be pure excitement for what lies ahead. Excitement for the unknown. Excitement for tracking, monitoring and logging every little seemingly insignificant detail.

Why is this so important? It's because we must start this journey consumed by excitement so we can leverage it to build proper habits at the onset. If we are genuinely excited about taking progress pics every two weeks, practicing posing regularly, tracking macros daily, logging training sessions and documenting our journey, we will, by default, build those behaviors into daily rituals. They'll become a habit that compounds over months and yields a fantastic outcome.

If our excitement is lackluster, we'll feel obligated to track these various metrics, and the likelihood that we'll cut corners and shirk our responsibilities will be amplified. During this prep, there will be a time when our excitement wanes and our willpower is greatly diminished. When that time comes, we will be leaning on our habits, not our energy or motivation. If you have the proper habits in place, you'll continue making progress. If you don't, you won't.

There are over seven billion people on this planet and every single one of them wants to look good. Nobody would complain if they woke up one day and had six-pack abs and defined arms. The desire to look good for oneself and others is hardwired into our DNA through years of evolution and natural selection. This desire has only been intensified since the advent of social media and our ability to compare ourselves to others constantly.

An Instagram model can attract millions of followers simply by the curvature of her ass—is that normal? My answer is that humans want to look good, period! Yet of the seven billion people walking around right now, I think it's safe to say that the vast majority don't resemble anything close to a Greek statue. The rock-hard abs and bulging biceps have given way to a fluffy beer belly and sagging moobs. Why?

If everyone desires to look good, why do we see the exact opposite in reality? The answer is: ambition and desire are not enough. Many people want to compete and look like sheer perfection, yet few ever grace the stage. We do not rise to the level of our ambitions; we fall to the level of our systems. Re-read that last sentence and let it sink in.

The habits we establish in Phase One form the baseline for this entire keto contest prep system, so don't take any of these steps for granted. Pour your all into every single one of them. Give it 100%. The only way to honestly give anything your all is to love what you're doing, truly. Love for something is directly correlated to your excitement for it. Be excited about the growth you are about to experience as an individual in modern-day society. Be enthusiastic about the fact that of the seven billion people walking around on this planet, you will be one of the few with purpose. You are leaving a life of mediocrity to pursue one of greatness. Of those seven billion people, you will be a warrior, mentally and physically hardened through the trials that lie ahead.

Be excited about becoming a f*@king SAVAGE!

[2]
PHASE TWO: ESTABLISH YOUR PROTEIN THRESHOLD

Welcome to Phase Two! As the title suggests, this one is all about establishing protein thresholds and involves a good deal of macro manipulation. We spent all of last phase laying the necessary groundwork to set us up for success. We determined our current baselines and calculated our initial macronutrient goals. This phase is all about manipulating those individual macros to obtain our desired outcome.

Referring to our prior analogy about knowing where to go, we now have our starting location and a detailed map with precise GPS coordinates. In this phase, we'll fire up the engine and hit the road. There will be a few detours and possibly some roadblocks, but we will still have a serious advantage toward our final destination.

What do I mean by "protein threshold?" I must have coined this term as it relates to the ketogenic diet because I never hear other coaches talk about it, and I'm constantly getting asked to define it in greater detail. Our individual protein threshold is simply our body's protein cap where any intake in dietary protein beyond that cap yields a less than optimal response.

Protein is an essential macronutrient and should not be taken for granted. It provides the building blocks necessary to add lean tissue, recover and optimize for contest prep; however, that doesn't necessarily mean it should be given a golden halo and consumed in excess. Like all things in life, there is a point of diminishing returns. The primary objective of this phase is to establish that cap.

It's important to note that no formula or equation spits out your exact protein threshold. This is a highly individualized metric and is influenced by various factors including age, sex, muscle maturity, training, hormones, genetics, environment, stress, lean mass and even personal preference. There are data-driven metrics that can point us in the right direction, but a good deal of this feedback will be internal. That means you're going to have to pay attention to how you feel and perform.

You'll learn to get in tune with your body and pay attention to yourself throughout this phase. For many people, this will be the first time experiencing something like this, it's okay to naturally lack a bit of perspective here. To be fair, how could you possibly know what you're looking to feel if you've never felt it before?

I'll do my best to describe precisely what metrics we'll be focused on and how to interpret relevant data. All it takes is practice: the more you go through it, the better you'll get. As you learn to interpret the feedback your body is giving you more accurately, you'll be increasingly more effective at making these dietary manipulations. You'll learn what changes need to be made almost by instinct, and knowledge of oneself to that degree is empowering.

Before we begin making these manipulations, I want to set an expectation for this phase. In working with hundreds of clients, I've noticed there tend to be two types of responses to the manipulations made throughout Phase Two.

One is a steady drop in body weight right out of the gate, which is likely due to the higher fat ratio combined with simply eating more consistent meals. Individuals who experience this initial drop are likely dipping into a slightly deeper level of ketosis than they were before and are flushing out excess fluids and inflammation as a result. It's not uncommon for some to experience keto-flu like symptoms due to this initial drop in water. For these people, I recommend ensuring that your electrolytes are in check by staying on top of your sodium and potassium intake to mitigate any adverse symptoms.

The other typical response is less motivating but shouldn't be viewed as unfavorable. Many individuals experience very little if any drop in body weight during Phase Two. This can be incredibly disheartening. After all, these people are also tracking all of their metrics, meal prepping, consistently hitting the gym and their macros and generally putting forth a ton of effort. To not see a drop in the scale weight is just not fair, right?

Realize that seeing a ton of physical, external changes should not be the expectation throughout Phase Two. This potential lack of change doesn't mean things aren't happening internally. The internal changes are what we are trying to prioritize here, and any external changes are just a bonus. Keep that in mind as you go throughout this phase, and don't get discouraged if you don't see a drastic drop on the scale. Just stay the course and know that you're laying the necessary groundwork to carry you through the later phases.

PHASE TWO OBJECTIVES

As we discussed earlier, the primary objective of this phase is to determine our protein threshold. As such, we need to gradually increase our dietary protein intake as high as we possibly can before we start to experience any adverse effects.

One of the keywords here is *gradually*; it makes no sense to spike protein too much too soon. If we do that, we'll be unable to determine the actual tipping point at which changes start to occur. Since this keto prep journey starts at a relatively low protein intake, we have quite a bit of room to increase protein. This increase in protein allows us to take advantage of a few different factors.

Protein has a higher TEF than the other macronutrients by about 15-20%. Basically, our body must burn more calories to break down protein and turn it into usable fuel. This is advantageous in a cutting protocol because it allows us to burn more calories simply by eating a specific macro group. This higher TEF is often why coaches advocate an incredibly high protein intake relative to other macronutrients.

On the surface, that makes intuitive sense, right? Eat more protein, burn more calories. Tada! Unfortunately, it's not quite that simple. As mentioned earlier, the increase in total caloric expenditure is actually quite trivial. There are other factors at play here, and at times, we'll benefit from having a lower protein intake relative to our dietary fat. That said, any temporary bump in total expenditure we can derive from a higher TEF as we increase protein throughout this phase is welcomed with open arms.

Another benefit to manipulating protein intake is that it simply provides a different stimulus to the body. There are times during prep where you will feel up against a wall and struggling without seeing much weight loss. Sometimes, a simple shift that seems to make no sense will make things move again. During a prep, your body becomes very resilient to the pressures applied to it. It fights to stay in homeostasis and not waver from the "norm" it knows. Providing a slight shift in how we are doing things often provides all the necessary stimulus to get the momentum going again. This increasing protein variable acts as a lever we can pull to generate that shift.

This phase also provides us with the opportunity to gain some much-needed perspective. It is best to experience how various macro ratios feel and how they affect your performance. We started this journey at an 80% fat ratio; how did that make you feel? Compare that to your overall feeling as you progress through Phase Two and your fat ratio steadily drops while your protein ratio simultaneously increases.

Do you feel better at a 75% fat ratio? How about a 70% ratio? What do you notice concerning your performance in the gym? Are you able to achieve a solid muscle pump and contraction with every rep? How is your endurance? Has your sleep been impacted positively or negatively? Do you feel more satiated with the increased protein? Do you prefer that, or did you feel better with less food volume and more calorically dense, fattier options? Has your mental clarity been affected? What about the actual numbers? Did your weight change as protein increased? What about measurements?

These are all worthwhile questions that you need to ask yourself with each week that passes. I can write the world's most extraordinary blueprint to ketogenic fat loss, but that won't change the fact that some people perform better at a higher fat ratio while some perform better with more protein. It's absolutely crucial that you learn your body well enough to pick up on these subtle nuances.

Phase Two will effectively prime the pump for the manipulations we'll make later in this journey. We are starting this prep at a higher fat ratio, and we'll likely end it at a relatively high-fat ratio as well.

Phase Two grants us the opportunity to leverage and benefit from higher protein, so take advantage of it. The higher we can effectively raise our protein now, the more runway we'll have to taper it later. Also, since we are increasing one macronutrient, our overall caloric drop is relatively slow. This effectively makes cutting calories much more sustainable and significantly more enjoyable. Please take advantage of your higher volume, protein-heavy meals now, because they won't be around forever!

PHASE TWO GUIDELINES

Now that you have a high-level overview of the objectives and expectations for Phase Two, let's get into the nuts and bolts. Our baseline calories and starting macronutrients from Phase One will be what we strive to consume throughout the entirety of the first week of this contest prep. How you organize this is up to you, but I prefer building this timeline in a spreadsheet that illustrates the dates and numbers I'm targeting. Each week will likely have different macronutrient goals, so organizing it in weekly increments works well. Feel free to format this however you like, but I've included a free spreadsheet that you are welcome to download and use. That spreadsheet is available at www.ketogenicbodybuilding.com.

Remember, we are starting at a higher fat ratio to promote a deeper initial level of keto adaptation at the onset. Protein will increase throughout this phase, so don't concern yourself with having low starting protein. The relatively high caloric intake at the beginning of this prep prevents any chance of muscle catabolism. It is honestly another great reason to start at or reasonably close to your maintenance caloric intake instead of a significant deficit. This is also why having a healthy caloric and metabolic baseline is critical.

If you have healthy caloric intake initially, there shouldn't be any risk in starting at a low protein ratio. That low percentage of protein relative to healthy caloric intake should still be within the realm of healthy, albeit on the lower end of the spectrum.

INCREASE PROTEIN

Every manipulation we make throughout this contest prep will be made in a deliberate, strategic manner. The same is true concerning our increasing protein during this phase. There is no need to make any aggressive changes if we've allotted enough time for this prep. Subtle changes are significantly more sustainable and much more informative.

Increase dietary protein by 5-10 g per week as you go throughout this second phase; any less than 5 g will likely be too insignificant a change to quantify and any more than 10 can cause too much confusion.

Ideally, you'll be able to keep your food choices the same every week and then tweak them slightly as the macro goals change. The average egg contains 5-6 g of protein, so a straightforward maneuver to titrate protein up by 5-10 g each week is to add an egg or two. This simple adjustment can be readily incorporated into the meal plan and its effects are easy to gauge.

DECREASE FAT

We increase protein throughout Phase Two, but not overall calories; it is a contest prep after all, and overall consumption still needs to trend downward. There isn't a whole lot of room to decrease dietary carbohydrates as those have already been dropped by default through this ketogenic protocol. That leaves one other macronutrient to manipulate: fat.

As we gradually increase dietary protein throughout this phase, we will simultaneously drop our dietary fat intake. Since protein contains about four calories per gram and fat contains about nine calories per gram, we will experience a net drop in calories if the two macros are manipulated at the same rate. For instance, an increase in 5 g of protein per week would increase 20 calories, but a corresponding 5 g drop in fat would yield a decrease in 45 calories. If the two happen simultaneously, the net effect on overall calories will decrease by 25 total calories. If you were to make the same adjustments but in 10 g increments, the general reduction in calories would be 50 calories. A 25-50 calorie drop each week may not sound like a ton, but it has a compounding effect.

Dropping by so few calories each week will likely not result in a massive drop in scale weight in the very beginning, but it will make this entire process significantly more sustainable. It's much easier to mentally prepare yourself to remove an egg or two from your next week's meal plan than it is to slash several hundred calories and have to remove an entire meal. The more sustainable this process is, the more likely you are to adhere to it for the entire prep. That adherence combined with the compounding effect of these 25-50 calorie adjustments is where the magic truly happens.

WEEK BY WEEK

Continue this process of gradually increasing dietary protein while simultaneously decreasing dietary fat. If you want to take a more conservative approach and have time to go as slowly as possible, feel free to stagger the macro shifts.

An example of this would be increasing protein one week by 5-10 g but doing nothing to dietary fat. The following week you can drop fat by 5-10 g but leave protein constant. This is a much slower iteration of this process and usually not necessary unless you know you're going to be prepping for 30 weeks or more and have a bit more weight to lose than is optimal for starting the prep. The typical 5-10 g macro manipulations simultaneously on protein and dietary fat should be ideal in most scenarios. This second phase lasts for several weeks and is excellent for familiarizing how our body responds to the varying fat ratios at different caloric intakes.

TRACKING METRICS

It's imperative to track as many metrics as possible as you go through this phase, particularly if you don't experience a significant drop in scale weight. If you have stagnant weight loss, it's much easier to embrace the process anyway if you're able to see other shifts such as measurements or changes in body composition. I recommend breaking these metrics into specific intervals and then tracking them consistently without fail.

Track your body weight daily as soon as you wake in the morning after using the bathroom. This morning weight will fluctuate depending on hydration, sleep quality, inflammation, stress, what you ate the night prior and hormonal cycle, but it is still a significant data point. Please don't get discouraged by the daily fluctuations. As we said before, these numbers aren't inherently good or bad; it's simply data.

It's optimal to weigh in daily rather than just once a week because daily measurements allow you to track your weekly average. The important thing here is to determine the average rate and direction you are trending over time. The consistent daily data also gives us a ton of insight into how your body responds to the various manipulations you make.

For instance, if your scale weight jumps up several pounds overnight, take a step back and take stock of what happened the previous day. Did you over-consume sodium? Did you train legs and are now experiencing some temporary inflammation and water retention? Has your cycle started? These are all worthwhile questions to have a general pulse on.

Daily weigh-ins allow us to make more informed decisions and manipulations throughout prep. Don't let weight fluctuations become a negative feedback loop that messes with your head. Approach the morning weigh-ins like a scientist interprets experimental data: the numbers are just numbers.

I like to consider other metrics in addition to morning weigh-ins. A simple daily mirror check is a great way to see how your body is responding to your weekly macro manipulations. Look in the mirror every morning for any subtle changes. Does your stomach look flatter? How is your vascularity? Do you feel like your skin appears a bit thinner? Hit a pose or two and observe your muscle fullness. Has it improved since the week before?

It can be hard to see changes if you're seeing yourself every day, but make it a point to observe yourself to spot subtle changes. As I've gone through this prep system over the years, I've noticed that when I start seeing particular veins in my shoulder caps and legs that I'm under 8% body fat. When I see striations in my glutes, I know that I am sub 5% body fat. Pay attention and you'll be surprised at how much insight your body can give you.

Additional metrics to track on a bi-weekly basis can include tape measurements, body fat tests and standardized pictures. Using a simple seamstress tape, measure the circumference of certain body parts every other week and log them in a journal to see how things are moving. This can easily be done with the help of a second pair of hands, so enlist your spouse, friend or family member if possible. Measure the circumference of your neck, shoulders, chest, arms, waist, hips, thighs and calves, all while relaxed. If you notice changes as compared to prior weeks, you'll know that your body is responding to dietary manipulations.

A bi-weekly body fat test done with a non-invasive InBody scan or skinfold caliper is also great data. Measuring every two weeks or so allows enough time to pass to see measurable changes and can provide solid feedback on our body composition independent of scale weight. Another metric to keep tabs on every week or two is your overall strength towards specific compound movements. I like to track my strength in bench, squat and deadlift to ensure that I'm not experiencing any significant dips as my calories decline.

You've likely heard the saying, "a picture tells a thousand words." That couldn't be truer when it comes to contest prep. Taking standardized progress pictures every two weeks is one of the best habits you can form throughout this journey. It may be a pain in the ass, but commit to it at the onset and don't waiver.

Try and take these pictures in the same room under similar lighting conditions each time. I recommend doing so first thing in the morning before eating a meal and before you train. Don't try to get a great muscle pump and take the most Instagram-worthy photos possible; that isn't the point.

Once you've taken pictures for a few weeks, compare your body changes over time. Do you see any differences? Any more separation in your hamstrings? Any more detail in your triceps? Any less fluff in your lower back?

If you have access to a DEXA machine and have financial means, it's also a good idea to get an accurate body composition analysis every month or two. This certainly isn't a requirement, but it gives you precise feedback on how your body responds throughout prep. With any of these testing modalities, keep in mind that your lean mass is certainly subject to change based on the fluctuations you are experiencing in fluid retention, food volume and inflammation. Most of these tests are not great at accurately determining changes in actual muscle mass within a very short time period.

PROTEIN THRESHOLD INDICATORS

So what does reaching your protein threshold look and feel like? Typically, you'll begin to experience a combination of GI distress, increased blood glucose, decreased blood ketones, lower quality sleep, a decline in overall energy, bloating, water retention, a plateau in weight loss and diminished mental clarity and focus.

Experiencing any one of these in isolation doesn't necessarily mean you've reached your threshold, so keep that in mind as you're analyzing your body's feedback. Many people show one or two signs and automatically assume they've reached their threshold and prematurely move to the next phase. There is no rush here. Take your time and let what is happening unfold so that you can fully grasp the context of what your body is telling you. I encourage you to stay in this phase a week or two after truly reaching your protein threshold to solidify your transition.

Truly paying attention to all forms of biofeedback is vital here. Since everyone will have a highly individualized protein threshold, there isn't a formula or equation for a black and white calculation. Explore all possible factors when you're analyzing these various feedback points.

For instance, say you're experiencing a plateau in weight loss and feel like you're holding some extra water with a bit more inflammation than average. As a result, you're more bloated than usual and assume that all of this must mean that you've reached your protein threshold. Upon closer inspection, you realize that you've just hit your menstrual cycle. This would confound your feedback points. In that situation, I would suggest remaining in Phase Two for a bit longer to ensure that your hormonal cycle isn't playing a role.

Many of the signs and symptoms of a protein threshold can also be experienced after a week of travel and being in a high-stress environment with sub-optimal sleep. Try to be consistent with your macros and meal planning, and don't work off a weekly average with your macro and calorie goals. Try and get within 5 g of your target macros every single day.

Ideally, you'll keep your foods consistent throughout the week to remove any variance there. If you feel like you're nearing your protein threshold, eat the same thing for a week to ensure that the food itself isn't adding any adverse symptoms. Make it a point to remove the noise from your life, and control for as many variables as you can when homing in on your protein threshold.

The above reasons are why I like to track blood glucose and ketones. I typically don't track these metrics in normal day-to-day function, but it's valuable for Phase Two and throughout the prep. As protein levels increase and dietary fat decreases, you'll reach a tipping point in which gluconeogenesis seems to intensify and ketone production dips. This results in a corresponding rise in blood glucose and a drop in ketone levels. For me, that measurement observed with other symptoms independent of confounding variables is a reliable indicator that I'm nearing my protein threshold.

During my last competition prep, I started at a caloric intake of 3,445 calories at a bodyweight of 177 lb to provide context. My initial fat intake was 305 g, and I started at 155 g of protein. I stayed in Phase Two for about 10 weeks, during which I was manipulating dietary fat down by 10 g a week and increasing protein by 5 g a week. I had a significant caloric intake to start with, so I opted to be more aggressive with the dietary fat manipulations. By the end of the ten weeks, my daily macro goals were 215 g of dietary fat and 200 g of protein. That put me at a 68.7% fat ratio and marked my final week in Phase Two. My dietary protein was nearing a 1:1 ratio with my fat intake, and I was experiencing symptoms that told me I had reached my threshold.

PATTERN RECOGNITION

In working with hundreds of clients over the years, I've become acutely aware of specific patterns and trends related to how the average person responds to dietary manipulations. Everyone has a highly individualized protein threshold, but I've learned when to anticipate hitting those thresholds based on past evidence experience. For instance, I've noticed that males tend to respond better than females to increasing protein and decreasing dietary fat for a bit longer. While a woman may reach her protein threshold when her total caloric intake comprises 70-74% fat, a man may not reach his until 65% of his calories are coming from fat.

Again, these percentages are certainly not set in stone. I've worked with clients who were complete outliers from this average. However, overall, I've noticed that men can typically avoid many of the adverse effects of Phase Two for a bit longer than most females. This is primarily due to the hormonal implications a decreasing fat ratio can have on female competitors.

The average "tipping point" occurs when you near the 1:1 ratio of protein grams to fat grams. We started this journey with 80% of our calories coming from dietary fat. Over several weeks of gradually increasing protein while decreasing fat, we've gotten closer and closer to this 1:1 ratio. Ideally, you will become very in tune with how your body responds to these manipulations and can accurately gauge when enough of them are occurring to move confidently into the next phase. On the other hand, if you're completely removed from your body and don't know how to interpret the feedback it's giving you, try to reach this 1:1 point first. If you do this, you'll be able to have at least the odds in your favor of what the average threshold ratio is.

PHASE TWO MINDSET

Phase Two is going to exercise your patience muscle above all else. Always remember that this entire prep protocol is a long-game approach to sustainable body recomposition. It's incredibly effective and surprisingly efficient, but you're not likely to experience any massive shift in scale weight at any one specific time. Every manipulation we make has a purpose and helps set the stage for ongoing success. Phase Two is crucial because it allows us to increase our dietary protein in the context of a net decrease in calories. We are trying to determine our protein threshold, which involves determining the point at which our body starts to experience some degree of adverse effects. These negative effects don't mean the protocol isn't working, and this slow or negligible drop in scale weight doesn't mean the system is flawed. Again, it's all about patience.

If you expect to look show-ready after a few weeks in Phase Two, you'll be sadly disappointed and will likely throw up your hands in despair. Don't! This is the phase where we start manipulating macros and shift calories every week. It's exciting to be able to start moving things around because it stimulates our imagination, but we also often hold many unrealistic expectations. After all, a few weeks (or even a few months) of dropping dietary fat and increasing dietary protein isn't going to miraculously turn you into a chiseled, world-class competitor.

Don't be so adamant about getting shredded that you rush through this phase and move on to Phase Three prematurely. Every step is critical and deserves your utmost respect and attention. Use this phase to build the proper habits of meal prep, macro tracking, sleep and training that will carry you through the rest of the prep with solid momentum. Also use this time to set expectations with your friends and family. They want to get together and have a cookout? Fine, no problem—you'll just bring your prepped meals. Even though this is the beginning of prep, it's the foundation of all future success. If you build a solid foundation, you'll kick ass. If you don't, you'll crumble and fall in the later stages.

The Phase One mindset was all about focusing on excitement for what lay ahead. Phase Two is the beginning of the journey. Don't flame out in a matter of weeks simply because you're not experiencing massive drops in scale weight or nothing seems to be changing. To give some perspective, during my last prep, I was in Phase Two for 10 weeks and my weight only dropped 5.4 lb in that time!

The whole time, I nailed my daily macros, didn't miss training sessions and became the definition of discipline and consistency. Did that tiny 5.4 lb drop discourage or demotivate me? Hell no! I was on a freaking mission. Now, *you're* the one on a mission. This phase sets the groundwork for all the success that follows. Don't fool yourself into thinking that you'll have time to adjust later and that you can get away with more mistakes now. You committed to this on day one. You're already in the trenches. Stay there and dig deep. Commit.

[3]
PHASE THREE: TAPERING MACROS

Congrats for making it this far! You've got more discipline than the average individual who gives up after a few weeks, but this phase will test that discipline, so keep those blinders on. Phase Three involves tapering all your macronutrients. We established your protein threshold in the last phase, so there's no need to continue increasing protein. Now that we've found that intake, we'll start tapering protein as well.

Wait, what?! We spent all that time bumping up protein just to drop it in Phase Three? It probably sounds a little pointless, right? Even if it sounds pointless, understand this: our personal thresholds and ideal macronutrient ratios are constantly in flux throughout prep. They fluctuate based on our total caloric intake, body fat percentage, hormonal changes and metabolic changes, so it stands to reason that our macro ratios and protein thresholds should also move accordingly.

Total caloric intake starts dipping more rapidly in this phase now that we are titrating both dietary fat and protein down. The lower calories get, the greater the benefit from the increasing fat ratio that results from decreasing protein intake. Remember, fat is where we get our energy. As we get leaner and leaner, we'll have less body fat to tap into for energy and less to help regulate our hormones and metabolism. All of this is more reason to rely heavily on our dietary fat to keep these variables healthy.

Phase Three is one of the most straightforward phases of this contest prep: we are simply tapering our macros. Even so, don't let that simplicity fool you into thinking this phase will be easy. In all honesty, this is one of the most challenging phases to power through.

This is when the contest prep starts to become difficult and the "grind" really kicks in. Calories are dropping, hunger is increasing, strength is waning and motivation is tested. This is a depletion phase, and you'll figure that out pretty quickly. Throughout this phase, you'll be in a deep enough deficit to lose that "filled out" look that makes being in the off-season so appealing, but you won't yet be lean enough to get excited about looking like you are show-ready.

This is the purgatory phase in which you experience more hunger, less energy, and look "flat" and depleted. Recognize that now and set your expectations accordingly. I've described the transition from off-season to stepping onstage as the "Full to Flat to Freaky" metamorphosis. This phase is the "Flat" phase. Embrace it!

PHASE THREE OBJECTIVES

As I mentioned earlier, this phase is all about tapering both our protein and dietary fat macros. It's going to be a bit different for everyone, but the majority of you will find yourself in this phase after about one to three months of dieting. By now, we will have established our protein threshold, gone beyond the tipping point of our caloric maintenance and are starting to put the pedal to the metal on our caloric deficit. Since protein and fat will both decrease in this stage, we'll likely see a faster drop in total weekly calories than we experienced in the prior phases. This means hunger will probably start ramping up and the test of our mental fortitude will be a bit tougher. This is where we see what you're made of.

This phase will likely be the most prolonged phase of your prep, so prepare for a bit of monotony. Consistency is key in Phase Three. After the first few months of dieting and consistently applying pressure, your body is primed to be in a heightened fat-burning state. It's safe to say that most of your adipose tissue will be burned in Phase Three if you adhere to the protocol and continually apply pressure. Your body constantly adapts to the manipulations we are making. As you decrease calories, your body's metabolism slows to follow suit. By continually dropping calories a bit every week, we can stay ahead of this adaptation and ensure that body fat continues to decline.

There may be periods that you seem to plateau during this phase. Don't let that discourage you. If you keep applying pressure via weekly macro drops, your body will eventually be forced to adapt and your overall composition will improve. Don't let the temporary fluctuations in weight loss or the "flat" look associated with it make you deviate from the protocol and the planned macros!

There is nothing fancy about this phase. Nothing is exciting. Take pleasure in knowing that this phase and its lack of novelty is what causes most competitors to veer off track and falter. Be an outlier. Be the one that doesn't waver from the plan but rather illustrates extreme discipline and consistency. Take progress pictures and measurements on a bi-weekly basis throughout this phase. Seeing those changes, as small as they may seem, will keep you motivated to stay the course.

Since your dietary protein will be reducing weekly, you'll likely experience an uptick in your blood ketone readings and a corresponding dip in your blood glucose. Towards the end of Phase Three, you'll be in a significant deficit and the increase in circulating blood ketones will help ward off many of its adverse effects. The anti-catabolic effect of the ketones will help you maintain lean muscle tissue, and because ketones can cross the blood-brain barrier and energize your cognitive function, you will be kept out of "zombie status."

The Phase Three equivalent in traditional bodybuilding nutritional protocols is often categorized by meager calories and a food selection that includes incredibly lean sources and low-calorie fillers such as rice cakes. Traditional competitors in this stage begin to lose all semblance of physical performance and mental cognition. It's what gives bodybuilding a bad name.

Following a super low-fat approach, competitors begin to experience significant fluctuations in hormonal function, satiety, libido and mood. I'm not going to suggest that all of that can be entirely avoided by following a ketogenic outline. Still, I can confidently say that many of those adverse effects can be significantly reduced. In all honesty, the increased blood ketones and decreased blood glucose kick many competitors' mental functions into overdrive.

Have you ever experienced a period of heightened productivity during an extended fast? A similar level of heightened awareness and cognitive function is present during this stage in our ketogenic competition prep. While your competitors are floundering around like zombies, you can experience a heightened state of mental awareness and cognitive productivity. I'll take the latter, please.

PHASE THREE GUIDELINES

The pages that follow will break down the exact manipulations you'll want to make to truly optimize your body and brain and get the most out of this phase.

As with all phases, do *not* rush through Phase Three haphazardly. Phase Three is where you will lose most of your body fat, so embrace the simple fact that you'll likely be in this phase for the most extended period—no sense in rushing off to the subsequent phases even though they are a bit more exciting. Suppose you implement this protocol flawlessly in Phase Three. In that case, you'll effectively build the necessary momentum to power through the remainder of this prep like a freight train and keep you trending in the right direction.

If you squander this phase, you'll likely be met with plateau after plateau in later phases. Give this phase your all, and you'll look shredded as hell onstage come show day. While this phase isn't the most exhilarating, it's crucial in priming your body for Phase Four and everything that it entails.

Although Phase Four will see the introduction of ketogenic caloric refeeds, those refeeds will be totally and utterly useless if your body is not lean and depleted enough to absorb and make use of them. That leanness and depletion happens in Phase Three. If you half-ass this phase, there will be no benefit from the refeeds in the next phase, so embrace it entirely.

DECREASE PROTEIN

Now that we've established our protein threshold, the next step is to decrease daily protein intake week after week. Since we've been dropping dietary fat in previous phases, I like to slow down the decrease in fat slightly at this point and be a bit more aggressive with the drop in protein. Depending on how much time you have left before you step onstage, I suggest dropping protein somewhere between 5-15 g a week. You can also alternate between those amounts depending on how much time you have left and how quickly your body responds. If you're seeing continual progress week after week, slow things down a bit and only drop by 5 g. If you are coming up on time and don't see the response you were hoping for, bump it up to 10-15 g a week.

A quick word of caution on the more aggressive 15 g decrease: I do *not* recommend going that fast unless you started at a significant caloric intake. I had a few weeks during my competition prep where I was a bit more aggressive with my drop in protein and decreased by 15 g a week, but I also started my prep at 3,500 calories and had plenty of runway to work with. If you are beginning much lower on the caloric spectrum, do not rush the process and cut your protein too quickly.

DECREASING DIETARY FAT

Remember, we will still be dropping dietary fat during this phase as well as our protein. Since we are coming out of Phase Two and are likely at our lowest fat ratio as a percentage of total calories, I like to be a bit more aggressive with the protein drop than the fat to increase my overall dietary fat ratio.

What is the benefit of that? As I mentioned earlier, ketones are incredibly anti-catabolic and higher circulating blood ketones can contribute to better lean mass retention in the context of a caloric deficit. At this stage in prep, calories are getting very low and ketogenic caloric refeeds are still yet to come. At this stage, your body may want to start catabolizing hard-earned muscle, which nobody wants. By transitioning to a higher fat ratio, you can minimize those adverse effects and preserve as much lean tissue as possible. Though the goal is still to drop total calories and decrease dietary fat, it's important to do so at a slightly slower rate than your decrease of protein.

Athletes commonly experience a dip in blood ketones and an increase in blood glucose throughout Phase Two. The exact opposite effect should happen in Phase Three. Our decreasing calories combined with an increasing fat ratio should only amplify circulating blood ketones and maximize the body's efficiency with fat oxidation.

DECREASING DIETARY CARBOHYDRATES

Since we started this journey at a whopping 20 g of total carbs there likely isn't much room to taper those further. However, if you so choose, feel free to whittle those down to 15 g or even 10 g or lower at this stage. At this level of fat-adaptation, you likely place the protein and fat macros in higher regard than the calories allocated towards your carbohydrates. Feel free to chip away at what little remains if you have it to spare.

HOLD MACROS CONSTANT

There may be times when you could benefit from not dropping a particular macronutrient for a week or two, such as when your fat ratio is low and you want to increase it but have little caloric runway. In those cases, you may benefit from not dropping fat grams for a week or two. This will slow the rate of your caloric decrease, but it will prolong your prep time and enable you to gradually bump up your fat ratio by the corresponding drop in dietary protein.

All of this adds to why giving yourself a ton of time is worthwhile. Similarly, if your body responds to your manipulations better than you hoped for and your weight is dropping steadily with improved composition, you may benefit from tapping the brakes. I don't usually recommend not dropping any macros, but don't feel the need to double down and cut calories if it's not necessary. There's no need to down-regulate your metabolism if you see the desired outcome at a higher caloric intake.

MEAL PREP AND NUTRIENT DENSITY

The meal tweaks in Phase Three are honestly pretty easy. In Phase Two, you have to get creative with macros and find ways to increase one macronutrient while simultaneously dropping another to result in a net caloric loss. Phase Three is simply dropping both, which removes quite a bit of complexity.

Your hunger will likely reach a new level in Phase Three, especially in the tail-end. Because of that, it's worth your while to make nutritional manipulations that preserve your satiety as best as possible. You won't be able to escape the hunger entirely, so set your expectations accordingly. Even so, you can use certain nutritional and psychological hacks to make this phase more sustainable.

One is to simply use the most nutrient-dense and bioavailable sources of food you can. If your body is receiving an adequate supply of vitamins and minerals, you'll experience fewer cravings.

In my earlier bodybuilding days, I focused solely on food volume because I equated volume with satiety. That was a huge mistake. I'd have my protein and fat source and then pad it with a massive bolus of low-calorie lettuce or shirataki noodles in the hopes that it would fill me up. It did fill me in the sense of being incredibly bloated, but it did very little for my satiety. It only amplified my hunger.

If you eat a ton of vegetation or high fiber foods with your very nutrient-dense foods, the fiber works to reduce the absorption of those nutrients. This sounds contradictory to what we were raised to believe, but it's true. If you're in a caloric deficit, your body wants to use every morsel of food you consume for day-to-day function. As a result, you'll likely experience a significant decrease in the amount of waste your body produces. Get ready for fewer trips to the bathroom in Phase Three!

When this happens, know that it does *not* necessarily mean that you're constipated and in need of fiber; in fact, I would argue that high-volume fibrous foods are the worst thing to consume at this stage. Instead, try to prioritize the most nutrient-dense options you can find, such as organ meats. There are more micronutrients in a 100 g serving of beef liver than any vegetable you'll find on the grocery store shelves, and the beef liver will top off many of your body's nutrient demands without leaving you with a distended midsection.

MEAL FREQUENCY

Since total caloric intake wanes significantly in Phase Three, it makes sense to manipulate our meal frequency a bit. Intuition suggests that we should spread our calories out throughout the day with several smaller meals. Traditionally, this is thought to keep our metabolism elevated and enhance our ability to burn fat. It's also supposed to keep us satiated and craving less food. This couldn't be further from the truth!

Small, frequent feeding intervals constantly elicit a blood glucose response resulting in a release of insulin. On a ketogenic diet, the constant demand for insulin is reduced because dietary carbohydrate intake is significantly lower. All the same, feeding in general results in some degree of insulin release—even just thinking of food, smelling food or chewing gum results in what's called the cephalic phase of insulin secretion. This cephalic phase secretes enough insulin into the bloodstream to cause a physiological response that increases hunger and cravings. What does all this mean? It means you'll likely benefit from a much shorter feeding window and an extended fasting period.

As calories get lower, overall food volume also decreases significantly. Rather than chasing higher volume, nutritionally void food sources like we discussed earlier, prioritize the most nutrient-dense sources of food you can find and consume those foods in a shorter feeding window. This contradicts pretty much all the "bro wisdom" you might receive as you go through your bodybuilding fitness endeavors but trust me on this one. My first several competitions were done following IIFYM protocols, and I would eat six or seven meals a day full of carbohydrates and high-volume veggies and lean meats. I was starving all the time and never felt satisfied, which contributed to me spiraling out of control and falling into a pattern of disordered eating.

After I started a ketogenic diet, I removed all carbohydrates, but I left many of my lousy dieting principles intact. I incorporated many high-volume veggies and bro dieting "hunger hacks," such as zero-calorie sweeteners and shirataki noodles, which resulted in constant cravings because of the cephalic phase of insulin response. I pulled out all the stops during my last competition prep and removed all high volume, nutritionally void fillers and sweeteners. I consumed the highest quality, most nutrient-dense sources of fat and protein I could find such as organ meats, wild game and grass-fed/finished beef.

As calories got lower in Phase Three, I transitioned from eating two or three meals a day to just one larger meal. Much to my surprise, this reduced my hunger cravings and made the entire prep significantly more sustainable.

One Meal A Day (OMAD) is a great way to accommodate decreasing calories in Phase Three. From a physiological perspective, you'll be experiencing far fewer fluctuations in blood glucose and insulin, resulting in far fewer cravings and hunger swings. From a psychological perspective, I've found it much more satisfying to consume one large meal that truly satisfies you than multiple smaller meals that leave you wanting more.

By only eating once a day, you won't spend nearly as much time thinking, planning and preparing your meals, which is incredibly liberating. Spending less time thinking about food does two things. First of all, you won't experience the cognitively induced cephalic phase of insulin response multiple times throughout the day. Secondly, you won't waste nearly as much time and will have an increase in productivity.

Won't eating just once a day lead to a massive amount of muscle loss? No! The increased fasting window will also contribute to an increase in circulating blood ketones: as we discussed earlier, these are incredibly anti-catabolic. By eating lower volume, more nutrient-dense foods, your body will experience increased nutrient absorption. That coupled with the expanded fasting window and up-regulation in ketone production yields something counterintuitive but compelling: less hunger, better muscle preservation, increased cognitive function, fewer distractions and more sustainability! I don't know about you, but it all sounds pretty appealing to me!

INCREASE CARDIO

Earlier in this book, I mentioned how calories and cardio should have something of an inverse relationship. You don't want to start prep by doing a massive amount of cardio just as you don't want to start with a massive cut in calories. You want to leave yourself enough caloric runway from which to taper. The inverse is true with cardio. You want to start with minimal cardio so that you have enough cardio runway to increase it over time as needed. The bulk of your compositional changes should come from your dietary manipulations; however, as your calories decrease and your body tries to adapt, you may experience periodic plateaus.

To bust through these plateaus, we either manipulate macronutrients further or bump up the cardio. As we get farther into prep, our ability to manage macros becomes more difficult as there are fewer calories to work with. Fortunately, since we started with minimal cardio, we still have that lever to pull late in the game.

Phase Three is generally the longest phase of prep, and it also tends to include the lowest caloric intake. It's where most fat loss occurs and also includes the majority of cardio manipulations. To keep things standardized and systematic, I recommend slowly titrating cardio to prevent plateauing. It's good to keep applying increased pressure to ensure that you maintain the momentum you've built. This isn't possible if you started your journey with a ton of cardio, so again, let me stress that you *don't* want to start with obscene amounts of cardio.

As mentioned, the Stairmaster is my preferred form of cardiovascular activity. It makes standardizing this process even easier because level 10 on the machine is always level 10. There are never any fluctuations. Suppose you find yourself doing a form of cardio that is more flexible and subject to your mood. In those cases, you'll likely experience volatile shifts in intensity as you get lower in calories.

An example of this would be hill sprints. As your calories get lower, your ability to standardize the intensity of your hill sprints will decrease. This will happen subconsciously, and you won't even be aware of it; but it's the last thing you want to happen. The Stairmaster, on the other hand, won't lie to you. Level 10 is always level 10.

For illustrative purposes, let's imagine starting a prep with a minimal dose of cardio consisting of 10 minutes on the Stairmaster at level 10 twice a week. Imagine that you maintained that intensity throughout Phase Two and started ramping up cardio at the onset of

Phase Three. We have three different levers to pull when it comes to ramping up our cardio. We can increase the time, frequency and intensity. An example of a sustainable increase in cardio would look something like this:

> Baseline: 10-minute session @ level 10 2x/week
> Week 2: 12-minute session @ level 10 2x/week
> Week 3: 12-minute session @ level 12 2x/week
> Week 4: 12-minute session @ level 12 3x/week
> Week 5: 14-minute session @ level 12 3x/week
> Week 6: 14-minute session @ level 14 3x/week
> Week 7: 14-minute session @ level 14 4x/week
> Week 8: 16-minute session @ level 14 4x/week
> Week 9: 16-minute session @ level 16 4x/week
> Week 10: 16-minute session @ level 16 5x/week
> Week 11: 18-minute session @ level 16 5x/week
> Week 12: 18-minute session @ level 18 5x/week
> Week 13: 18-minute session @ level 18 6x/week
> Week 14: 20-minute session @ level 18 6x/week
> Week 15: 20-minute session @ level 20 6x/week
> Week 16: 20-minute session @ level 20 7x/week
> Week 17: 22-minute session @ level 20 7x/week

If you'll notice, none of these three levers were pulled at the same time within the same week; instead, only one of the three metrics changed in a given week. Doing this allows your body to acclimate to the increase in cardiovascular duration, intensity and frequency in a sustainable manner. The exact breakdown of your cardio duration, intensity and frequency could differ from this depending on your fitness and preferred form of cardio, but this is an excellent example of what it could look like.

Notice that the time spent doing cardio in this example is relatively short—just 10-30 minutes per session should be sufficient for most individuals. If you're spending hours and hours each day doing cardio, then you likely didn't give yourself enough time for prep, didn't start at a healthy composition, aren't implementing an effective resistance training protocol or aren't correctly manipulating your macronutrients. Cardio is a tool to be used throughout prep. It shouldn't be viewed as your primary weapon but rather your sidearm to achieve the composition you're looking for.

RESISTANCE TRAINING

I know how hard it is to maintain your heavy lifts and intense resistance training sessions in this phase. Calories are low, motivation is waning and the feeling of depletion is more prominent than ever. If you're used to being in a caloric surplus and are always focused on building, it's very discouraging to feel weak on movements that you usually bust through without breaking a sweat. In a surplus, training sessions seem to float by as if you were in a wonderland. You can turn up the music and get lost in your thoughts. The PRs come effortlessly, and you're in a constant state of flow, one with the weights and lost in the moment.

That isn't the case this far into the prep journey. The PRs come few and far between, if they come at all. The 45lb bar feels as heavy as 225 did a few months ago. You no longer get lost in the music and float through your workouts—not even close. Now, you have to mentally prepare yourself for every new exercise, every single set, every damn rep! Rather than counting the different exercises you have planned in excitement, you count down the sets you have left before you can justify ending your training session. You start every session exhausted and leave every training session crawling on your hands and knees.

Sure, maybe I'm exaggerating just a tad—there will still be days when you feel like a million bucks. Soak in those days and hold on to them tightly because they will be few and far between during the last few weeks of Phase Three.

I may be a bit biased, but I have absolutely no doubt in my mind that a well-formulated, nutrient-dense, ketogenic diet is the healthiest dietary protocol for competitive athletes deep in competition prep. Compared to other dieting philosophies, keto ensures the most lean muscle mass retention, healthier levels of hormone regulation and more overall sustainability. However, don't fool yourself into thinking that this will be a walk in the park. This phase of competition prep is incredibly difficult regardless of the type of diet you're following. Your strength, motivation and endurance will all take a hit.

I know it's easier said than done, but you must continue lifting as hard and heavy as you possibly can. Don't sacrifice form and risk injury but do try and maintain the same volume and intensity you were implementing while at a maintenance intake. You'll likely experience a dip with particular exercises and movements but fight it as best you can. Remember, the heavier you train, the more reason your body has to retain the lean mass you've built!

Resistance training is one of the single best things you can do to prevent muscle wasting during a caloric deficit. As calories drop, your body looks for sources to catabolize and fill the void left by your decreased fuel intake. If you start training with drastically less intensity and lower resistance, your body will recognize that there's no demand for that muscle. From an evolutionary survival standpoint, it makes no sense for your body to carry around that extra lean tissue that isn't being used; instead, your body reasons that it's better to tap into that reservoir that is keeping your metabolic rate revved up.

I don't like the idea of trying to "trick" our bodies. Our body is smarter than we think. Even so, within the context of this phase, we *are* trying to "trick" our body because we know there's a light at the end of the tunnel.

Instead of tapping into our body's muscle reserves for fuel, we must work to retain as much of that lean mass as possible and keep our metabolism functioning at a high rate. The best way to do that is to continually train hard and heavy. Muscle preservation is paramount throughout Phase Three when calories are low and you haven't yet introduced ketogenic caloric refeeds. When it gets tough, remember your "why." Remember what put you on this path to begin with. Double down on your desires, exercise extreme discipline and train like the bodybuilder that got you this far in the first place!

TRACKING METRICS

The decreased calories, slowed metabolism and constant sacrificing of social gatherings and festive parties of Phase Three can be overwhelming. By now, you will be nearer to show day than ever, but you won't look like a bodybuilder just yet. As you notice your "flat" look along with your hunger ramping up and your strength plateauing, it will weigh heavily on your mind. *Am I doing this right? Am I going to look the part on show day? Is this worth it? Should I just take a day and relax and eat some cinnamon rolls?* Hell no!

The point of all this is just to point out that our minds are liable to play tricks on us in Phase Three. Still, recognize that this is the darkness before the dawn stage and embrace it.

The more you can do to keep your mind straight, the better. One of the best things for that is to track all your physical metrics. I recommend doing this on a bi-weekly basis throughout the entirety of the prep, but it's especially critical at this stage. Every two weeks, take updated progress pictures and measurements and do a body fat test to measure your compositional changes. As your mind and willpower start to waver, these metrics will keep you motivated to stay the course.

Many of my competition preps have had me totally disheartened and discouraged by Phase Three, so I understand how hard it is. The sheer length of the prep and the time spent at maximum effort and discipline start to pull at your willpower—and willpower is a finite resource, you know. If you are constantly tapping into it without topping it off, you will not have the strength required to prevail. Watching your progress via these tracked metrics is a tangible way to top off your willpower tank. Though there will be weeks where the measuring tape reads the same, your weight is constant and the changes in your pictures are minuscule. But there will also be weeks when everything seems to shift dramatically. Measure your stats bi-weekly, expect the fluctuations and be objective with your results.

CONCLUDING PHASE THREE

To put it simply, the end of this phase should have you looking freaking shredded! You'll likely look incredibly depleted and flat, but you should be carrying significantly less body fat than you were at the onset. There will still be quite a bit of polishing and refining to do in the stages ahead, and the ketogenic caloric refeeds of the next phase will undoubtedly assist in that. Still, you mustn't move on to Phase Four's refeeds prematurely.

I know you're hungry. I know the thought of a ketogenic caloric refeed is making you drool right now as you read this sentence, but seriously—grab a napkin, wipe your mouth dry and buckle up. Advancing into Phase Four and implementing ketogenic caloric refeeds too early will do more harm than good. Push beyond the point of discomfort and dig deep here. Give it your everything.

Many novice competitors make the mistake of thinking their peak week protocol will create a massive shift in how they look. They assume they are simply "holding a bit of water," and the refeed manipulations combined with water and electrolyte tweaks will miraculously reveal a world-class physique. Don't fool yourself.

You're not just holding a little extra water. If you don't look impressive by the end of Phase Three, you will not look exceptional on show day. There is a significant difference between looking impressive and needing a little refinement vs. simply not being conditioned enough to be competitive. If you do not see some exceptional conditioning by this stage, you should consider staying in Phase Three for even longer. What if you're running out of macros? In that case, you should consider reverse dieting and cycling through these phases again later after your metabolism has improved and you can start from a better baseline. I harped on that message relentlessly at the beginning of this book, so you can't say I didn't warn you!

If you've followed the protocol flawlessly and are looking shredded, I commend you! You're likely leaner than you've ever been before. It's likely that you're seeing veins and striations you didn't even know existed—and you're also probably hungry and depleted and wanting it all to be over despite being excited and anxious for what lies ahead. Congratulations! You haven't made it out of the woods yet, but you've navigated the thickest part of the forest.

If you've done everything correctly, you are now likely starting to experience some of the adverse effects associated with a down-regulating metabolism. Your libido may be waning, or your hair and nails may be growing more slowly. Sometimes, it may feel like you're struggling through every rep. On a scale of 1-10, your hunger is probably close to a 12. That's good. It means your body will soak up every morsel of nutrients we provide in the next phase when introducing the ketogenic refeeds.

Transitioning into Phase Four is all about timing. If you start implementing refeeds too soon, your body will soak up the calories but be hesitant to keep dropping body fat. That means you'll likely plateau, and your progress will come to a grinding halt. If you time it just right, the refeeds will elicit a much more favorable response. Your metabolism will up-regulate, and you'll bust through any potential plateaus. The weekly refeeds will make the low overall calories much more sustainable, and you'll be able to keep chipping away at your macros. Your training will benefit, and so will your outlook.

Having something to look forward to each week will do wonders for your mental attitude, which will in turn make the whole process even more sustainable. If this describes you, I'll see you in Phase Four!

PHASE THREE MINDSET

In short, this essence perfectly illustrates what people call the "grind" in the sport of bodybuilding. Training becomes a chore rather than an enjoyable way to spend your time. Nutrition becomes dull as your meals get smaller and smaller, and your cravings for various flavors and more volume intensify. Your mind begins to plague you with doubt and insecurity, and you start thinking that maybe bodybuilding just really isn't worth it. The mindset you'll have to rely on in Phase Three is psychological resilience.

Psychological resilience is the ability to cope with crises and return to baseline quickly, whether those crises are mental or emotional. The "resilience" part is where you use certain processes and actions to boost your strength and protect yourself from the potential damages of external stress. This is appropriate, because Phase Three is one crisis or stressor after another.

For whatever reason, the stars never seem to align for contest prep, and the universe seems to be conspiring against you. In all honesty, what's really happening is a result of your weakening willpower and mental fortitude. After being in prep long enough to be deep into Phase Three, it's safe to assume that your relationships are likely being tested. Your spouse is probably more excited about prep being over than you were for it to begin! With less fuel coming in, simple day-to-day tasks like picking up the dry cleaning now seem like huge undertakings, and anything outside of your regular routine is considered a massive inconvenience.

The reason you've been able to survive this long is because of your uncanny ability to structure routines that help you accomplish the tasks at hand—whether that means training, cardio, meal prep, your job or anything else! By this stage, everything in your life has become a formula. However intense it may be, I view this as a necessary transition if you are to complete prep and maximize your full potential, but it's a transition that comes with compromise.

Standardizing your exercise, nutrition and mindset so much can inherently distract from other areas of your life. That distraction is what results in psychological crises.

Your ability to turn to psychological resilience is going to be your saving grace in Phase Three. Understand what is happening. Recognize that your temper will likely be a bit shorter. Embrace the fact that this prep was your decision, and no one else should be negatively affected by it.

Have perspective and know that other people have gone through much more challenging things. This may be the hardest thing you've ever endured, but the universe doesn't revolve around you. You are just a tiny speck, and your existence is a blip in time. Make the most of that blip and conduct yourself in a manner that compliments the brevity of life. Accept that the hardships you are currently enduring do not define you. They are simply moments in your life. Be stoic and remember that this, too, shall pass.

[4]
PHASE FOUR: INTRODUCING KETOGENIC REFEEDS

Now is the moment you've been waiting for: refeeds! Before your excitement turns into frenzy, let's pause for a moment and discuss how we can leverage refeeds as a tool to fuel further success.

In traditional bro dieting and IIFYM dieting protocols, refeeds consist of a surge in calories that typically come from dietary carbohydrates with some additional fat and protein. With a conventional prep, by now, your dietary fat is deficient and your carbs are also reasonably low while protein has remained relatively high. With most protocols, the tapering of carbs and fat has left you looking depleted as well, and your glycogen stores have run dry. Your hormones and metabolism have taken a hit and your cravings are off the charts.

In that context, having a traditional refeed with a bolus of carbohydrates and some additional fat replenishes those glycogen stores, fills out your muscles, gives you a "fuller," more vascular look and satisfies your cravings and hunger for a bit. Traditionally, you would rely on carbohydrates for energy if you weren't in a state of ketosis. The additional carbs would understandably and profoundly impact your energy. But since we're on the complete opposite end of the spectrum with our ketogenic approach to competition prep, we aren't going to be implementing carb-heavy refeeds.

Remember, as we discussed earlier, there is no inherent benefit to deriving energy from dietary carbohydrates once you're deeply adapted to a ketogenic lifestyle. We will be implementing a ketogenic caloric refeed, but it will comprise a strategic increase of dietary fat and protein. We'll also manipulate our electrolytes slightly, which I'll walk through in great detail.

Ketogenic caloric refeeds are included during the final stages of our prep, somewhere between the last two to six weeks. They will *not* have such a drastic impact to miraculously transform you from a fluffy, unconditioned athlete to a chiseled competitor capable of winning the world title. Do not assume that these refeeds will be your saving grace if you're out of shape going into Phase Four. These are used to optimize the final stages and add some polish to your physique. Don't implement them before you are ready!

A correctly implemented ketogenic caloric refeed can help you optimize your physique and overall mental and physical health in various ways. They have a temporary benefit on your metabolic rate since an increase in calories helps rev up your internal furnace.

After months of constantly dropping calories, your metabolism inevitably will down-regulate. A temporary spike in those calories can cause a favorable metabolic response and stoke the flames. Recognize that I said it could have a temporary benefit on our metabolism, with the keyword being temporary. We are still in a net caloric deficit by quite a bit, so don't anticipate a massive up-regulation. That said, any temporary stoking of your metabolic flames is much appreciated at this stage in the game.

By Phase Four, your body and mind are both likely exhausted along with your energy and mental fortitude. Implementing ketogenic caloric refeeds has the additional benefit of providing a temporary mental break from the constant pressure you've been under. Make no mistake, these refeeds are *not* a diet break, and they certainly aren't a free-for-all to let you eat whatever your little heart desires. They are calculated and designed with a specific purpose in mind. However, as trivial as it may be, the simple increase in calories provides us with something to look forward to and get excited about.

Excitement is incredibly welcome and unusually empowering at this stage in the game. In Phase Four, you may find yourself clawing for any foothold you can to keep yourself moving forward and see your prep through to the end. These refeeds can be the foothold that helps you keep grinding.

From a physiological and psychological standpoint, these refeeds bump up your average caloric intake for the week, allowing us to continue dropping caloric intake on every non-refeed day. This prolongs your deficit and enables you to continue lowering body fat and improving your physique. Your temporary bump in metabolic rate coupled with this continued drop in overall calories allows you to bust through any late-game plateaus and keep making progress.

This prep implements ketogenic caloric refeeds during peak week in Phase Five. Thus, Phase Four allows the opportunity to refine that protocol and optimize it. By having several weeks to hone in on macronutrient ratios, electrolyte manipulations and specific foods, we can test, tweak and perfect an ideal peak week protocol. As such, we'll try and structure the refeeds in Phase Four as we intend to implement them during peak week. Consider Phase Four a trial phase for peak week and give it all the attention and dedication it deserves.

PHASE FOUR GUIDELINES

There is a ton of confusion and ignorance on the topic of refeeds. The tricky part about incorporating refeeds correctly is that you must be objective about how it's impacting your body. This is hard to do in the tail-end of competition prep when your hunger and desire to eat are significantly amplified.

It takes a ton of willpower to grant yourself more calories, enjoy every single bite, wake up the following day, look at your physique objectively and decide that you should reduce your intake for your next refeed. Who wants to eat less at this stage in the game? If you are working with a trainer or have a gym partner that can shoot you straight and be honest, that is great! The more honest sets of eyes you have looking at you, the better. Still, having a trainer is a luxury many of us do not have, so I'm going to walk you through this section as if you have to do everything yourself. I'm going to teach you what to look for and how to time and implement your refeeds correctly so that you can genuinely get dialed in and optimized.

Let's start with a reiteration of the point I made in the last section. Refeeds are *not* effective if implemented too soon! This point bears repeating again and again to dissuade any of you from jumping at the opportunity to eat more food when you're not ready for it. You need to be incredibly lean—damn near stage lean—to truly take advantage of refeed benefits. You can still benefit from refeeds if they are implemented too *late* in a prep, but you will only be setting yourself back if you implement them too early. To clear up any confusion, allow me to paint a picture of the ideal time to start introducing refeeds.

The ideal candidate for Phase Four refeeds is in the tail-end of their prep. Their show is only a few weeks out, likely between two to six. They've been hitting their macros flawlessly and their body has responded well to the steady drop in calories. Due to macro manipulations in Phase Three with the ever-decreasing fat and protein (protein at a slightly faster rate than dietary fat), they are likely at a relatively high fat ratio (probably somewhere between 75-80% of their total caloric intake), and their total calories are definitely on the lower end of the spectrum.

Total caloric intake is individualized based on sex, age, lean muscle and overall metabolism, but it's safe to say it will likely be sub-2,000 calories for most men and likely sub-1,500 calories for most females. Due to the lower intake compounded over the past several months, their metabolism has down-regulated to preserve energy.

Their NEAT is at an all-time low, and they don't fidget or exert themselves near as much as they did at the beginning of this prep.

Their training has stayed steady, and they've likely been able to maintain most of their heavy lifts in the gym, but every rep is much more of a struggle. Lower calories have taken a toll on their hunger and the thought of food is often top of mind but still manageable, especially if the calories they are consuming are incredibly nutrient-dense and absorbed fully.

Their hormones have been impacted negatively due to the months of dieting, so libido is likely down a bit, and they are a bit moodier than usual, having an attitude and a slightly shorter fuse. They are incredibly lean, ideally within a few percentage points of their target body fat, but they look pretty "flat." If their electrolytes are dialed in properly, they can probably still achieve a decent pump in the middle of a training session, but that pump is a fleeting phenomenon. Most of the day, they look flat and emaciated. Vascularity is visible when flushed, such as during a training session or after a hot shower, but that is about it.

Speaking of hot showers, these are incredibly appreciated because this individual spends most of their day feeling quite cold. Even if the room is a normal, comfortable temperature, they feel freezing. This constant coldness is another indicator of down-regulated metabolism. If this all sounds like you, congratulations! You're in the correct phase and ready for the refeeds! If not, please do yourself a favor and return to the previous section in Phase Three.

DIALING IN ELECTROLYTES

Before we calculate our refeed macros, let's touch on electrolytes. As we all know, electrolytes play a massive role in ensuring we can achieve a solid pump, maintain energy in the gym and day-to-day life, avoid headaches and muscle cramps and function properly. We also know that having the proper equilibrium between our sodium, potassium and hydration levels is what allows our body's water retention to stay within a healthy range.

If that equilibrium is out of whack, you're likely going to retain a ton of excess fluids and look very soft and puffy due to all the water retention in your subcutaneous layer of skin. This day-to-day fluctuation in water retention produces slight fluctuations in our daily scale weight and is an entirely normal process. However, as we get leaner and leaner, these fluctuations become much more visually apparent and can profoundly impact the way we look.

I recall one instance during a 2017 contest prep in which I was in the later stages and was craving brussels sprouts for whatever reason. I ate a small bowl of these sprouts and felt compelled to cover them with an excessive amount of salt. I woke up the next day and stepped on the scale, and almost fell over in astonishment. I jumped up eight pounds overnight!

Before I allowed myself to go batshit crazy and blame myself for ruining my entire contest prep endeavors, I leveled with myself. I thought about what I had done the day prior that could have contributed to this massive spike in weight. I soon remembered the brussels sprouts covered in salt and put my mind at ease. My electrolyte equilibrium was thrown off, and my body retained a ton of additional fluid as a result. I simply dialed my electrolyte intake back and my body flushed out all of the excessive fluid. I was back down to my average weight within 48 hours.

We will manipulate our electrolytes slightly during our Phase Five peak week. Phase Four and all the keto caloric refeeds involved in this phase should be treated as trial runs to test the effectiveness of our refeed protocol in preparation for peak week. As such, we will manipulate our electrolytes slightly in this phase as well. Before we have any hope of managing our current electrolytes and monitoring our body's response to that manipulation, we need to establish a solid baseline.

We must track our sodium, potassium and water consumption throughout the entirety of this phase to truly get those baseline numbers dialed in. Hopefully, you've been monitoring your sodium intake intermittently throughout the prep thus far and you have a basic understanding of what ratio your body responds well to. If not, we have some catching up to do.

In my experience, most people incorporating a well-formulated ketogenic diet tend to respond well to a 2:1 ratio of supplemental sodium to potassium. What do I mean by supplemental? If you're following a ketogenic diet, you're likely consuming a considerable amount of meat, possibly some seafood, some amount of nuts, avocado, veggies, eggs and some dairy. All these foods have a fair amount of potassium, so you're ingesting a solid dose of this vital element through dietary means.

Ideally, you're avoiding processed foods that contain an excessive amount of added sodium. Most of our whole, single-ingredient foods are very low in naturally occurring sodium. As such, it stands to reason that we'll need to supplement a bit more sodium than potassium, thus the 2:1 ratio of supplemental sodium to potassium.

The actual number will vary greatly depending on your size, activity level, perspiration and other factors, but an excellent place to start is around 4,000 mg of sodium and 2,000 mg of potassium, though you can titrate up or down from there depending on how your body responds to that intake. It's important to realize that our bodies are smart and can establish equilibrium at a higher or lower level if the ratio is intact. I've noticed that as I get into contest prep, I crave salt more and more. As such, I tend to increase my potassium intake to follow suit and maintain that healthy equilibrium.

As calories get lower and lower, you may find yourself drinking more fluids to try and curb your appetite. This increase in hydration will likely have an impact on your electrolyte equilibrium. If you hyper-hydrate, your body will respond with increased urination and your kidneys will flush out much of your sodium and potassium. For this reason, I encourage you to have a pulse on how much fluid you're consuming daily and adjust your electrolyte intake accordingly.

TRACKING SODIUM, POTASSIUM AND FLUID LEVELS

So, how does someone go about tracking sodium, potassium and fluid levels without going crazy and pulling out their hair? There are a few things you can do to simplify the process. As far as water goes, I recommend just getting a large water jug and drinking that throughout the day. I shoot for a gallon a day, and I don't like constantly filling jugs, so I just grabbed a one-gallon stainless steel Yeti jug.

Another way to go about it is to simply purchase a one-gallon Berkey water filter. Fill it up at the beginning of the day and use it for all your coffee, tea, water and hydration needs. If you drain it by the end of the day, you'll know you've hit your mark. It's also all filtered, which is a bonus.

As far as sodium goes, I like to keep things super simple. I recommend using an old seasoning container that you have lying around and fill it with an entire day's dose of sodium. Sprinkle it on your foods and in your drinks throughout the day as needed until it's empty. Using this method, you only measure out your sodium once, so you're being accurate and consistent. A quarter teaspoon of Redmond Real Salt contains about 500 mg of sodium. If you're shooting for 4,000 mg of sodium throughout the day, that will equate to about two teaspoons of Redmond Salt. Speaking of Redmond Salt, they released an electrolyte blend that has a pre-mixed 2:1 ratio of sodium to potassium. You could use that to keep things simple and ensure that your numbers are always in check.

As far as potassium goes, I'd recommend using either potassium citrate, potassium chloride or a combination of the two. Dose it with your sodium throughout the day instead of all at once. You can keep things simple using a sodium/potassium blend similar to the Redmond Re-Lyte blend mentioned above, or you can opt to purchase it separately and dose it alongside your salt.

If you do go the blended route, make sure to account for the ratios because all blends are not created equal! One thing found to be very beneficial is Upgraded Formula's liquid nanosized potassium chloride. This supplement uses nano potassium, which means that the particle size of the potassium is smaller than your red blood cells to ensure better absorption. You can likely get away with supplementing less of it simply because your body will absorb it more thoroughly. If the powdered forms of potassium leads to GI upset, this liquid version used in smaller dosages may be the way to go.

The relationship between sodium and potassium in your body plays a major role in the level of intracellular and extracellular water you are holding, so this topic is very important. Track your fluid intake, sodium and potassium levels throughout Phase Four and get those numbers optimized!

MINIMIZE VEGGIES

Another critical point to keep in mind on refeed day is that we want to minimize or eliminate our intake of vegetables and high-fiber foods. Even if vegetables and higher volume foods sound more appealing than ever, they are the last thing you want to consume to optimize your appearance on the day after a refeed.

Regardless of how well your body assimilates and digests veggies, you'll likely experience some degree of bloating and water retention—two things you want to avoid. Since the Phase Four refeeds are supposed to test out our peak week protocol, I would advise against any vegetable intake or nutritionally void, high-volume foods on the day of the refeed. In fact, I often eliminate these foods starting two days before the refeed to fully ensure that they've cleared through my system and are no longer a threat to optimizing my appearance.

CALCULATE REFEED

So, how do you go about calculating your refeed amount precisely? I recommend starting on the conservative end of the spectrum. You can easily add more food on the next refeed if your body responds exceptionally well to the first trial run; however, it's much more difficult to take food away if we start too aggressively.

First, take note of your current macronutrient intake. This will likely be your daily macro goals at the end of Phase Three. Most people's caloric intake will be pretty low, and the fat ratio will likely be somewhere between 75% and 80% of your total calories coming from dietary fat. For illustrative purposes, we'll examine my personal intake for Phase Four during my last competition prep.

Now, it's important to note that my competition season was pretty long, so I started introducing refeeds a bit earlier in the process to prolong the Phase Four period. As such, my first refeed came in when my fat ratio was only around 72%, and my calories were still relatively manageable. If you're doing your first show or are only peaking for a single performance, I would start these refeeds closer to the 75-80% as mentioned above, when your calories are definitely on the lower end of the spectrum. Back to the example:

My daily macros before introducing the refeed were 150 g of dietary fat, 120 g of dietary protein and 12 g of total carbohydrates. That put me at a total caloric intake of 1,878.

Total Calories: (150 x 9) + (120 x 4) + (12 x 4) = 1,878

(150 x 9) = 1,350 total calories
1,350 / 1,878 = 0.7188
Fat Percentage = 71.88%

A good conservative approach to calculating our initial refeed amount is to increase our caloric intake by about 30% of what we are currently consuming. Using this example of 1,878 calories, that would look as follows:

1,878 x 30% = 563.4
1,878 + 563.4 = 2,441 Total Calories

In this example, a 30% increase in our current caloric intake would yield an additional 563 calories. Therefore, our refeed day will grant us a total caloric intake of 2,441 calories.

If you've been dieting for quite some time, as I'm sure you have, that extra 30% increase sounds downright delicious! Now that we know how many more calories we'll be consuming, how do we determine the macronutrient breakdown of those calories? Generally, your protein intake will be at an all-time low during this phase. To make that relatively low protein intake more sustainable, I like to bump up protein intake during these refeed days. As such, I recommend increasing your total dietary protein up to a 1:1 ratio correlated with your lean mass.

In my case, during my last prep, my lean mass was about 150 lb, which means I would bump up my total dietary protein on refeed day to equal 150 g. I was already consuming 120 g of protein a day, making that a 30 g increase in protein. The remaining calories can be allocated to dietary fat.

Lean Mass in pounds = Refeed Protein in grams
150 LBM = 150 g of protein

Total Refeed Protein - Current Protein = Additional Protein
150 - 120 = 30 g added protein
30 x 4 = 120 calories allocated for protein

Now that we know how much we're increasing protein, simply subtract the caloric load of protein from the total increase in calories and add the remainder to dietary fat:

563 Refeed Calories - 120 calories of protein = 443 calories for fat
443 / 9 = 49.2 g of dietary fat

To simplify our macro tracking and keep things in 5 g increments, I will round the 49.2 g of dietary fat up to 50 g even. Based on these calculations, our total macronutrient breakdown for our first refeed will look like this:

Fat: 150 + 50 = 200
Protein: 120 + 30 = 150
Carbohydrates are held constant between 0–20 g

BEST PRACTICES

Now that we know precisely how much we're increasing calories and their exact macronutrient breakdown, let's talk a bit about the foods we should use to comprise those macros. As I mentioned earlier, we want to avoid a ton of vegetation or high-volume foods that could result in unnecessary bloating and water retention. Ideally, you'll only use foods that you know your body responds well to; this is not the time to introduce new variables. Choose foods that are easily broken down by the body and absorbed.

An example of this would be to opt for ground beef rather than steak because ground beef is going to require less time to assimilate. Opt for fat sources that you know your stomach handles well.

In my experience, ground beef and eggs are relatively foolproof and rarely result in any bloat or stomach discomfort. If you've included dairy throughout your prep thus far with zero adverse effects, feel free to leverage that as well.

Feel free to get creative and use your bump in macros to make meals that you want to eat, just do so within the range that you know your body will respond well to. Prepare foods that are easily tweaked and tracked so that we may dial in your ideal peak week protocol.

I've come to love ketogenic "fathead" pizzas for my refeed meals (I've included the recipe in the appendix of this book)! My body responds well to the ingredients and they are very calorically dense, so I don't experience any unnecessary bloating. If you can handle dairy in quality cheese, I would highly encourage you to try the fathead pizza as a refeed meal.

I prepare the crust with three simple ingredients: almond flour, cheese and a single egg. I top the pizza with ground beef, possibly some pesto and my secret weapon: anchovies! Anchovies are incredible for delivering a massive bolus of sodium with zero unnecessary volume. The average can of anchovies contains between 1,000 and 2,000 mg of sodium, which is exactly what I try and increase my sodium intake by on refeed day.

PROPER ELECTROLYTE MANIPULATION

If you are as lean as you should be at this stage in your contest prep, every minor tweak and manipulation has the potential to make a noticeable difference in the look and feel of your physique. This concept holds true regarding how full and vascular you look as a result of sodium manipulation.

Loading or cutting sodium is typically discussed in peak week protocols; still, since we are using this phase to test our body's response to refeeds and develop our ideal peak week protocol, I'll dive into it now. Our primary objective in optimizing our electrolyte equilibrium is to force as much of our body's water into muscle cells as possible and leave very little in the subcutaneous layer between the muscle and skin. The more water we carry in our subcutaneous layer, the softer and less vascular we look.

Our body naturally carries most of our total water intracellularly, but the massive fluctuations in consumption, electrolytes, body fat and various hormones throughout prep can shift extracellular retention up or down. As is true with most changes in our body, we fight to maintain some degree of homeostasis.

Just as our body "wants" to maintain a certain weight and body fat, it also wants to maintain a certain intra- and extracellular water retention ratio. Many peak week protocols based on bro science can backfire catastrophically and force water retention to fluctuate in an incredibly unhealthy and even dangerous manner. For instance, if you drastically cut sodium intake and water consumption to flush out any subcutaneous water, your body is going to fight to maintain homeostasis and regain a sense of equilibrium.

As such, your aldosterone hormone that governs water retention will increase, and your kidneys will start working hard to reabsorb more water. Since your body will fight to maintain a natural water retention ratio even if you cut water or take a diuretic, the balance between your intracellular and extracellular water will likely stay the same. This result is less fluid volume in your actual muscle cells and, therefore, less size and ability to get a great pump onstage. You'll look even more flat and emaciated, which is the last thing we want!

Just as our body wants to maintain homeostasis with water, it also wants to maintain homeostasis with blood serum sodium levels. If the sodium in your blood rises or falls far outside ideal levels, you could die! As such, our bodies tightly regulate the sodium circulating in our bloodstream at all times. If sodium increases, our bodies decrease the secretion of the aforementioned aldosterone hormone to excrete sodium; the same is true on the other end of the spectrum.

If you drastically cut your sodium intake, aldosterone increases so your body can reabsorb more sodium through the kidneys. For this reason, we can reset our equilibrium at a higher or lower intake of sodium depending on what we personally crave and respond best at. Keep in mind that sodium and potassium share a correlated relationship, so if you increase sodium, you'll likely need to have a corresponding increase in potassium and vice versa.

NOTES ON EQUILIBRIUMS

If our bodies naturally gravitate to an equilibrium, what is the purpose of manipulating electrolytes in the first place? It's a worthwhile question, and the answer deserves a deep understanding.

Our ability to re-establish an equilibrium set point doesn't happen instantaneously. As we increase or decrease our sodium intake, it can take between 24 and 48 hours for our bodies to regulate themselves and return to homeostasis. That window can be leveraged to achieve a temporarily enhanced physique. The problem with this is that many coaches don't understand the biomechanics behind this equilibrium, and they tend to operate in the extremes.

Many of the peak week protocols prescribe several days of sodium depletion and water cutting leading up to the show. This drastically ramps up aldosterone and makes our bodies incredibly susceptible to retaining fluids. However, if you're not consuming any fluids during that time, there is no sodium or water to be absorbed and your serum levels dip. Not only is that incredibly dangerous, but it also results in a drop in your blood pressure, which certainly is *not* advantageous for bodybuilders trying to maximize blood flow for a great pump. This depletion phase is often followed by a drastic and sudden increase in sodium or water right before the show. This can shock your system and leave you feeling downright terrible, but it also doesn't give your body near enough time to re-establish an equilibrium. As such, we do "fill out"—but not in a good way.

Rather than looking full and hard with paper-thin skin, you look like an inflated water balloon or the Goodyear Blimp! After months and months of hard dieting and training, the last thing you want is to blow it during peak week by incorporating these ill-advised and utterly ineffective sodium and water manipulations.

The best thing you can do is come in freakishly lean and in shape, totally independent of any electrolyte or water manipulations. If you are looking great, you'll do amazingly well due to your hard work and dedication, not some crazy, miraculous peak week manipulation. Still, there are a few things you can do with electrolytes to add an enhanced level of "polish" to the fantastic package you're already bringing to the stage on show day.

As it relates to electrolyte and water manipulations, you need to understand this: make *small* changes! Just as we've made gradual manipulations to macronutrient intake throughout this prep, we will also make conservative changes to our electrolytes. Also, please realize that the look we can achieve with manipulating sodium intake is only temporary. You will re-establish an equilibrium point after a day or two, so our intention here is to "peak" for that short period in time when you'll be onstage.

SODIUM LOADING

So how do we go about peaking? Before our body's regulation and reestablishment of fluid levels and electrolytes, we have a short period to optimize for a specific look. That "look" is often achieved by a slight and temporary bump in sodium the evening before the show, followed by a steady consumption of sodium and a moderate intake of fluids on show day. What is going on here at a cellular level?

By increasing our sodium slightly above our current body's "set point," we can force a bit more extracellular water from the subcutaneous layer of skin into the actual muscle cells to give us that volumized, shredded look. This will provide us with a slight increase in blood pressure for a better pump and a more vascular look. The increase in intracellular fluids combined with the slight rise in blood pressure and the paper-thin skin yield an amazing physique that can do some serious damage on show day! That is the look we are striving for.

From an electrolyte standpoint, I would increase sodium on refeed day by 500-1,000 mg to start. I recommend the bulk of that day's sodium be introduced in the evening hours. This grants us more time to maintain that look on show day since shows are typically in the afternoon and evening hours. We can gradually titrate that sodium intake up as needed throughout Phase Four, depending on how our body responds to the sodium load. It's safer to start on the lower end of the spectrum and increase rather than starting high and decreasing. I've found my sodium load "sweet spot" to be around the 2,000 mg mark on refeed day—though keep in mind that is the amount sodium increases by, *not* the total sodium intake for the day.

Using myself as an example, my daily sodium intake throughout

Phase Four is between 4,000 and 6,000 mg. I've found the 2,000 mg increase to be most effective for me, so that would put my total sodium intake for the refeed day up around 8,000 mg on the high end. These numbers are *not* universal, which is why tracking your electrolyte levels daily throughout Phase Four is so important! Figure out your daily intake and then experiment to see what sodium load your body responds best to.

POTASSIUM LOADING

I would be remiss if I didn't touch on potassium here. Many ill-informed peak week protocols involve a potassium "loading" phase while simultaneously (and drastically) cutting sodium. This is done in the hopes of flushing out excess fluids and acting as a diuretic. Unfortunately, it doesn't work—and it's pretty dangerous.

The relationship between our body's serum sodium and potassium levels drives the electrical synapses in charge of powering our cells. This relationship is responsible for most functions in our nervous system; it is even what allows our muscles to contract. If the relationship between our sodium and potassium levels is extremely compromised and potassium levels far exceed sodium, you run the risk of hyperpolarizing your cardiac cells. That hyperpolarization can cause your heart to stop beating. It doesn't take a medical professional to diagnose the fact that that isn't good.

Rather than playing around with electrolyte levels through crazy loading and depletion phases, let's just dial in our ideal equilibrium and make subtle tweaks to optimize for a particular look. The 2:1 ratio of supplemental sodium to potassium that we talked about earlier still applies here. Our bodies seem to respond quite well to that ratio, so there's no need to deviate from it significantly.

As we increase our sodium a bit on refeed day, you may want to bump up your supplemental potassium a bit as well to follow suit. You likely won't need quite the increase that we are doing with sodium. Remember, the goal is to elicit a favorable response from the slight increase in sodium. While we are increasing sodium by 500-1,000 mg to start, I would probably increase potassium by about 100-300 mg. By keeping these electrolyte levels in check, we can avoid all the potential risks associated with excessively low or high serum sodium and potassium levels.

ANALYZE REFEED IMPACT

Since Phase Four grants a window of opportunity to test our peak week protocol, treat these refeeds with as much seriousness and attention to detail as you would in your actual peak week. Later, we'll incorporate refeed meals and electrolyte manipulations the day before the actual show to optimize nutrient absorption and intracellular fluid retention required for peaking. As such, treat the day after these refeeds as your pseudo show day.

Most competitions are scheduled on a Saturday, so we'll assume our refeed will occur the evening before on Friday. Try to get most of your day's allotment of calories toward the back half of the day so that you'll be able to capitalize on the changes throughout the following day.

If you've been at a significant deficit for any length of time, you'll likely notice some changes in how your body feels soon after consuming the refeed. I experience an increase in my body temperature, and my vascularity and fullness improve within 20-30 minutes of the refeed meal. I notice a profound impact from the sodium load in that same timeframe as well. It's essential to be conscious of all of these changes and take note of them to adjust the following week's refeed based on your findings. If you want to gather the data, I'd recommend the following protocol:

> **Friday Morning:** Weigh-in as usual. Gather some baseline blood markers such as a BHB blood ketone test and a blood glucose test. Take baseline pictures and measurements against a standardized background with set lighting.

Friday Evening: Consume the refeed meal containing the majority of your day's calories. Be sure to include the initial increase in refeed day sodium of 500-1,000 mg above your baseline. Enjoy the bolus of food and appreciate the novelty in eating something different and more substantial after months of dieting. Be present and take stock of how the increase in calories and sodium makes you feel.

Do you feel bloated? How about satiated? Do you feel like you've opened the floodgates and have the urge to binge? (If so, don't do it!)

How are your energy levels? Do you feel like your skin is tighter? Do you feel incredibly thirsty from the extra sodium in your meal? Does your entire body feel warmer than usual? I encourage you to go for a short walk after this refeed meal. The movement will help with your digestion and get the blood flowing a bit more. The increase in blood flow will help move the increase in calories and sodium throughout your bloodstream a bit more efficiently—nothing crazy, just a leisurely 10- to 20-minute walk around town.

When you get back from your walk, take note of how you look. Consider taking some follow-up progress pics to see if you can see a difference in your composition. Observe yourself in the mirror. Do you notice more vascularity, thinner skin and more of a "pump?" Drink a bit more water if you need to but try to avoid chugging too many fluids. Keep your water intake reasonably consistent with what you've done on the days leading up to this refeed. Go to sleep and see if the increase in calories improves the quality of your slumber.

Saturday Morning: Wake up and step on the scale as usual. Did the refeed cause your weight to increase, or do you see an unexpected drop in the scale weight? Retake your measurements and see if there is a difference. Observe yourself in the mirror. Do you look "dryer" and crisper than you did the day before when you first woke up? Do you feel incredibly parched or normal?

Take some updated progress pics in the standardized setup with the same lighting as before. Hit all your mandatory poses and treat this photo update with the same seriousness as you would the show day itself. As you go through your poses, you'll likely experience a bit of a pump and will notice an increase in blood flow. That's great! The pictures will likely continue to improve as your pump heightens.

How do your muscular contractions feel as you hit different poses? Do you feel soft and flaccid or hard and grainy? Compare the pictures you just took with the ones you took on Friday morning. Do you see a tangible difference?

This is the protocol I would recommend every week going forward. We are in the home stretch now, and every little manipulation makes a big difference. Your composition and overall appearance will start changing more noticeably on a weekly basis now. As such, take each week seriously and capture the changes in pictures and measurements. We will gradually increase calories and sodium as needed and add more sodium on the refeed days if that yields a positive outcome. Take these updated progress pictures as outlined to have a solid feel for how your body responds to refeed manipulations.

FURTHER MANIPULATIONS

In monitoring how your body responds, you may notice that the initial 30% increase in calories simply isn't enough to elicit the response you're looking for. Perhaps your body soaks up that 30% immediately and you see a benefit, but the noticeable effects have dissipated by the following morning.

Try increasing the refeed amount with each week that passes; I've seen a positive outcome from as much as a 50% increase in calories from baseline. The challenge here is in being truly objective and not simply hungry. At this stage in the prep, we all crave more calories. The question is, would those extra calories produce a better look or just a more satisfied belly? Be honest with yourself and analyze the pictures.

Another strategy is to implement a consecutive two-day refeed. Since fat is absorbed and assimilated so much slower than carbohydrates, it takes quite a bit longer to see its effects on your overall composition. This became evident in working with many of my female clients. I would trial them through a traditional Friday refeed strategy with the intention of them peaking on Saturday. However, I would notice that they looked better on Sunday. After further experimentation, I found that the most optimal strategy was to start the week's refeed on Thursday rather than Friday. I still recommend backloading most calories on Thursday. Depending on how they looked after that Thursday refeed, I would either increase calories further on Friday's refeed or be a bit more conservative. Having a slightly more extended period at the high calories seemed to give their bodies the necessary time to absorb and reflect the benefits of the refeed meals. With this longer refeed period, I still recommend only manipulating sodium on Friday.

This is a perfect example of how individualized this process truly is. Everybody is going to assimilate dietary fat and protein at slightly different rates. Everyone is going to absorb and reflect the changes in their supplemental sodium and potassium differently as well. There is no such thing as an online calculator and mainstream resource that offers the optimal solution for everyone. This is honestly why one-on-one customized coaching exists. You can use the principles I've laid out thus far to get pretty damn close to perfect. However, recognize that you're going to need to get in tune with your body, track the data, monitor your manipulations and make necessary tweaks to "peak" in a manner best suited to you!

There is one more point I'd like to make regarding further refeed manipulations. As you've likely noticed, refeed calories have been increasing week after week in Phase Four. That does not necessarily mean overall calories have been increasing. Phase Three saw a continual decrease in both protein and dietary fat macronutrients; that decrease in fat and protein still applies here in Phase Four. Calories increase on the actual refeed day, but the overall average weekly intake may still decrease depending on how aggressive you are with your refeeds.

The temporary increase in energy intake on refeed day makes these ever-decreasing weekly calories much more sustainable from a mental and physical perspective. If you still have more body fat to lose, I encourage you to keep reducing calories from fat and protein as we illustrated in Phase Three. The addition of the refeeds in Phase Four may help you sustain the lower calories while also pushing you through any potential plateaus. The only situation in which I would recommend *not* continually decreasing overall calories would be if you peaked early on or hit your caloric floor and cannot safely go any lower.

In these situations, you simply want to hold steady up until show day. Maintain your daily caloric intake and continue manipulating refeed macros and electrolytes as needed while analyzing the effects as you prepare for peak week. I want to point out that it's not healthy or sustainable to try to maintain a low caloric intake for any significant length of time. There are many moving pieces in prep, and it can be hard to know how your body will respond over several months of dieting. However, as you get better and better at this process, you'll be able to time things much more efficiently, and you'll be able to peak at the proper time without having to try and hold steady or maintain for weeks on end.

Unnecessary time spent maintaining a low caloric intake is

simply not optimal. That time could have been used to build more muscle while at a caloric surplus or even maintain a healthier metabolic and caloric intake for a longer time before transitioning into a steep deficit.

CHANGES TO TRAINING

We will manipulate our training slightly during peak week, but I would caution against it during the trial refeeds in Phase Four. Doing so can prevent you from gaining 100% clarity on how your body responds to things, which is important to have during peak week. Phase Four is still go-time, and the last thing we need to do is skimp on our training intensity.

If you make a change, I suggest slightly increasing intensity. From a physical standpoint, we'll be able to take advantage of the bump in calories from the refeeds. Psychologically speaking, we'll be able to finish strong and know we gave it our all during the homestretch leading up to the show. This doesn't mean you should kill yourself on every set for the next few weeks, but it does imply that you leave no stone left unturned and cut no corners.

Don't neglect your training, skip cardio or go through the motions. Train with intention and intensity. Be able to step onstage confidently, knowing that you couldn't have done any more than what you have.

From a technical standpoint, I encourage you to structure your training so your most demanding training day falls on the day after your keto caloric refeed. For most people, this will be a leg or back day. Time your split so that you can take full advantage of that surge in calories and fuel and put it to good use.

Believe it or not, the show day and your time spent onstage posing are incredibly physically demanding. The nerves combined with the burning stage lights, the competition and the need to hold a fully flexed pose for an extended period will leave you exhausted. Imagine your training sessions are an embodiment of your future stage presence. Give it your all, hit your reps, go to failure and contract your muscles fully.

After training sessions, take the time to go through all of your mandatory poses again. Flex in the mirror and hold your positions for an extended time. Try to force as much blood into your muscle tissue as possible. The progress pictures you took earlier were taken immediately upon waking without a pump. How do you look now with a pump? Is there a significant difference from before? How you look now will be similar to how you'll look onstage after you've had the time to pump up backstage.

Are you pleased with the look? How is your vascularity? Are you holding a ton of water? Did the refeed meal have a noticeable impact? Be conscious of these subtle differences and monitor them with each trial refeed we implement in Phase Four.

PHASE FOUR MINDSET

Phase Four is the final push in competition prep. You've been incredibly strict with your macros and meals for months on end. You've been diligent with your training. You've kept your cool, and you've been incredibly patient. What type of mindset do you need to possess to excel in Phase Four? To be honest, it depends on the kind of person you are.

You'll need to adopt a different type of approach if you're the type that is prone to ease up at the end versus the kind who is likely to overdo things and burn out. Imagine you're in a race. Once you round the corner and see the finish line, do you need to run even faster, or do you drop your speed to a less taxing intensity and coast through to the end? If you give it your all and sprint to the finish, you are liable to collapse to the ground as soon as you cross the line. I don't want you to collapse at the end of this prep because, quite frankly, the show day isn't the "finish line." You can't afford to collapse.

What if you're the one to coast to the end? Is that better? Not exactly. You certainly don't want to ease up and squander your time in the final weeks before the show. The last thing you want is to be filled with regret on show day, thinking you could have done more.

Self-awareness is so crucial here. Be honest with yourself. What kind of behavior do you typically illustrate when something you've been working incredibly hard on seemingly comes to a close? Do you burn out or are you invigorated to keep going?

I could quickly write a motivational blanket statement in this section that appeals to the masses, but the problem with those is that they can be incredibly damaging if you lack the perspective necessary to apply them and be okay afterward.

Perhaps I can provide more clarity with a story.

During my very first competition prep in 2012, I lacked perspective. I wasn't aware of the depths of hell my mind could descend to. I rounded the corner and saw that I had a few weeks left before peak week, so I convinced myself that I could do anything for those few weeks. I made the mistake of assuming absolute suffering should be a direct by-product of pushing it as hard as possible to the finish line.

I cut calories even further, way beyond what was healthy. I increased my cardio time on the Stairmaster exponentially. The absolute hell that I created for myself manifested most prominently in my training; it was where my obsessive-compulsive disorder kicked in. If 10 reps were good, 15 were better. I'd hit 15 reps and then decide that I only deserved to step onstage if I could muster the strength to hit another 10. I'd be at 25 reps, and then darkness would take over. I envisioned someone holding a gun to my head or my family's heads and demand that I double the reps or else they would get a bullet between their eyes.

I'd somehow find the strength to reach 50 reps, literally crying in pain and quivering in agony. I'd do another few more reps to keep the visions at bay, and then I'd fall off the machine, crawl to a corner and puke before composing myself enough to move on to the next exercise and repeat the process.

Why am I telling you this? I'm telling you because I want to be completely transparent. Strange things happen in a contest prep when you're incredibly depleted and your metabolism is downregulated. The safety buffer between your physical body and your mind is much thinner. The pressure you apply to your body transcends the physical and enters your subconscious. That's why it's so imperative to be self-aware.

The last thing I want is for any of you going through this competition prep to endure the hell I created for myself in 2012. Granted, I didn't know what I was doing with my nutrition then. I wasn't aware of my OCD, I didn't have any guidance or mentors, and I had no coach and no plan. My intention is for this book to be that guide for you. I want to give you that perspective so that you know what is possible and feel empowered to be completely honest with yourself. Know what tendencies you have. Understand how you approach and respond to stressful situations and develop your plan accordingly.

I wholeheartedly encourage you to push beyond your limits. Give this prep your all (plus a little more) so you can gain that perspective. Competition prep is an excellent opportunity for personal growth and development because you get to experience something challenging and push through it. Adversity is a great thing, but it's best to base your decisions on your strategy and the feedback your body and mind give you. Analyze how the refeeds are impacting you through an objective lens.

Ramp up the cardio and the training but not so much so that this entire journey becomes miserable. Competition preps are supposed to be hard, and they are supposed to push you beyond your self-perceived limitations. They are *not* supposed to be a self-induced hell. I want the outcome of this prep to yield a net positive for you, not a net negative. Don't set yourself up to fail by choosing a non-sustainable path to burnout.

[5]
PHASE FIVE: PEAK WEEK AND SHOW DAY

Peak Week. Just the words themselves sound almost sacred! Up until now, it has probably seemed like this moment would never come. Now that it's here, it probably seems like it came without warning and snuck up on you! Hopefully, you've put in the work up to this point and you look the part. If so, congratulations are in order.

Regardless of the placing, you've done something amazing with your life! You've accomplished something that less than 1% of the population has achieved. You've pushed yourself physically, mentally and emotionally to your limits—probably harder than you've likely ever been pushed before. You've likely seen some incredible growth in character and resilience, and nobody can take that from you—certainly not a judge sitting across from you at a bodybuilding competition! For that reason alone, I'm incredibly proud of you. I'm honored to have played a small role in your journey.

What now? Well, to be honest, all the hard work is done as far as competition prep is concerned. The reverse diet certainly isn't easy, but we'll talk about that later. Let's be present and focus on the here and now. Optimizing for peak week and show day is, and should be, a relief. If you've put in the work up to this point, you're able to enjoy the fruits of your labor and coast into the show.

Throughout this week, we will scale back on our training and the intensity of our cardio. We'll continue to implement the ketogenic caloric refeeds. We'll focus on reducing as much stress and anxiety as possible, so feel free to spoil yourself with a massage, some sauna time, plenty of rest and meditation or whatever else fits your fancy. Truth be told, if you don't look great now, you're not going to be able to miraculously change a few things and look like a Greek god or goddess in a week. That wouldn't even be realistic. However, if you've pushed hard up to this point, followed the protocol and look the part, you'll be able to take a step back and breathe this week.

It's counterproductive to ramp up the intensity of your training and cardio at this stage, because the acute inflammation can cause you to hold water and look worse on show day. If you're incredibly stressed and anxious, you'll also retain unnecessary fluids. This is one of those rare situations where it pays to do less and relax more, so enjoy it! The hard work has already been done!

Still, this doesn't mean you should book yourself a vacation to the Bahamas and sit on the beach drinking keto cocktails all day. There is still work to do, and attention to detail is paramount at this stage in the game. We don't want to deviate so far from what we've done the past several months that our body goes into shock and responds poorly. We want to maintain our current routine and timing. Continue to wake up, eat, train and sleep in a similar way to what you've done throughout prep; just don't kill yourself on any of it. I will take the following chapters and lay out an incredibly detailed peak week and show day protocol. Take notes and prepare yourself for what is to come.

SETTING EXPECTATIONS

For whatever reason, peak week and show day have spawned some of the strangest and most inadequate training and nutritional protocols.

These unorthodox techniques and practices likely originated from some small grain of truth, like many things in life: electrolytes need to be tweaked, water intake needs to be monitored, training should be adjusted and macros can indeed be manipulated to elicit a specific response. In general, however, the pendulum has swung so far in the opposite direction of what is optimal and even necessary. My objective with this section is to paint a picture of what *not* to do during peak week. It all starts with expectations.

The worst thing that can happen during a competition prep is that you go into the journey with the wrong expectation and then feel let down or betrayed when things don't work out as you planned. Misaligned expectation can result in despair and turmoil in relationships, business deals, career goals and bodybuilding competitions, so let's be honest with ourselves.

Many contest prep coaches fill their clients' heads with delusions of grandeur and assure them that they are "holding a bit of water" and will flush it out during peak week. Let me be perfectly clear: if you are coming into peak week out of shape, you are holding body fat, not merely water weight. No "bro-tocol" peak week magic is going to change that.

The beginning of peak week should see you looking pretty darn close to what you envision yourself looking like onstage. Take your sex, experience and competitive category into consideration. If you're a male going into an open bodybuilding category, you better look pretty damn striated, shredded and crisp on Monday going into peak week. You may, in fact, be holding a bit of water. Perhaps there needs to be a bit more work done with your electrolytes. The refeed should undoubtedly help fill you out a bit, but you should look absolutely amazing on Monday! If you're expecting a miraculous change to occur over the course of five days, you're in for a rude awakening.

I'm not saying any of this to discourage you or sway you away from stepping onstage; I'm laying this out to set a realistic expectation. Peak week does not change you. It simply amplifies what you already have. If you're already shredded and look amazing, it amplifies that. If you're still super soft and holding too much fat, it will likely amplify that as well.

Review what the last few weeks of Phase Four brought to the table. Did the refeeds reveal a better version of yourself? Or did you feel like you were going backward? What happened in Phase Four is a precursor to what is about to occur as we transition into Phase Five.

If you're being completely honest with yourself and are not happy with the package you're bringing to the table, you have a few options. If your calories are within a healthy range, you can continue dieting down and select a competition that falls on a later date. If your calories have bottomed out and you're approaching burnout, I highly encourage you to take some incredibly detailed progress pictures and maybe even schedule a professional photo shoot. Use this as an opportunity to document how you look and feel at the apex of this prep so that you can gain the perspective and compare against it next time. Transition into a building phase and cycle back through this program when it's more feasible for you.

A third option could be simply stepping onstage anyway to gain the experience. I know several people who jumped onstage when their bodies had no business up there from a competitive standpoint, but their minds needed that experience. I can totally respect that decision as well.

If you've put in the work and need the closure of seeing it through to the end come hell or high water, by all means step onstage and strut your stuff! I competed against a gentleman one year who was clearly out of shape and did not pose a threat to my placing. I couldn't help but wonder what he was doing there. I later found out that he'd had multiple surgeries that year and lost a ton of weight and wanted to use the bodybuilding competition as a vehicle to celebrate that. His story was incredibly inspiring, and I was proud to share the stage with him! I'm sure he didn't expect to win the title. Instead, he simply wanted the experience. In instances like that, I say go for it! I just encourage you to have the right expectation going into it.

There is a dark side to this on the opposite end of the spectrum as well. I've known individuals who were absolutely shredded and had peaked perfectly talk themselves out of competing. Their view of themselves had become skewed; they overanalyzed their physiques, convinced that they weren't ready. This stems from a lack of self-awareness and improper expectations as well.

I almost allowed this to happen to myself during my very first competition. The night before the show, I looked in the mirror and convinced myself that I wasn't ready. I was on the verge of calling the whole thing off and resuming everyday life. The reality was that I was utterly shredded and had peaked just fine. My mother, of all people, talked some sense into me, and I regained my composure and committed to seeing it through to the end.

Recognize that we are never perfect and that our vision of an ideal physique will likely be just beyond our grasp. That's okay. In this scenario, the best thing you can do is commit and follow through with what you've worked so incredibly hard on for the last several months of your life. You'll continue to get better and better as you cycle through these phases. How you look at this show is not a fixed representation of you, and this isn't your entire life. This is just a moment in your life, a life that will continue to get better and better if you keep working on yourself. Enjoy this moment and make the most of it. It's part of the journey.

PHASE FIVE GUIDELINES

If you genuinely capitalized on all the opportunities Phase Four had to offer, Phase Five should be reasonably straightforward. This week, we get to replicate what we learned in the last phase—and this time, it counts!

Human nature is such that we consciously know when it's game time or purely practice. This week is game time. Maybe you were a bit lax with your electrolyte measuring in the last phase. If so, get it dialed in now. Perhaps you fudged a few macros here and there last week. There's no time for that now.

This is the moment you've been training for the past several months. Be present, soak it all in and don't take anything for granted. As I mentioned earlier, you can coast this week if you've put in the work up to this point. Coast does *not* mean you can be sloppy. On the contrary, I hope you take this week to double down on the accuracy and precision of every manipulation you make.

The only objective of this phase is to get you optimized for show day itself. To have you peak with perfection and do so in a healthy manner. Take these following chapters and combine them with your knowledge of yourself and your physiology. Apply the principles in the pages that follow along with the work you've done up to this point to create a masterpiece!

TRADITIONAL PEAK WEEK

We've already covered refeeds and electrolytes in-depth in the last phase, but I'll touch on them again briefly to reemphasize their importance as it relates to peak week. Before I do that, I'd love to examine a classic example of what *not* to do—no matter what you've heard on bodybuilding forums or in the athletic folklore.

PEAK WEEK (CARBS, WATER AND ELECTROLYTES)

Traditional bodybuilding wisdom suggests a sodium and water loading phase about a week before show day accompanied by a shift to depletion workouts designed to burn through all muscle glycogen. Carbohydrate intake is significantly reduced to maximize glycogen depletion, which is followed up with a sodium depletion, a corresponding spike in potassium and a drop in water intake in the few days before stepping onstage. Generally, this is when coaches encourage their clients to backload carbohydrates to super-compensate muscle glycogen stores and fill them out further.

This strategy is touted as the ideal way to "dry" you out further and ensure you aren't holding on to any excess fluids while also maximizing your pumps and vascularity. Combine this protocol with the use of diuretics, stimulants and the everyday stressors of peak week, and you have successfully created the ideal environment for physiological failure! If you hear any semblance to this method from your coach or fellow competitors, tune them out and run the other way!

Let's break this down even further, starting with the depletion and loading of dietary carbohydrates. If you're reading this book, it stands to reason that you are interested in following a ketogenic contest prep protocol. Regardless of your reasoning, you're here, and you want to do this as a ketogenic athlete. Congrats! Now, let me highlight a specific point.

You do *not* need dietary carbohydrates to peak for a bodybuilding competition if you are genuinely fat-adapted! I am amazed at how many competitors are willing to stay strict keto throughout their entire prep and then become convinced that they must introduce carbs during peak week to maximize their physique for the stage. This is not true. In reality, it's the worst thing you could do.

As I repeated numerous times in Phase Four, peak week should *not* include any new variables. The addition of new variables will likely negatively shock your body and elicit a poor response, which is the last thing we want during the final few days before competition—and this couldn't be truer when it comes to reintroducing carbohydrates.

Carbs are typically loaded during the final few days to supersaturate muscle glycogen, but if you're fat-adapted and have been for a while, your body is going to use significantly less glycogen during your day-to-day training. The slight amount used is replenished quite efficiently through your regular ketogenic diet in the absence of carbohydrates. What does that mean? It means your stored muscle glycogen will be at levels similar to your carb-dependent competitors. Combine that with the fact that your reduced training intensity throughout peak week provides ample time for your body to replenish muscle glycogen.

As such, there is absolutely no need or benefit to introducing carbs. You won't "fill out" any more, and you run the risk of looking soft onstage due to the retention of excess fluids and unbalanced electrolytes. Better to play it safe and steer clear of the carbs altogether.

What about the relationship between fluid levels and sodium depletion and loading? Surely we would benefit from that, right? I don't want to repeat myself too much, but I do want to highlight a few simple facts. Firstly, as far as water is concerned, we want as much intracellular fluid as possible. This will result in a fuller, harder look and will yield a great pump onstage.

For this reason, the last thing we want to do is cut our water intake and dehydrate ourselves. What possible good could that do? I am amazed at the number of competitors convinced they need to cut water intake to look more shredded onstage. In all reality, the exact opposite is true. Our entire body comprises about 60% water. Our brain is about 80% water. Our heart is about 75% water and our muscles are 70-75%. Why in the world would we want to deplete those vital organs and tissue of the fluid that they contain? Don't do it!

You don't want to chug a liter of water immediately before stepping onstage simply because you don't want to be stuck having to pee or look like you have a full stomach of water. Other than that, stay consistent with your fluid intake throughout the entirety of peak week! Stay hydrated, establish your baseline intake and don't deviate from it. There's no sense in making a healthy sport incredibly unhealthy by unnecessary dehydration, which will inevitably result in a less impressive physique.

That said, we want as little fluid extracellularly in the subcutaneous layer of skin as possible. This is where electrolyte equilibrium comes into the picture. Remember that your body naturally disperses water intracellularly. This dispersion is subject to change during compositional changes, fluctuations in electrolyte intake and hormonal shifts, as is often the case during prep.

Our bodies always fight to maintain a homeostatic setpoint, but they often lag a bit behind the initial stimulus. If you cut sodium intake and water consumption, your body will respond by increasing your aldosterone hormone, which will send a signal to your kidneys to reabsorb more water and sodium. If you increase sodium significantly, your body decreases the secretion of aldosterone so that you flush out more fluids.

Our body's uncanny ability to return to a healthy baseline is a unique survival mechanism and proof that we shouldn't try and tamper too much with these biological systems. However, a *slight* tweak here or there during the final stages of a competition prep can elicit a favorable response. There's no need to dehydrate yourself or massively shift your blood serum sodium levels.

What does a slight change look like? Simply a temporary bump in sodium and potassium the night before the show. Remember, it can take between 24 and 48 hours for our body to regulate and return to homeostasis. If we time things correctly, the show day can fall within that 24- to 48-hour window, and we can leverage these hormonal shifts and fluctuations in fluid retention to step onstage looking a bit sharper.

This should not be a guessing game! As mentioned in Phase Four, it's paramount that you know and understand your daily sodium and potassium intake. The more accurate you are in knowing your baseline and thresholds, the more confidently you can tweak things to elicit the desired response. If you tested out refeeds and played with slight increases in sodium on refeed day during Phase Four, you likely know what your body responds best to.

In working with my clients and years of self-experimentation, I've found that it's only necessary to increase sodium intake on refeed days between 500 and 2,000 mg above normal intake to elicit the desired response. To maintain a proper ratio between sodium and potassium, I would also encourage you to increase potassium intake slightly as well. The increase in potassium doesn't have to be too aggressive, maybe only increasing 100-300 mg above the normal intake.

This targeted increase in sodium temporarily forces a bit more extracellular water into the muscle tissue and bumps blood pressure slightly. The corresponding result yields a more impressive physique with seemingly thinner skin, fuller muscles and increased vascularity.

Keep in mind that this is a brief look! As soon as your body catches up to the manipulations, the dispersion between intracellular and extracellular water will return to normal. You'll still look amazing, but you won't have quite the appeal that you do on show day. That is why the art of "peaking" for a show is a short-term process—a singular moment in time. Your body isn't designed to maintain that look indefinitely.

PEAK WEEK REFEED MEAL

To maximize your potential during that 24- to 48-hour window, you must implement a refeed meal that your body responds well to. Again, this is where we lean on the knowledge gained during our self-experimentation throughout Phase Four.

In Phase Four, we started with a 30% increase in caloric intake on refeed day and titrated up from there depending on how our body responded. After doing that for a few weeks, you likely have a solid idea of what caloric intake and macronutrient ratio your body prefers. On average, I've noticed this intake to be around a 30-50% increase in calories from a typical day. I've also noticed that the macronutrient breakdown for these refeeds tends to range between 70% of total calories coming from dietary fat up to 85% of calories coming from dietary fat.

This is an incredibly individualized process, so it would be unwise for me to throw in a formula here and expect it to allow anyone to peak perfectly.

This individuality goes beyond macronutrient ratios and total caloric intake. It bleeds into the dietary choices made toward the actual foods on refeed day. It's crucial to choose easily absorbed foods that don't contribute to any gastric distress or bloating.

Generally speaking, this means zero vegetation and fibrous foods.

Often, people experience acute inflammation from dairy products, so that may or may not be something you want to exclude. I have no issues with dairy, so I leave the cheese and heavy cream in my diet during peak week. I recommend choosing sources of protein that you know your body responds well to and can break down easily.

For this reason, I tend to default to a quality ground beef and egg mixture since they tend to cause the fewest issues for anyone.

As far as dietary fat is concerned, I recommend choosing sources you've used in the past and that you tolerate well. There is no sense in risking the consumption of 4 tbsp of MCT oil if it forces you to become a slave to the porcelain god for the next several hours. I do not suggest consuming a massive bolus of rendered fat either, as this may have a similar effect.

As always, avoid vegetable oils as your primary source of dietary fat. On average, saturated fats tend to invoke less GI distress than unsaturated fat, so I would recommend choosing meat sources that are high in fat rather than adding a ton of oils to your meals. I've had quite a bit of success with a 75/25 or 80/20 ground beef blend, raw beef suet, heavy cream, Keto Bricks, egg yolks, various nut butter and fatty pork sausage. A bit of olive oil or avocado oil is excellent, but I wouldn't make them your primary source of dietary fat now, during peak week. Ideally, you will have already experimented with these various sources of dietary fat in Phase Four and know what works for your body.

Dietary carbohydrates are a moot point since they are not necessary. However, since dietary fiber is technically classified as a carbohydrate, I'd love to touch on it briefly. As we mentioned in Phase Four, you want to keep fiber to a minimum when optimizing your refeed meal. A large bolus of fiber results in varying degrees of fermentation in your gut that can lead to bloating. We don't want that!

To play it safe, I recommend cutting all high-volume fibrous foods for about 72 hours before stepping onstage. That way, you've got plenty of time to clear it from your system, and there is no risk of the fiber drawing more fluids into your intestines and disrupting your electrolyte balance. I know we are super low on calories at this point and your hunger is rampant. Saying goodbye to high-volume foods will be challenging, but it's a worthwhile decision and it's for a finite period. Let the excitement of stepping onstage be more appealing to you than the allure of a large bowl of food.

Some competitors lean on fiber to stay regular and ensure their bowel movements are predictable. If you've been fat-adapted for any significant length of time, you've likely noticed that dietary fiber is not required to stay regular and avoid constipation. However, many people prefer to leave some dietary fiber in their nutritional protocol and fear removing it entirely during peak week will result in unnecessary bloating, constipation or other digestive issues.

If you're having any problems with your bowel movements in the days leading up to a show, you have a few options. First, ensure that you are adequately hydrated and your electrolytes are in check. Those two variables have a tremendous effect on your regularity; you can increase supplemental magnesium to get things moving if need be. Another option is to incorporate a cup of black coffee. Having the coffee poops is a real thing whether you admit it or not, and a well-timed cup of coffee may just do the trick to get your pipes flowing.

Put all of this together, and what do you get? Depending on your macronutrient needs and caloric intake, you have several different options. For illustrative purposes, I'll map out what a typical refeed day looks like for me:

> Soon after waking, I'll have a fatty coffee with a combination of heavy cream, butter or MCT oil, depending on how many macros I have to work with on that given day.

> I'll follow an OMAD approach and save most of my calories for the refeed meal itself, or I'll have an incredibly light meal prior to the refeed meal. That first meal could include a few

hard-boiled eggs and a few pieces of bacon— something easy to digest and nothing that would weigh heavily on my system.

The refeed meal itself is much larger and calorically dense. This meal is typically consumed in the evening hours the day before the show and contains the lion's share of calories for the day. You can keep it super simple and hit your macros using nothing more than ground beef, eggs and whatever dietary fat you choose. I like to create something that tastes amazing and gives me something to look forward to, so I generally opt for a keto fathead pizza, which I described earlier. I'll also include a Keto Brick with the refeed meal to increase my intake of dietary fat; they are high in stearic acid and don't seem to cause any digestive issues for me.

I can tweak the portion sizes and food choices depending on macronutrient targets, but this basic layout is my go-to for refeed days. The anchovies provide an excellent source of sodium. The ingredients in the fathead pizza fill me out but create zero bloat, and the brick gives me all of the dietary fat I need from an energy standpoint without weighing me down. Feel free to experiment with the foods you put in your refeed meal and find what works well for you, but definitely give this setup a try!

PEAK WEEK TRAINING MANIPULATIONS

There are definite changes you'll make to your training throughout this peak week protocol. If you recall, we did not manipulate our training during Phase Four so that we could squeeze the most out of refeed calories from a performance standpoint. We still want to optimize performance, but the definition of performance has shifted during this phase. Now, we are less concerned about training intensely to maximize fat loss and retain muscle. Currently, our primary performance metric is achieving a particular physical look.

In traditional contest prep peak week protocols, you'll often see coaches prescribe a ton of depletion workouts in the weeks leading up to peak week, followed by a total elimination of training altogether during peak week itself. You'll see the exact opposite end of the spectrum as well, and people will be going for PRs on squats the day before stepping onstage. Both methods are wrong, and as is true with many things in life, the answer lies somewhere in the middle.

You've been training consistently throughout this entire contest prep. Training is part of your routine, and your body has acclimated to it. Your maintenance calories are built into it, your electrolyte intake, your hydration, your sleep, everything! If our primary objective for peak week is to optimize our physique while manipulating as few variables as possible, how could it make sense to remove one of those variables entirely?

Training forces blood into the muscle tissue and delivers nutrients from your food consumption and the supplements you're taking. That blood flow and muscular stimulation also maintains the intracellular water balance we talked about earlier. It keeps you looking full and jacked rather than flat and soft. We want to amplify that full and jacked part, but don't let the pendulum swing so far in the opposite direction that you try to increase the intensity even further during peak week.

First of all, any fat you could lose and muscle you could gain has already been established; there's no sense in trying to catch up on lost time at this stage. There is an inherent risk of lifting incredibly hard and heavy in the days leading up to show day. Training is excellent in that it provides a form of acute inflammation that triggers the body to adapt. This adaptation takes the form of muscle growth.

As you know, building substantial muscle is a very long process, but temporary inflammation is very acute. Like most forms of inflammation, training results in a temporary increase in fluid retention as a protective mechanism. This is fine in the grand scheme of your bodybuilding career but not optimal in the context of the days before stepping onstage. The last thing you want is for all your definition to be washed out by fluid retention from an insane leg day the night before!

Knowing all of that, what should you do? I like to lift as I have been throughout the entirety of my prep until about Tuesday, assuming the show is on Saturday. I'll frontload the heavy compound movements I don't want to miss like deadlifts and squats and train those early in the week. I'll rearrange my training block the week before as necessary so that my back day and leg day fall on the Sunday, Monday or Tuesday preceding the show. That way, I can train those body parts hard and heavy per usual without any manipulation until Wednesday.

Starting on Wednesday, I recommend reducing the intensity a bit and cycling through a few additional body parts so your training is more like a circuit. At this stage, we will have recently trained legs, so you can skip the lower body and do a well-rounded upper body circuit. On Thursday, you want to decrease the intensity even more and add some simple leg movements for blood flow. A full-body circuit would work well here.

On Friday, the day before the show, decrease intensity yet again and hit another full-body circuit. At this point, you could accomplish your training using only resistance bands or light dumbbells. We certainly aren't trying to hit any new PRs at this stage in the game; we are just focused on blood flow and stimulation.

Depending on where your show is located, you may have to travel and stay at a hotel. I encourage you to invest in a set of resistance bands for this exact situation. You don't need much to get the blood flowing, but you do want to make sure you're able to activate your muscles and keep them full of blood, water and nutrients. I do recommend finishing off each training session with a solid posing session. The post-workout posing forces even more blood into the muscle tissue and conditions your mind for how hard it may be to pose onstage with the heat from lights and the energy from the competitors.

PEAK WEEK CARDIO MANIPULATIONS

I like to keep cardio reasonably consistent up until the Thursday before the show. I use the Stairmaster as my cardio equipment of choice, and I'll typically train in 20-minute sessions. Depending on how aggressive I am with my cardio during the latter half of my prep, I may not even incorporate it during peak week. Still, I find that the average mindset of a competitor in the final week of prep tends to gravitate toward the extremes, so it's not likely that you'll want to skip out on all cardio entirely. The more demanding objective will be to ensure you don't overdo it and kill yourself on the cardio.

A good rule of thumb is to cap yourself at that 20-minute mark; there's no need to exceed 30 minutes of cardio per day. Again, I recommend sticking with the Stairmaster or some other stable form of cardio. To minimize any unnecessary water retention brought on by acute training inflammation, I recommend skipping the intense cardio on the Friday before the show. A casual walk should be all that is necessary—no need to kill yourself on the Stairmaster 24 hours before stepping onstage.

While I don't classify my casual walks as intended cardio sessions, I think they play an integral role in the prep and can afford some much-needed reflection time during peak week. I highly encourage you to set aside some time every day during peak week to simply walk for a mile or two. No defined step count goal, no set pace and no specific calorie burn goal—just simple walking. These walks accomplish a few things. First, they allow better blood flow and help regulate blood sugar levels. They also contribute to NEAT activity and will get you outside and into some fresh air.

Most importantly, they give you some time to be alone with your thoughts and reflective toward this entire journey. Don't squander this opportunity by listening to loud music or a podcast. Simply be in the moment alone with your thoughts, introspective and acutely aware of your surroundings. My walks during peak week have always been some of my most transformative during prep.

I gain a clearer perspective of my surroundings, and I appreciate the blessings I have in life. I become increasingly aware of who I am and who I want to become. I gain a deeper appreciation for the people in my life who have supported me, and I make it a point to acknowledge their support. These walks act as a time of meditation and reflection. You can float through them as if on a cloud. Leverage this opportunity more for the mental and cognitive benefits than the physical ones.

I suggest going on these brief walks either immediately before your largest meal or shortly after. I prefer to walk before my meal as a way to escape the constant thought of food and consumption. I'd force myself to focus my attention on life outside of the dinner plate and the macros I was about to ingest.

Focusing on something that you inherently know is more important than the food itself has a great way of sustaining you through periods of minimal food intake. When you allow your mind to highlight areas of your being that are more important than the food itself, the thought of food doesn't take hold of you and become overpowering.

If you go on a walk after consuming your meal, you'll benefit from the stabilized blood sugar and absorption that moving your body post-consumption provides. Since you will have just eaten, you'll likely not be fixated on food during your walk. Instead, you'll be able to turn your thoughts toward gratitude and appreciation.

You'll be able to take stock of your day and what you did well or need to improve upon. You'll be able to prepare for the next day and everything that it holds. You'll be able to embrace peak week and be grateful for the opportunity it presents. In either scenario, I encourage you to be present. Don't walk for the physical benefit. Walk because your mind and emotional state will benefit from it immensely!

PEAK WEEK POSING

With the decrease in training intensity throughout your peak week protocol, you should have more time for posing practice, so take advantage of it! Every manipulation we make will be subtle, but it will have a noticeable impact on your physique daily. Macro tweaks, training intensity, electrolytes, travel to the competition venue and sleep quality all have a tangible impact on how you look.

Generally speaking, these subtle changes aren't that noticeable in day-to-day life. Such is not the case during peak week. Your body is running in real-time at this stage in the game. There is no built-up fuel reserve and there is no safety buffer. What you manipulate has a direct, corresponding effect on how you look, and it's increasingly noticeable. As such, make it a point to take notice!

Practice posing every single day throughout peak week. I like to hit a few poses immediately upon waking first thing in the morning after using the restroom and weighing in. This allows me to get a feel for how my meal the night prior impacted my morning composition. Do I look dry and grainy, or do I look watery and puffy? These are all questions that can be answered with a simple mirror check first thing in the morning. Based on your body's feedback, you can adjust things that day to deliver feedback that you can observe the following morning.

The bulk of my posing is done after training. Since training intensity is reduced, I fill the leftover time with posing practice. Posing post-training has a few advantages. First, you'll have forced plenty of blood into your muscles and will have a great pump, which will mimic what you'll likely look like onstage.

The other advantage of practicing your poses post-training is that you will likely be slightly fatigued.

It's hard work hitting all your mandatory poses in front of a panel of judges! The more you can pre-exhaust your body before running through your routine, the more you'll be able to prepare for what lies ahead on competition day. People who have never competed have difficulty understanding the physical demand of flexing every single muscle in your body with maximum control and fluidity for multiple minutes onstage. Rest assured that it will kick your butt, so the more you can prepare for it, the better! Judges can instantly tell the competitors who put in the work and practiced their posing religiously from those who neglected that aspect of the competition prep. If you are onstage shaking like a leaf, completely exhausted, it's likely that you won't place well.

I've seen multiple competitors who were absolutely shredded with flawless conditioning and perfect symmetry throw it all away in the final hour by not delivering on their posing. Don't be that person! Put in the reps with the posing practice just as you do with nutrition and training.

I recommend practicing posing every single day of peak week, preferably post-workout. Have a second set of eyes on you if possible. Ideally, you'll have a partner, coach, training buddy or friend who can offer unbiased feedback about how you're looking and what can be improved.

Since you won't have a mirror onstage, practice posing without one as well. Try and record your poses with a camera and watch the playback afterward. This is often much more insightful than any feedback you might get from the mirror alone. It's easy to hit perfect poses that highlight our best body parts when looking in a mirror; practice revealing those same strong points without one so that you can replicate it to the judges on show day! I'll go into the actual poses later in the appendix, but suffice it to say that your body and mental resilience will all benefit from you hitting the poses every day throughout this week.

I also recommend hitting a few poses right before going to bed. This affords you a clear representation of how your body has soaked up various inputs throughout the day (your electrolyte intake and final meal, in particular). Are you looking tight or bloated? Have the calories from your last meal absorbed into your system and are you seeing a freakish level of vascularity in your extremities? A simple mirror check at night before going to bed doesn't take more than a few minutes and can provide you with a ton of feedback. Compare how you look at night with how you look first thing in the morning and adjust throughout the day as needed.

PEAK WEEK STRESS

Stress ramps up our production of the cortisol hormone which can increase our level of extracellular fluid retention. Clearly, you don't want that to happen during peak week. Anything you can do to decrease your level of stress is worth your while here. This is the underlying reason why we have scaled back our training intensity: decreasing physical stress and acute inflammation and removing excess fluid retention. Mitigating stress goes beyond our training manipulations alone. We need to ensure that we aren't mentally and emotionally stressed throughout this week as well.

Peak week is the pinnacle of what you've worked so hard on for the past several months. So much is riding on it. Our minds automatically go toward that realization and emphasize the event's outcome, and we are led to stress about it. This does more harm than good. Eustress is a moderate or normal psychological stress generally thought of as being advantageous as it heightens our senses. Eustress toward competition day is a good thing. It keeps us on our toes and brings us excitement. Something is wrong with you if you're able to float through this week with no excitement and no anxiety. How can we toe the line between positive eustress and negative, overreactive stress throughout this week?

Shifting your focus toward mindset and being present is key at this stage. We've talked a lot about mindset throughout this book, but it truly goes beyond the psychological and has physiological implications. If you're incredibly stressed throughout peak week, you'll retain a ton of excess fluid and you won't look your best onstage.

If you harness the power of your mind and adopt a healthier relationship with your thoughts, your likelihood of minimizing stressors and peaking on show day becomes exponentially more likely. As such, let's dive into some of the practical techniques you can use to mitigate unnecessary stress throughout this week.

The casual walks I mentioned earlier can and should be leveraged as a method to mitigate stress. Use that time to be present and meditate on what you are going through and why, to visualize the entire week in advance. Visualize traveling to the venue, your circuit training, your preparation and the refeed meal. Visualize waking up the day of the show, going to the competitor meeting and learning about the federation, promoters and your fellow competitors.

Visualize being backstage, stepping onstage and running through your mandatory poses and routine. Visualize the celebratory meal afterward. Do it all in great detail and play everything through over and over in your mind. The more you run through it in practice, the fewer surprises you will face in actuality. That kind of visualization is one of the most empowering things you can do. This simple action will reduce your stress levels exponentially and put you in a stabler frame of mind for the real thing.

Visualization goes hand in hand with meditation. Some people benefit tremendously from daily meditation and mindfulness. For me, this mindfulness took the form of my visualization practice; however, if you currently incorporate a form of daily meditation, I highly encourage you to double down on that practice throughout this week. It's easy to let your mind wander into fear of the unknown during peak week. Work to maintain control of your thoughts throughout this week.

Prioritize quality sleep! Proper rest and recovery do wonders for both your body and mind, both of which are paramount during peak week. I'll often wake up several pounds heavier following a morning of poor sleep. This is a clear indicator of stress and inflammation, and you should do everything in your power to minimize the risk of a poor night's sleep. We all inherently know that sleep is crucial, yet so many of us fail to prioritize it. Having proper sleep hygiene is simple; it just takes discipline. The following is a list of techniques I incorporate into my nightly routine to optimize my sleep quality. Feel free to experiment with these and add to it if you find something else that works well for you.

Stop eating at least two hours before going to bed.

I'll often fall asleep faster if I eat a large meal immediately before going to bed, but the quality of my sleep is significantly diminished if I do. I've made it a point to finish my meals at least two hours before bedtime, and that has done wonders for allowing me to get deeper sleep and more REM cycles throughout the night.

Turn the thermostat down to 65 degrees or lower an hour or so before going to bed.

This allows my body to acclimate to the colder temps before crawling into bed and sets the stage for a better night's sleep. Thermoregulation is one of the single most significant things you can do to optimize your sleep quality.

Use mouth taping to improve deep sleep.

This one may sound a bit strange, but it works. As you sleep, it's common for your mouth to open slightly. In doing so, your tongue is likely to move and partially block your airway. As such, you'll start snoring or subconsciously shifting to resume better air control. This is similar to a mild form of sleep apnea. By simply taping your mouth shut, your tongue will stay stationary, and you'll be forced to breathe through your nose. As a result, you'll likely fall into a deeper sleep faster and stay there longer. After doing this every night for over a year now, my sleep quality has drastically improved. I use micropore tape to avoid any irritation to the skin.

Avoid screens and stimulants.
Common sense tells us to avoid stimulants such as caffeine before going to bed, but digital stimulation such as movies, TV and staring at your phone screen in bed should also be avoided. If you absolutely must look at a screen, I suggest doing so through the lens of a pair of blue-light blocking glasses. One thing I've found to be incredibly valuable is replacing the screen with a novel before bed. A simple 20 minutes of reading something fictional and stress-free can help you relax at the end of your day and prime your body and mind for sleep.

Sleep aids and supplements.
I don't use any sleep aids or supplements. I've played around with various CBD products and melatonin supplements, but I honestly can't tell a difference with them. Some people swear by their efficacy and if that is the case for you, by all means, keep using them. I've gotten the most benefit from simply following the steps above and doing so in a consistent manner to help prime my body and mind for optimizing my sleep.

TRAVEL STRESS

Sitting in a vehicle all day long can cause significant water retention, specifically in your lower limbs. The change in pressure from walking on the ground to flying in a plane can bring on massive fluctuations in fluid retention. The options for quality food are significantly diminished at gas stations and airport terminals. It's easy to skip your water intake while traveling (which will, in turn, skew your electrolyte equilibrium). You'll be away from your regular gym setting, and most hotel gyms are minimally equipped. Sleeping outside of your home setting often results in a subpar night's rest.

In short, there are a ton of variables associated with traveling any significant distance, and I have seen the stress of simply traveling to a venue ruin the look of many a competitor. Working around these factors and stressors and optimizing through them to protect your peak week is a challenge, but it can be done.

If you are lucky enough to live near the venue that will be hosting your show, you will likely be able to bypass many of these issues; however, that is not often the case. Competitors traveling in will be forced to adapt and be flexible.

Competitions usually happen on a Saturday, and competitor weigh-ins often occur the Friday evening before. I've found it to be significantly more convenient to get into town a few days before weigh-in to allow my body time to acclimate to changes and flush out excess fluid brought on by travel. Many competitions are hosted at casinos or conference centers that offer hotel stays. When given the option, I always recommend staying at the host hotel. Though it may be a bit more expensive, it generally reduces stress significantly. The tanning, hair and makeup and competitor check-ins are often available at the host hotel, reducing your transit time and streamlining the entire process. In a perfect world, that host hotel will also have a decently equipped gym or one nearby so you can do some simple circuit training.

Speaking of training, it's always a good idea to time your light, peak week circuit training sessions in a way that flushes out excess fluids from travel. I like to arrive at the host hotel on a Tuesday or Wednesday before a show, and one of the first things I do after unpacking my bags is head to the gym for light circuit work.

As far as food is concerned, you're best off preparing it all in advance and bringing it with you—though this can also pose a challenge, especially when flying to your destination. I've been known to pack a massive Yeti cooler backpack with a five-day supply of food and struggle through TSA by explaining what I'm trying to do. That can be a headache for sure, but it's worth it to provide you peace of mind. I also encourage competitors to call ahead to verify that their hotel room has a refrigerator and microwave. Nothing is worse than having several days' worth of food packed and ready to go only to discover that there is no way to keep it cold and fresh at the hotel.

Many people have a hard time sleeping at hotels because there are more lights and more noise. Whenever I'm staying at a hotel, I follow the tips above and I also go out of my way to unplug every device that has an indicator light. If I can't unplug them, I throw a shirt over them to block out illuminated buttons and displays. I'll also put in earplugs before drifting off to sleep. The last thing I want is to be jolted awake by some person's three-year-old running down the hotel hallway at 1 am!

When traveling during peak week, the best thing you can do is be as proactive as possible. Pack more than you need and leave nothing to chance. Get there early and budget enough time to move through the process with intention and minimal stress. Control everything you can and take the travel portion of this journey seriously. Give your body time to acclimate at least 48 hours before stepping onstage whenever possible.

FEAR OF THE UNKNOWN DURING PEAK WEEK

Throughout peak week, you'll be analyzing your body constantly and hypersensitive to how you look, feel and perform. This transcends the physical realm and gets into your mentality as well. At this stage, it's easy to start questioning your abilities. Imposter syndrome throughout peak week is a constant threat, and it can easily gnaw at you in the back of your mind. Don't let it!

Fear of the unknown is your biggest challenge throughout your first peak week. We gain confidence and clarity in life through perspective and experiences, and whether this is your first competition or simply your first ketogenic competition, rest assured that you will be all the better for going through it, no matter what happens. You've gained another layer of perspective that will help add to your confidence and self-awareness. Don't let the fear of the unknown loom over you and add extra stress to your body and mind. Breathe in and brace yourself for a new experience. You've done everything right.

PUTTING IT ALL TOGETHER

Because we've covered so much ground in this chapter, for the sake of clarity, I'm putting all these tips in a visually appealing format that is easy to follow. The more simplified this operation, the less likely we are to miss something and make a stupid mistake. After all, we are operating on minimal calories at this point, so the more we can reduce decision fatigue, the better!

What follows is a play-by-play of what a typical peak week protocol could look like. There may be a few changes depending on when you leave for the show venue, what your personal macro and electrolyte manipulations consist of and whether you've opted for a single-day refeed or a two-day refeed protocol, but this is a good place to get started:

Monday:

Nutrition: Consume the standard meal and macros you would have as a target intake via the competition prep protocol.

Water: Consume the regular water intake you have throughout this prep. Make sure you are well hydrated.

Electrolytes: Consume the regular electrolyte intake you have throughout this prep, likely somewhere within that 2:1 to 2.5:1 ratio of sodium to potassium.

Training: Frontload the majority of your heavy lifts into the early part of this peak week, with some of them done at the end of the week prior. Monday could be the final heavy leg day in your rotation, as an example.

Cardio: Final push for intense cardio is early on in this week. You should be incredibly lean at this point and only using cardio as a way to coast into the desired conditioning during peak week. You should be able to maintain the cardio intake you've been doing up to this point. A standard example would be 20 minutes of steady-state cardio on the Stairmaster.

Posing: Run through all poses post-training and practice without using the mirror. Make sure your routine and T-walk are flawless.

Other: Go for a casual walk in the evenings to get in more movement and blood flow and to prepare yourself for what lies ahead.

Tuesday:

Nutrition: Consume the standard meal and macros you would have as a target intake via the competition prep protocol.

Water: Consume the regular water intake you have throughout this prep. Make sure you are well hydrated.

Electrolytes: Consume the regular electrolyte intake you have throughout this prep, likely somewhere within that 2:1 to 2.5:1 ratio of sodium to potassium.

Training: This will likely be your last heavy training day. I recommend a heavy back day or something similar. You could also ease into the circuit at this point and start rotating between different body parts, lifting at about 70-80% of the intensity you usually do.

Cardio: You should be able to maintain the cardio intake you've been doing up to this point. Again, this likely consists of 20 minutes of steady-state cardio on the Stairmaster or something similar.

Posing: Run through all poses post-training and practice without using the mirror, again emphasizing your routine and T-walk.

Other: Go for a casual walk in the evenings to get in more movement and blood flow, as well as prepare yourself for what lies ahead. Gather all your necessary travel items, food and supplements and pack them before departure.

Wednesday:

Nutrition: Consume the standard meal and macros you would have as a target intake via the competition prep protocol.

Water: Consume the regular water intake you have throughout this prep. Make sure you are well hydrated.

Electrolytes: Consume the regular electrolyte intake you have throughout this prep, likely somewhere within that 2:1 to 2.5:1 ratio of sodium to potassium.

Training: Implement an upper-body circuit at this point, though you can throw in an exercise or two for the lower body. Still, you should be getting plenty of leg stimulation from the cardio, especially if you are using a Stairmaster or any form of incline movement. Cycle through all your different body parts and focus on getting a great pump and pushing blood flow. Lift at about 50-60% of the intensity you usually do.

Cardio: You should be able to maintain the cardio intake you've been doing up to this point. Again, this likely consists of 20 minutes of steady-state cardio on the Stairmaster. If you look spot on, you can start scaling back the cardio a bit at this point; if you usually do 20 minutes, do 15 instead.

Posing: Run through all poses post-training and practice without using the mirror. Make sure your routine and T-walk are flawless.

Other: Go for a casual walk in the evenings to get in more movement and blood flow, as well as prepare yourself for what lies ahead. If you want to get settled in early, I recommend arriving at your host hotel or venue on Wednesday. Get settled in at your new location, go for a walk and try and time your training and cardio to happen after you arrive (if you arrive early enough in the day).

Thursday:

Nutrition: If you're implementing a two-day refeed, factor that into Thursday's nutrition. If not, follow the standard meal and macros you would have as a target intake via the competition prep protocol. If you are consuming any veggies, I would remove them at this point. You may sacrifice some volume in doing so, but this will ensure that you don't hold any extra water in your intestines that can cause bloat onstage.

Water: Consume the regular water intake you have throughout prep. Definitely don't try and do any crazy water cutting or loading!

Electrolytes: Consume the regular electrolyte intake you have throughout this prep, likely somewhere within that 2:1 to 2.5:1 ratio of sodium to potassium. (This may be tweaked slightly if you are doing the two-day refeed, but it probably won't change much on this day.)

Training: Run through your full-body circuit. Depending on your location, whether you are at a typical gym or working out of a hotel room, you may have minimal equipment. Try and stimulate every muscle group and get a good pump. Target about 30-40% of the intensity you usually do.

Cardio: You'll be decreasing or removing cardio at this point. A simple 10-minute session on the Stairmaster is all that's needed here.

Posing: Run through all poses post-training and practice without using the mirror, making sure your routine and T-walk are flawless.

Other: I recommend being at the host hotel or venue no later than this point in the week. This helps your body acclimate to a new environment and flushes out any water retention from traveling.

Friday:

Nutrition: Implement the refeed strategy outlined earlier in this chapter. Backload the majority of your calories for later in the day. Feel free to have your fatty coffee or a light meal in the earlier hours—something minimal that won't sit heavy on your stomach. I usually have good luck with a simple fatty coffee, hard-boiled eggs and a few slices of bacon. Most of the macros will come from the refeed meal that I recommend consuming a few hours before bed. I've had tremendous success with the keto fathead pizza recipe, but hopefully you know exactly what your body needs at this point. I don't recommend consuming any fibrous veggies at this point—you don't want to risk fluid retention or bloat.

Water: Consume the regular water intake you have throughout this prep. Make sure you are well hydrated, and don't try any crazy water cutting or loading! The extra sodium in the refeed meal may bump up your thirst slightly. Feel free to quench that thirst, but again, don't try to water load.

Electrolytes: Increase your electrolyte intake based on what amount has proven well for your refeeds throughout Phase Four. Generally, this is somewhere between a 1,000-2,000 mg increase in sodium above baseline. Increase potassium slightly to follow suit. If you're implementing the fathead pizza as a refeed, I highly recommend topping that pizza with a can of anchovies to help hit the sodium target.

Training: Run through your full-body circuit. Depending on your location, whether you are at a typical gym or working out of a hotel room, you may have minimal equipment. Try and stimulate every muscle group and get a good pump. Target about 20-30% of the intensity you usually do. Most of your pump will likely come from the posing practice after training.

Cardio: You'll be decreasing or removing the cardio at this point. A simple five- to 10-minute session on the Stairmaster at low intensity is all that's needed.

Posing: Run through all poses post-training and practice without using the mirror. Make sure your routine and T-walk are flawless.

Other: Go for a brief, casual walk after your final refeed meal for better circulation and distribution of the nutrients you just consumed. Focus on relaxing, being present in the moment and being with the people surrounding you. I recommend you journal this experience and document the process. I highly encourage filming yourself talking about your expectations and the journey up to this point on the Friday before stepping onstage. Regardless of your placing, you'll have that video clip to look back on and appreciate. Set yourself up for success with a great night's sleep.

Saturday:

Saturday is show day, the moment we've all been waiting for. As such, it gets its own entire breakdown. Continue reading for a detailed breakdown of how to optimize for show day!

* * *

SHOW DAY

MORNING OF THE SHOW

If you're anything like me, it will be hard to sleep in because you'll be too excited. The day is finally here! The moment you have dedicated the last several months of your life to has arrived! Time to rise and conquer!

I recommend waking early and being incredibly deliberate in everything you do on show day because the last thing you want is to be rushed or reactive. Most competitions will have a morning competitor meeting to go over rules and regulations and introduce the show sponsors and organizers. This varies from show to show but usually happens somewhere between 8 and 10 am. The show itself starts shortly after that morning meeting.

To be in the right headspace for the day, I like to wake up around 3 or 4 am and meditate or read for 30 minutes or so before doing anything else. I'll drink a cup of coffee while I journal or vlog the feelings I'm experiencing. I do that because reviewing those materials *after* show day has been incredibly transformative for me and many other competitors.

You are okay to have a fatty coffee made with heavy cream, butter and MCT oil if you like—some initial fat in the morning will help get the digestion moving and give you some energy to start the day. Before drinking anything though, I do a preliminary mirror check to see how the previous night's refeed affected my morning composition. Ideally, the extra calories and sodium will have been soaked up and absorbed, filling us out and leaving our skin paper-thin. Hopefully, you're not holding onto any excess fluid in your ankles and wrists, and your vascularity is on a whole new level!

The increased sodium the night before has a way of ramping up your thirst, so feel free to quench it with a glass of water, but avoid trying to chug water at any point on show day. We want to stay hydrated, but we don't want to drink so much that it sloshes around in our stomach or "spills over" into our subcutaneous layer of skin.

Spend the first few hours of the early morning preparing your mind and body for what is to come. Do so in the comfort of your hotel room, away from the distractions of other competitors and people. This is your time to focus and visualize the coming day's events. Make the most of it and remove any possible distractions.

SHOW DAY NUTRITION

Today's nutrition is a bit different than any other day. We don't have a set of target macros we have to hit. Instead, you'll want to observe how you look throughout the day and adjust your intake as needed to optimize for when you step onstage.

Every show is a bit different, and it's often a mystery as to when your specific class and division will step onstage. Some shows have a morning pre-judging show and a "finals" show at night that showcases your posing routine and hands out awards. For the sake of illustration, we'll assume your pre-judging round starts in the morning and has you onstage at 11 am. We'll assume the night show begins at 4 pm and has you onstage at 5 pm.

Assuming that, I recommend getting a light meal in during the morning hours. If you have your fatty coffee soon after waking, you should be able to have ample time to eat an hour or two later (at approximately 6 am, for example). Avoid anything that will sit heavily on your stomach or cause digestive issues. I tend to gravitate toward something simple, like hard-boiled eggs and a few pieces of bacon. This will provide fat and protein and shouldn't create bloat. Sprinkle a bit of salt on your eggs for some sodium as well.

Up to this point, everything you consumed during competition prep has comprised larger quantities and fewer meals. By keeping calories condensed and having less time between feeding sessions, you've improved your fasting windows and regulated your blood sugar more effectively. On the day of the show however, you want to avoid any large boluses of food.

Instead, small feeding sessions spaced every 1.5 or 2 hours are optimal. This gives you the flexibility to adjust on the fly, which is helpful since your scheduled onstage time will likely change. It also ensures that you have a steady flow of dietary fat for energy and a small dose of protein and sodium to continue filling you out and keeping your electrolyte balance in check.

After the first meal, I recommend eating something small every hour or two until you step onstage. In traditional bodybuilding nutritional protocols, this tends to be a rice cake with either peanut butter and jelly or honey. Typically, this rice cake dessert provides sugar and fat and helps fill out the competitors without causing any bloat. Since we follow a ketogenic prep protocol, we will skip the rice cake and opt for something that gives us a fat, protein and a bit of sodium. Enter the Keto Brick!

This is the exact reason I formulated the Keto Brick back in 2017. I needed something that was calorically dense and didn't cause any bloating or discomfort. It provides a hefty dose of dietary fat and a moderate supply of easily absorbed protein. It also contains quite a bit of sodium to help ensure a proper electrolyte equilibrium on show day. I wouldn't recommend an entire Keto Brick every few hours; instead, break it up into quarters and have a small portion every one to two hours before going onstage. If you aren't using Keto Bricks, you could also eat something like a spoonful or two of nut butter to satisfy that need for dietary fat and some protein.

If your show is organized and everything is running smoothly, you'll likely have coordinators backstage helping with the timing. There will typically be a group of competitors onstage, a group of competitors "next up" and a group of competitors pumping up. Try and time things so that you consume your last bit of Keto Brick or fat source about 30-45 minutes before starting your pump-up circuit. That should give your body ample time to absorb the nutrients that will hone your optimal onstage look.

It is essential to stay hydrated throughout this entire process, so there's no need to water load or cut water. Drink normally, meaning quench your thirst and have water as needed throughout the day of the show without going overboard. You'll be consuming a steady stream of sodium in whatever food source you opt for backstage, so hydration is crucial to maintain your electrolyte equilibrium. If everything is properly balanced, your body will take those extra fluids and suck them into the actual muscle tissue instead of spilling them into your subcutaneous layer of skin. As such, your muscles will look fuller and your skin will appear thinner, which will showcase even more vascularity.

In addition to water, make sure you're getting enough sodium and potassium. I'm a big fan of the liquid nano-sized potassium on show day simply because it won't likely result in any GI discomfort or bloat —because you definitely don't want disaster pants right before stepping onstage. Using the bathroom in your posing trunks and a slippery layer of tanning solution is a nightmare in and of itself!

The hourly or bi-hourly feeds should last through the prejudging show. Depending on show specifics, you may have an hour or several hours between prejudging and the night show. If you have more than three hours, I recommend getting some solid food in you. A small bowl of ground beef with an egg or two should be perfect—you don't need anything too big. Getting a dependable source of protein and fat in will help fill you out for the night show. Add a bit of sodium to this meal, too.

More generally, try to consume roughly the same, or slightly higher, amounts of sodium on show day as you typically do the week leading up to the show. For me, this is around 4,000-5,000 mg. As mentioned, to meet my intake goals, I fill an empty seasoning container with the salt for the day and sprinkle it on my meals every time I eat. If you begin to look a little puffy, scale back on the salt and water. If your body is soaking everything up and you look a little flat, bump your calories up slightly and add a tad more sodium and fluids. Everyone's body is different, and there's no one-size-fits-all plan for show day. You'll have to monitor your body and adjust as necessary.

If you have the time between the prejudging and the night show, take advantage of the small meal mentioned above. About two hours after that, go back to the small incremental intakes of the brick or other fat source every one to two hours. Continue this protocol until about 30-45 minutes before pumping up before the finals and awards and make sure you're staying on top of your hydration and electrolytes. I can't stress that point enough!

Follow this simple protocol regarding show day nutrition. You'll be able to optimize all variables with minimal risk of any adverse effects like "spilling over" or not filling out. Most of your nutritional manipulations will take place the day prior on the ketogenic caloric refeed. If you leveraged the time optimizing your refeed in Phase Four, you should know exactly how your body will respond to this week's refeed, macro ratios and sodium intake. The more variables you can remove, the better! You should go into the peak week with 99% certainty about how your body will respond to your refeed. That remaining 1% will fluctuate depending on the variables the show throws at you that you couldn't possibly plan for.

To control for as many variables as possible, bring all your meals, water, pre-measured salt and anything else you may need backstage with you. Don't depend on anything or anyone and keep your show day nutrition safe and straightforward. Only consume foods you know your body responds well to and keep everything convenient and pre-measured in single-serve containers.

Know your body enough to recognize when it can tolerate a bit more food and sodium and when it has had enough. If you're unsure, be conservative. It's better to look a tad flat but absolutely shredded than it is to be too aggressive in your eating and spillover because that will wash out all your definition and vascularity. This is much harder to do in the absence of carbs, but it's still possible with too much food, salt and water intake. Play it safe on show day and enjoy the process! You'll be able to celebrate with a big juicy steak after finals (but more on that later).

SHOW DAY ROUTINE AND TRAINING

There's no need to kill it in the gym the day of the show; all of that work has been done already. By this point, you likely have your first coat of tanning solution on (if you are doing a spray tan). You certainly don't want to risk messing that up by getting all sweaty. Any training you do today will be incredibly light, focused just on increasing blood flow. Posing onstage is an intense workout on its own, so don't pre-exhaust yourself before that. As far as activity goes, I recommend keeping it incredibly light and simple on the day of the show.

Upon waking, go to the bathroom and perform a simple mirror check. Your skin should be paper-thin, and you shouldn't be holding any fluid in your ankles. Hit and hold a few basic poses and see how quickly it takes blood to flush into your muscles. A few minutes of posing in the mirror should elicit a noticeable difference.

It's worthwhile to go for a leisurely morning walk. This isn't to get a last-minute cardio session in and burn any more fat. The morning walk simply helps get blood flowing in the legs and ensures that the nutrients flow into every muscle group. I like to do this walk alone, often before anybody else is awake. Use this time to meditate and be alone in your thoughts before the excitement and energy of the day ensue. Get some fresh air and be at peace with your thoughts before any distractions enter your mind.

Once you're at the venue, the only "training" will be a brief pump before hitting the stage and the actual time spent posing. Don't overthink the "pump-up" time. Most shows break up competitors into four groups: the group onstage, the group about to go on, the group pumping up and everybody else. Figure out where you are in the lineup and plan accordingly. Most shows have staff backstage who help coordinate these groups and give competitors plenty of notice about when they will step onstage.

Competitions often feel like organized chaos. The estimated time it takes for one division to get through their routines is often much longer or shorter than the time that was planned for. Expect this and plan for it. Nothing is set in stone on show day. You may be told that you have 30 minutes before stepping onstage and still have to wait for an hour and a half! Don't stress the small stuff—just take things in stride and enjoy your day!

The space allotted for competitors backstage varies significantly from venue to venue. I've competed at shows where the backstage area was no more than a big closet, with very few dumbbells or pieces of equipment for pumping up. I've also competed at venues where the space was limitless and the backstage equipment could have furnished an entire gym. To be ready for either case, I highly encourage you to bring your own set of resistance bands.

Keep your pump-up circuit simple, and don't try and go for any new PRs. The fat source should help fill you out and you should get a great pump pretty effortlessly, especially if you're incredibly lean and had a good refeed the previous day. I recommend a simple circuit with every exercise falling in a 10- to 15-rep range. This routine could look something like the following:

- 15 air squats
- 15 dumbbell or banded rows
- 15 pushups
- 15 bicep curls
- 15 tricep extensions
- 15 lateral raises
- 15 shoulder presses

Run through this giant set in a slow and controlled manner. Focus on contracting your muscles throughout the entire range of motion and then repeat the process. Run through 3 sets of that rotation in your allotted pump up time. That should give you some solid blood flow and get your vascularity showing.

When the coordinators move you from pump-up to "next up," you'll likely be stuck in a hallway or behind the stage's curtain. Personally, I don't like to lose my pump during this limbo period, so I fill it with some additional bodyweight exercises. I'll crank out a few more pushups or bodyweight isometric movements to ensure that my muscles stay stimulated until I step onstage. One of my favorite techniques is to simply hold myself in the downward position of the pushup exercise.

By isometrically holding myself in the eccentric or "negative" position, my chest, arms and even legs all get engaged. Doing this also brings my heart down to the level of the rest of my body, which makes its job of pumping blood even easier. By simply holding this negative pushup position, I'll get a massive blood rush and step onstage with a super solid pump.

POSING ONSTAGE

People that suggest bodybuilding isn't a physically demanding sport have clearly never experienced the work required to be an excellent bodybuilder. Most of the work is outside the arena, in the gyms and the kitchen, but don't think for a second that the time spent posing onstage is a walk in the park.

Simultaneously flexing every single muscle fiber in your entire body while hot stage lights beat down on you is no joke! Being sleep-deprived, stressed out and having at least four months of caloric deficit under your belt is an incredibly taxing feat of strength and willpower.

Posing requirements vary between different divisions. Men's physique, women's bikini and women's figure will typically have fewer mandatory poses. Most require a frontal shot, side pose and rear pose to showcase symmetry and proportions. These are typically structured in a way that involves a symmetry round, one pitting you against other competitors. You'll likely have to hold various poses for a minute or so each, so it's imperative to have adequate conditioning.

During your solo routine, you'll be able to cycle through different poses throughout the motion of your T-walk from one end of the stage to the other. Physique, bikini and figure won't require you to hit traditional, muscular flexes like a front double bicep pose; however, you'll want to showcase your entire physique in a way that looks effortless, so mind-muscle connection and complete conditioning are fundamental.

Classic physique and bodybuilding require many more mandatory poses to showcase individual body parts, shape and muscularity. Because there are many more poses to run through, these divisions typically require more time onstage spent flexing every fiber in your body. There will be a symmetry round to showcase your front, side and rear poses followed by a mandatory posing round to demonstrate the front double bicep pose, lat spread, side chest and other mandatory poses.

These divisions often allow for your own unique posing routine as well, in which you can showcase your preferred poses to a personalized song and routine. Depending on the size of the show, the classic physique and bodybuilding divisions often include a "posedown" before announcing placings and distributing the awards. This is simply a head-to-head battle with the other competitors in which house music is played and everyone poses at will.

This round is used to hype up the audience and allow for an unstructured "freestyle." It's also an excellent opportunity for competitors to stand next to one another and showcase their strengths. These posing sessions require strenuous effort, and the judges can easily distinguish between competitors who have put in the work and practiced their posing and those who haven't.

You want to maintain an aura of confidence and calm composure while running through your poses, and this is nearly impossible if you're out of breath and struggling through each pose. Anticipate this and step onstage with confidence and intention. Walk up with the same game face you have when walking to the bar for a set of squats. You know what needs to be done, and you are prepared for it. Give it all you've got and hold nothing back!

Note: For more detail, there is a dedicated section on posing later in the book.

SHOW DAY STRESS

Interestingly enough, I have less stress on show day than I do any other day of prep. How could that be? By show day, everything is done. The work is done and there are very few tweaks I can still do to substantially change the way I look.

I can't control the other competitors or how they look. I can't influence the judges and what they are looking for. And I've done everything possible to control the package I bring to the table. In knowing that, there simply is no need to stress. It's useless. Unnecessary stress will cause more adverse water retention and decrease your enjoyment of the entire day. That is pointless!

You've worked so hard for months on end for this day to happen. It's finally here! Don't throw it away by stressing about factors outside of your control. Breathe deep and be in the moment. Be incredibly present and soak in every single detail the day presents you with. If you are ahead of the day's events, give yourself time for every step and follow the protocol, there is no reason to stress.

Many competitors backstage will mill about, unsure what to do with all their nervous energy and excitement. They'll start pumping up too early. They'll work themselves into a frenzy. They'll eat too much food out of boredom, or they won't eat enough because they aren't paying attention. Don't fall into these traps!

To be aware and present, I spend my entire time backstage in a constant state of meditation. I find an empty corner away from everyone else and carve out a little "sanctuary" for myself. I prop my feet up on a chair and lay on the ground with a hoodie pulled over my eyes. By propping my feet up, I ensure that I don't retain any excess fluids in my lower extremities and the blood circulation to my head is improved.

It's often frigid backstage, so I bring along a heavy blanket and wrap myself up in it. I've even gone as far as to bring a small space heater with me to plug into the wall! It's vital to try and stay warm and improve blood flow on the day of the show, so I leave nothing to chance.

After carving out my little oasis, I put in earbuds and listen to a book on mindset or stoicism, or I put on a guided meditation. I visualize every single movement of my posing routine. I run through every mandatory pose in incredible detail in my mind before ever stepping onstage. I breathe deeply, and I relax.

I may stand out like a sore thumb when everyone else is hanging out and talking and I'm wrapped in a cocoon in the corner with my hood over my head, but that's okay. There is a time for camaraderie, but the moments before stepping onstage is not the time. Get in the zone and get your game face on. You are about to step into the arena. You are about to go to war. Prepare yourself accordingly.

SHOW DAY PLACINGS AND AWARDS

The night show or "finals" is when all placings are awarded. Most of the actual judging takes place during prejudging earlier in the day, but if the judges are undecided on a few competitors, they'll make their final decisions during the finals.

Many competitors start to relax their posing a bit at this point and don't take their time onstage quite as seriously. This is a huge mistake! Assume you're being judged until the very last moment you're awarded your placing and don't slack off. Maintain an aura of confidence and prestige at all times. You're constantly being observed, so act accordingly.

There will typically be another symmetry round comparing various competitors so the judges can finalize their decisions. There is also time the competitors can use to demonstrate their individual routines set to music. After the comparison rounds, personal posing routines and T-Walks, the award ceremony begins. If the show is small enough, everyone comes back onstage for a final run-through. If it is a larger show, only the competitors who place in the top 10 or top five may come back onstage for awards.

If there are multiple height and weight classes, there will be placings for each category and then an overall winner of the division. In the bodybuilding division, there are first-place winners of the lightweight, middleweight and heavyweight classes. Depending on how many competitors there are, sometimes there are even more classes.

Once first-place trophies have been awarded, the winner of each class battles it out for the overall title of that division. At this point, you're competing against the best of the best within their respective classes, and competition is fierce. This will often involve another symmetry round, mandatory round and posedown.

Before the awards are given, the judges will hand the announcer their final placing sheet tallying all the points. Generally, placings are recognized in reverse order; in other words, announcers will start with the lowest placing and work their way up. When it gets to the first and second awards, the announcer delays to build up suspense and excitement in the crowd. The top two contenders are often called to center stage. Rather than continuing the reverse order, at that point, the announcers will call out the first-place award.

There have been a few times I've stood center stage alongside another great competitor and the announcement seemed to drag on forever. Time stands still in those moments, and you hang on to every word that comes out of the announcer's mouth. Every day of prep will flash through your memory, and you'll pause to think if there was anything you could have done differently or better. If you've given it all you've got, you should be happy regardless of the placing; however, it is pretty damn cool when, after a tremendous pause, the announcer yells your name as the winner of the show and the overall title!

AFTER THE AWARDS

Once the stage lights dim, what do you do? It's typical for most competitors to celebrate with a hearty meal alongside their family and friends. I highly encourage you to do just that—but not yet. Don't rush offstage to the feast before you take a moment to soak in the silence of the venue after the chaos is done. Everybody is quick to rush out, but the food isn't going anywhere. Take your time.

One of my favorite moments of the entire prep is the few minutes I have by myself in an empty backstage pump-up room with the reality of the day still fresh on my mind. Breathe it in, and don't squander it. You've worked so incredibly hard for the last several months. You've sacrificed so much, and you've proven to yourself that you can do something you didn't think possible. Take a few minutes to relish that.

Walk through the pump-up room. Walk across the empty stage. Sit in the corner and meditate or pray for a moment or two. Your friends and family will understand you needing a moment or two for yourself. Take full advantage and burn the moment into your memory forever.

After that, breathe deep and smile. It's time to join your family and friends and indulge in a well-deserved meal! Most competitors don't hold back in the post-show celebratory dinner—no food is off-limits and quantity is of zero concern. Personally, I advise against this unrestricted approach to post-show meals. For the sake of perspective, I'll share my experience after my first competition back in 2012.

After the show, my family and I headed to Red Lobster to celebrate. I was following a bro-dieting approach back then and was in no way prepared to limit my carbohydrate intake. I decided to order two or three different entrees, three frozen lemonades and a couple of desserts for good measure. That may sound like a lot of food (and indeed, it was), but my leptin and ghrelin hormones were so screwed up that I had no issues whatsoever getting it all down. It certainly felt great in the moment, but I paid the price.

A few hours later, I found myself in incredible pain. I couldn't sleep, I couldn't puke, I couldn't crap, I couldn't do anything but curl up in pain on the floor of my hotel room. My body was so depleted from months of dieting that it refused to give up any of the food I consumed. That misery lasted all night long until it finally passed through my system the following day. I thought I was out of the woods, but the truth was my downward spiral had only just begun. When I returned home the next day, I decided to jump on the scale to see how my body had handled the meal. I was in utter disbelief when the scale said I was 20 lb heavier than my previous weigh-in.

I looked in the mirror, disgusted with myself and my lack of discipline. I didn't know it at the time, but I had suffered from a massive post-show rebound. My body spilled over and held on to all the extra water and fluids. My ankles were the size of my biceps and my abs were hidden behind a layer of blubber. I felt like I had taken the last several months of my life and thrown them out the window. It led to a vicious cycle of starving and binging and acted as a catalyst for my disordered eating, which lasted for many years.

I'm not suggesting that a haphazard, over-consumption post-show is guaranteed to result in a negative relationship with food that spirals out of control and results in an eating disorder; however, I can assure you that the story just shared is far more common than bodybuilders and figure competitors would like to admit.

I share it because I know what is possible if you forsake all the discipline you've put in throughout prep. It can screw with your mind and emotions more than you realize. The competition itself shouldn't be viewed as the "finish line" because there is no finish line. Truth be told, the post-show journey is just as much (if not more) of a mental battle than prep itself! Don't step off stage thinking what lies ahead is trivial. It isn't.

The next two parts of this book will detail how to optimize your reverse diet after the competition. Give those two phases the same attention to detail and respect you gave the last five phases. You'll be a much better athlete for it!

To be clear, I don't mean to be all doom and gloom. Celebrate your victory with a well-deserved meal and time with your loved ones —just don't eat like an ass. Don't forsake all your nutritional wisdom and dietary lifestyle choices and consume foods you know will ruin your health. If you've found success by leveraging the ketogenic diet throughout this prep, don't throw it all away for a binge-fest on sugar-laden desserts. At the very least, I encourage you to keep it keto. Keep eating foods you know your body responds well to. Do this, and I guarantee you'll feel great, physically and emotionally.

I'm a huge fan of Brazilian steakhouses post-show. Something about all-you-can-eat meat sounds especially tantalizing after a bodybuilding competition. Your body should also respond incredibly well to a massive bolus in quality proteins and fats at that stage! You can enjoy various tastes and textures and keep it all entirely within the realms of a ketogenic diet. Skip the desserts and keep the skewers of lamb and ribeye coming as long as you like.

If you want something sweet to eat, I totally understand and respect that. After every show, I've enjoyed a massive keto brownie covered in melted Keto Brick and stevia-sweetened syrup, drizzled in dark chocolate. It's a great way to round out the evening, and I don't have to feel guilty about eating it. Since it's homemade, I know exactly what ingredients are in it, and I know how my body will respond. It doesn't create a massive spike in blood sugar, and I don't crash afterward as a result. I recommend preparing something similar for yourself after the show. Eat as much protein and quality dietary fat as you like; just skip the carbs. If you must have a dessert, let it be one you've prepared yourself and that's in line with a ketogenic lifestyle.

THE DAY AFTER

The day after the competition is typically a Sunday, and I recommend treating it as a recovery day. You'll likely be traveling back from the venue and might have a lengthy drive ahead of you. If you have access to a gym, feel free to go in and put all those calories from your celebratory meal to use. It's awesome to see how your body fills out during a training session after a massive bolus of food the day before. Of course, don't feel like you *have to* train.

I like to treat Sunday as a day of reflection and simply do whatever I want to do. If I want to train, I train. If I want to sleep a bit more, I do that. If I want to take my time driving home and stop at a hole-in-the-wall restaurant to indulge in the local community, I do that. I don't typically eat breakfast, but I do like to on the Sunday after a show. Like the celebratory meal, I recommend keeping it clean and keto.

Take the day to relax and reflect on the day before. What did you love about it? What would you do differently next time? What were your strengths and weaknesses? Where can you improve?

After competing, your body and mind tend to relax and let go of all the stress and anxiety they've been holding for the past several months. You'll likely feel exhausted and incredibly energized at the same time. Fill your day with the activities that work well with how you feel, and break out of your routine in a healthy way—whatever that means to you.

By granting yourself a day of relaxation, you set yourself up for success in what is to follow. There are still two more phases of this journey, and the reverse diet is about to commence. By allowing yourself a pause in accurate macro tracking, consistent training and ruthless discipline, you give your body the break it needs. Get more sleep than you ever have before and be in complete peace. When you wake up the next morning, it's time to get back to work.

PHASE FIVE MINDSET

> *It is not the critic who counts; not the man who points out how the strong man stumbles, or where the doer of deeds could have done them better. The credit belongs to the man who is actually in the arena, whose face is marred by dust and sweat and blood; who strives valiantly; who errs, who comes short again and again, because there is no effort without error and shortcoming; but who does actually strive to do the deeds; who knows great enthusiasms, the great devotions; who spends himself in a worthy cause; who at the best knows in the end the triumph of high achievement, and who at the worst, if he fails, at least fails while daring greatly, so that his place shall never be with those cold and timid souls who neither know victory nor defeat.*

—Theodore Roosevelt

Teddy Roosevelt's "man in the arena" speech sums up my thoughts toward peak week and show day quite eloquently. This is the height of the summit, ladies and gents. It's the moment you've been training for. All along the way, people have likely given you their thoughts and unsolicited opinions. You've heard positive feedback, negative feedback and everything in between.

If this is, in fact, your first show, you lack the perspective going into peak week to know what to expect and how to plan. As such, you're more likely to hold on to others' opinions. Don't. *You* are the man in the arena. *You* are the one who put in the work and made the sacrifices. Nobody can take that away from you.

The words of an armchair quarterback or keyboard warrior should hold no weight over you. Any doubt from your family, friends and community should only strengthen your resolve. Supportive feedback is welcomed, but even that shouldn't determine your actions. You did this. You put in the work. Put your blinders on and stay focused. Have the mindset of a warrior going into battle, be incredibly resolute and live with intention. Every action you take from the moment you get up to the moment you lie down should be intentional. You are on a mission, and you are unstoppable.

Truth be told, training throughout this week is significantly lighter than usual. If you know you've put in the work and haven't cut any corners, your stress should be down as well. You're not trying to burn any last-minute body fat at this stage in the prep, and you're certainly not trying to build any muscle, either. The point of this week is to get organized, focus, optimize your mindset and be totally and completely present in the moment.

If you've done everything you need to, you can relax a bit and breathe a sigh of relief. After your last hard training session is done, the strain on your body should be significantly reduced. Reduce the strain on your brain as well. Rather than pondering what could or should have been different, focus on what is and take delight in it.

During my last prep, I would finish each training session, hit some poses and then head to a local park. I walked throughout the wooded area and took time to observe every tiny detail—the color of the leaves, the playful nature of the squirrels, the distant laughter of children. I would sit and reflect on the last several months of my life, knowing that everything I had done has led to this moment. I would soak up the scenery and ponder the meaning and significance of what I was doing. I would burn a mental image of how I felt into my memory forever. I would take nothing for granted and I would appreciate everything in its entirety. I encourage you to do something similar.

This clarity of mind and stoic demeanor is what I refer to as my "stillness." For whatever reason, at the tail end of competition prep while totally depleted and exhausted, you can let your guard down and get in tune with stillness. I encourage you to take the time to do so.

That seems a bit contradictory, doesn't it? I promise, it isn't. Observe any genuinely great performer, world-renowned athlete, educator, speaker or entertainer. Moments before they step into the center stage, they seem like nothing could phase them, positively or negatively. They are tranquil and stoic.

They are confident in who they are and their ability to perform in what lies ahead. When you know you've done everything right and you've put in the work, there is no need to fill your mind with unnecessary stress and anxiety. It only distracts from your ability to perform at a high level. Remove that angst, breathe deeply, be present, find your stillness and enjoy your moment of glory!

[6]
PHASE SIX: REVERSE DIET REFEEDS

Now that the show is over, you get to gorge yourself and consume everything in sight, right? Not exactly. The implementation of a well-structured "reverse diet" is crucial, but it is often overlooked. You've just put your body and mind through incredible strain, so how could it make any sense to remove all that discipline and consistency instantly? It doesn't! So many people make the mistake of deviating so far from their routine that their body backfires and their mind spirals out of control. This is precisely what happened to me after my first competition prep, as I wrote earlier.

There is nothing more frustrating than dedicating months of your life to achieving mental and physical excellence and then throwing it away in an instant because you don't have a vision of where to go next. Instead, I want to paint a very clear picture for you during the reverse diet. I want you to avoid the mental and physical heartache I suffered from disordered eating, negative physical rebounds and psychological mayhem.

Bodybuilding and figure competition can and should be a healthy sport. Setting yourself up for success post-show is the best way to ensure that your body and mind benefit from its rigors. A healthy reverse dieting phase will make the entire process sustainable and enjoyable as opposed to toxic and debilitating. Give the next two phases of this journey the same attention to detail as the first five, and I guarantee you will come out of this better than you went in. Neglect them and I guarantee you'll be beating yourself up for it in a few weeks!

The reverse diet is all about resetting your calories, metabolism and hormones at a healthy, sustainable level. As the saying goes, what goes up must come down. The same is true in reverse as it pertains to your nutrition. Your caloric intake, body fat percentage, lean mass, metabolic rate and hormone function are likely all down-regulated as a result of prep. Our goal in the reverse diet is to ramp them back up to healthy levels that you can sustain and improve upon until you transition into another cutting phase at some point in the future.

It's unrealistic to expect that you will sustain your show day conditioning indefinitely. That is not healthy, and it is certainly not optimal. Continuing to eat at a significant deficit can damage your metabolism and hormone function, but it's also sub-optimal from a muscle-building perspective. If you're training hard to build more muscle, you need to provide your body with the necessary fuel and building blocks to do it. This is a nearly impossible endeavor if you're in a deep caloric deficit.

The reverse diet is the "yin" to competition prep's "yang." You simply can't optimize one without optimizing the other. Both are necessary for achieving your optimal self, physically and mentally. Give the reverse diet the attention it deserves, and you'll have many more long healthy years of enhanced human performance!

PHASE SIX OBJECTIVES

I've broken the reverse diet into two separate phases, Phase Six and Seven of this journey. Phase Six is all about the manipulations you will make immediately post-show. We will continue leveraging the ketogenic caloric refeeds we implemented in Phases Four and Five. We will titrate both dietary fat and protein upward to fuel your body and reset your hormones and metabolism at a healthy, sustainable baseline.

The goal of the reverse diet is simple: ramp up metabolism and end with a higher caloric intake than you started prep with but end with an improved body composition from what you had at the onset. If we accomplish this, you'll be in a much better starting position for the beginning of your next competition prep with more muscle, less body fat and have more calories to work with.

Truth be told, there isn't a "gold standard" for reverse dieting. As a concept, it is not nearly as understood or implemented as cutting and fat loss diets are. It's sexy to talk about how much weight you've lost and show off your abs—not nearly as sexy to talk about weight you gained.

Social media content and nutritional wisdom related to bodybuilding tend to highlight fat loss and gloss over or entirely ignore reverse dieting. This lack of appeal results in competitors often glossing over these phases as well.

A simple Google search on reverse dieting gives a vague definition: "The act of slowly increasing your food intake after a calorie-restricted diet to promote long-term weight maintenance." In other words, it is the act of resuming your regular eating habits after a cut without gaining all the weight back.

Though that's true, it doesn't give us much definite direction about how to properly implement a reverse diet.

Some coaches recommend going back to maintenance calories instantly; others recommend slowly increasing calories week after week until you return to maintenance. Finally, other coaches never mention the term reverse diet at all and simply wish you the best of luck after the competition!

There likely isn't a one-size-fits-all approach to reverse dieting. It's going to depend heavily on your personal preferences and lifestyle factors. How much body fat are you willing to gain post-show and how quickly? You will inevitably gain some body fat back in the reverse diet, so accept that; however, the rate you gain it back is going to depend on the individual. Some people are willing to gain more fat early because they place higher value on eating more food, having more energy and returning to normalcy sooner. Others prefer to keep things tighter for longer and willingly stay disciplined throughout the reverse. You'll have to ask yourself where you belong on that spectrum and adjust accordingly.

Throughout this section, my goal is to show what I believe to be the optimal strategy for reverse dieting as it relates to this specific nutritional protocol and contest prep. So far, we've done everything differently than traditional bodybuilding tends to. It only makes sense that we would do things a bit differently with the reverse diet as well.

WHY IS REVERSE DIETING NECESSARY IN THE FIRST PLACE?

Throughout our evolutionary past, there were times when food was incredibly scarce. As such, we have a built-in survival mechanism: the down-regulation of our metabolic rate.

As food becomes scarce, our body reduces NEAT activity, turns down our internal thermostat and avoids unnecessary energy expenditure. These adaptations allowed our species to survive with little food intake. When you think about it, these adaptations make intuitive sense; if you don't have energy coming in, it's only logical to reduce your energy going out. We do this consciously and subconsciously by reducing our physical activity and becoming less active, and this happens with all mammals.

Think of a bear that hibernates during the winter months. During that time, food is scarce and bears survive by going into deep rest. Hibernation is simply a state of minimal activity combined with metabolic depression. This is often characterized by low body temperature, slow breathing and heart rate and a lower metabolic rate. This explains why your NEAT activity has likely reduced throughout prep and also why you are probably much chillier throughout the day

Unlike a bear, you haven't slept through most of this prep (hopefully). Your activity has likely dipped subconsciously, but we've fought tooth and nail to keep training hard, increasing our cardio and staying active. This is contradictory to what you would find in nature in our evolutionary past, which is one reason why the sport of bodybuilding is so unnatural!

It makes no sense to intentionally up-regulate our activity, train harder and eat less from a survival standpoint. This is also why you likely didn't see too many jacked and shredded troglodytes walking around in the past. I would guess that cavemen were probably specimens of health compared to most people today who follow a Standard American Diet (SAD), but cavemen didn't look like the statues of Greek gods that we try to emulate.

Another survival mechanism is to put aside processes not required for our own survival and livelihood, such as sex and reproduction. As such, it's not uncommon to see a massive down-regulation of our sex hormones during extreme caloric deficits. Pregnancy and childbirth are incredibly taxing on the female body. It makes little sense to maintain the pathways for pregnancy and delivery in the wild if you don't have your own basic needs met. This is one reason why many female competitors often lose their menstrual cycle during the tail-end of a prep. Procreation isn't nearly as taxing for the guys, but still, sex is usually not a high priority if you're fighting for survival.

Healthy body fat, adequate caloric intake and sustainable levels of environmental stress are all necessary for optimal metabolic rate and healthy hormone levels. These all decrease throughout prep, so now we need to ramp them back up.

One of the main benefits of leveraging a ketogenic diet is that dietary fat intake stays relatively high. Since fat is a significant regulator of hormone function, our hormones are likely in a much better place than they would be had we followed a traditional protocol significantly lower in dietary fat; however, that doesn't mean our hormones are in an optimal range. Any protocol that substantially reduces your caloric intake will put stress on your body and can cause a downregulation of hormones and metabolism. This is true across the board, regardless of macronutrient distribution. As such, any competitor coming out of a competition prep will benefit from a period of reverse dieting.

HAVE A PLAN OR PLAN TO FAIL—THERE IS NO "FINISH LINE"

If you view competition day as the "finish line," you have set yourself up for failure. Instead, think of show day as the peak of a summit. There has been a steady and gradual climb to get up and there will be an equally important, gradual descent to return to base camp (or in this case, baseline). If you view competition day as a finish line, you are much more likely to cross it and collapse in exhaustion (in other words, throw caution to the wind and pay no mind to your dietary choices). This will most certainly result in a negative rebound where you gain 20-50 lb quite rapidly post-show. This is what we want to avoid.

Fast weight gain brings with it a host of negative physical and psychological implications that suck the fun right out of this sport. Mitigating that risk through a well-formulated reverse diet is critical. Head into the cut knowing that the competition day isn't the finish line, and you will be setting yourself up for success.

Leptin and ghrelin are the "hunger hormones." They play a major role in managing your hunger and satiety. Like many other hormones in your body, they are totally out of whack immediately post-show! Therefore, relying on your body and its natural signals for intuitive eating is a bad idea. This is true even if you don't suffer from any form of disordered eating. Your body is simply not stable enough to reliably give you information about how you should eat.

Many competitors have tried to "listen to their body" and eat intuitively post-show. The problem is one can "intuitively" eat 10,000 calories in a sitting coming out of competition prep, which is far removed from any degree of normalcy. Rather than lean on intuition, I suggest having a plan that eliminates uncertainty and controls for variables. Like prep itself, the reverse diet should be structured and sustainable.

I don't want you to feel like you're going right back into another prep with strict tracking and obsession over macros. That takes the fun right out of it! The simple truth is that we aren't stepping onstage to be judged again during the reverse. There is no need to "peak" and no need to be perfect. I like to loosen the reins a tad during the reverse and allow myself a bit more grace and flexibility.

As with the prep, sustainability is key. The reverse diet should be simple and straightforward. To that end, I like to implement weekly "date nights" throughout the reverse in which I can eat something totally outside of the standard plan. This gives me something to get excited about and lets me experience flavors and textures I haven't had for months. Again, this is not a free-for-all restaurant buffet. Estimate your intake as closely as possible and have a plan!

As far as training and cardio go, the reverse diet portion offers a period of increased opportunity. With an increase in calories and energy, you'll likely find yourself performing better in the gym! You'll be able to slowly scale back your cardio so it's much less demanding. You should see an increase in strength, power and overall excitement for pumping iron as well!

The latter half of prep is often characterized by decreased energy, a lack of satiety and a corresponding increase in anxiety. This is a recipe for piss-poor gym performance. Even if you maintained your heavy lifts and total volume, training likely became a burden that you started to resent. That anxiety should lift now. Many of my best workouts have been immediately post-show in the weeks and months when I felt on top of the world.

Another benefit is you'll still be incredibly lean and thus much lighter than your off-season weight. This, combined with the increased fuel intake, results in an impressive power-to-weight ratio that yields great strength markers. Combine that with the fact that your muscle pumps and vascularity will be amazing, and you have a recipe for pure savagery in the gym!

As mentioned, the primary objective of the reverse diet is to reset your body's baseline to a better place than where it began. Ideally, you'll be able to end at a lower baseline body fat percentage while consuming a higher caloric intake. Follow that with a successful period of building lean muscle, staying in a healthy caloric surplus and keeping a healthy body composition and you'll be able to transition into another competition prep in the future with a huge advantage!

You'll likely have more lean tissue, a higher functioning metabolic rate and increased calories to start with, so more caloric runway at the onset and less body fat to shave off. Done correctly, you'll be able to look significantly better every time you transition through another cutting phase and step onstage. It's what makes this sport healthy and sustainable. You'll get better and better year after year as opposed to worse and worse. Congratulations, you've just discovered the fountain of youth!

Unfortunately, many competitors fall victim to the trap of overcompeting, neglecting the reverse diet and not allowing themselves to be in a surplus. Think about it: if you compete multiple times a year every year, you are almost certain to spend most of each year in a caloric deficit. We budgeted four to six months to diet down for this show alone. On average, it probably takes another two to three to bring calories back up to a healthy level—then it takes several more months for hormones and metabolism to stabilize at that intake. None of that period primes your body for building lean tissue.

For optimal muscle building, you need to be in a healthy caloric surplus, train hard while implementing progressive overload principles and have a healthy hormonal baseline. That is nearly impossible while constantly cycling between deficits and reverse diet cycles. As such, many competitors start to become more and more catabolic, wasting away and looking worse and worse every time they compete.

This leads to frustration and the introduction of performance-enhancing drugs to mitigate the adverse effects of over-competing. It's a slippery slope that I've always tried to avoid.

Falling in love with the sport of bodybuilding is fantastic; I just caution against taking it to an unhealthy extreme. By implementing a healthy reverse diet followed by a period of surplus that prioritizes muscle gain, you can improve the likelihood of making this a genuinely healthy sport. Remember: you must have the "yin" and the "yang" to optimize for either!

PHASE SIX GUIDELINES

Implementing a sustainable reverse diet will vary from person to person, but these are a great foundation. During the reverse, I subscribe to the "have a plan or plan to fail" mentality, but recognize that you don't have to be perfect. Adopting a more relaxed attitude now will encourage you to be much more rigid during your next actual prep—and this can be as simple as averaging out your weekly calories rather than obsessing over them day by day.

Before stepping onstage, I recommend tracking everything on a 24-hour revolving basis rather than averaging it over a week because it ensures consistency and minimizes performance risk. Of course, that is far less of a concern after the show is over. Feel free to have a calorie window or an average weekly calorie goal and aim for it.

This strategy may differ by individual. Some people binge one day of the week and convince themselves it's okay to starve themselves the remaining days as long as they hit a weekly average. That is *not* good! Be self-aware and recognize if you're likely to fall into binging tendencies. If so, avoid a weekly average protocol. As with anything nutrition-related, figuring out what is most sustainable is half the battle.

RAISE PROTEIN

This reverse diet is divided into two separate phases. This phase will leverage the ketogenic caloric refeeds we implemented earlier to help transition into higher caloric intake. We want to be strategic, so I still highly encourage you to track your macronutrient intake. If the idea of continued tracking and caloric restriction depresses you, let me give you something to be excited about. We are going to be raising protein—a lot!

For whatever reason, I'm often labeled the "high fat, low protein" guy within the ketogenic community. Truth be told, I'm not an advocate for low protein in general. I consider myself a "high fat, optimal protein" guy. I recommend keeping protein strategically lower for a finite period during the cut, but I always follow it with a significant increase. Protein is essential, and I'm not saying otherwise.

Now that the show is over, I recommend increasing your dietary protein intake in grams to however many pounds you carry in lean mass. A simple 1:1 ratio here works quite well for most people. This will come with a slight increase in bloating and a dip in blood ketones, but that is all right. Immediately after the show, you will likely find yourself in a bit of a feeding frenzy, and it's better to fill that void with quality protein, rich in vitamins and minerals. This jump will also provide a corresponding bump in overall food volume, which helps a bit with satiety while hitting specific macronutrient targets.

My last month of a competition prep often puts my daily protein intake somewhere between 75 and 100 g of protein (granted, with weekly ketogenic refeeds, which provide a protein bump). That said, 75-100 g is pretty low for me, as my lean mass is somewhere between 140 and 150 lb. When I start my reverse diet, I bump my daily protein intake up to 140–150 g to put myself back in that 1:1 range. This ensures that I don't have any unnecessary catabolic effects and gives me something to look forward to.

REVERSE PROTEIN THRESHOLD

Phase Two of this prep journey was all about discovering our unique protein threshold. We will likely experience something similar as we continue to raise protein in the reverse diet portion. There is absolutely an upper limit in protein for optimal consumption. This limit is often more subjective than objective, so it's important to pay attention to feedback from your body and control for as many variables as possible.

Depending on how low you took your calories throughout prep, you may not find your actual protein threshold until the final phase of this journey (Phase Seven). However, since we will be increasing protein quite rapidly throughout this phase, you will likely experience many of the effects of operating near that threshold.

Like Phase Two, possible symptoms of reaching that threshold include:

- GI distress
- Increased blood glucose
- Decreased blood ketones
- Less quality sleep
- A decline in overall energy
- Bloating
- Water retention
- Decreased mental clarity and focus

Of course, experiencing just one of these symptoms may not be indicative of anything. In general, I recommend pushing the envelope and eating as much protein as possible during the reverse diet and building phase, within the context of what is enjoyable and sustainable. If you feel terrible consuming twice as much protein as dietary fat, then don't do it!

In working with clients over the years, I've found that most people tend to level out near a 1:1 ratio of dietary fat grams to protein grams. This is typically sustainable and flavorful, with a wide selection of food available. Still, that 1:1 ratio depends on a healthy caloric intake, maintenance weight and body fat percentage. Though there will likely be some tweaks, recognize that somewhere near that 1:1 is likely where we'll end up. In the meantime, continue tracking your macronutrients and pay attention to any relevant biomarkers or biofeedback you notice.

CONTINUATION OF REFEEDS

If I were to summarize the primary objective of Phase Six as it relates to refeeds, it would look something like this:

> Increase weekly calories while simultaneously decreasing refeed calories. When the caloric intake throughout the non-refeed day exceeds that of the refeed day, phase out the refeeds.

It's a bit of an oversimplification, but it's truly what we will be doing throughout this phase. Ketogenic refeeds started in Phase Four and provided a specific catalyst to fill out our muscles and peak for show day. They also offered a psychological break by giving us something exciting to look forward to during a steep deficit. The physiological benefit was making our average weekly calories higher, which in turn made lower daily calories more sustainable. Now that we're increasing daily calories throughout the reverse, refeed days will eventually become obsolete.

We don't want to do away with them all at once because we are still in a reasonably significant deficit, even with the big jump in dietary protein. They also still provide a crucial psychological benefit in giving us a day (or two if you're following the two-day refeed protocol) to eat a bit more and include some increased variety.

Your refeed macros were likely the highest during peak week itself. Throughout the reverse, we will be decreasing refeeds from the peak week level, chipping away at dietary fat and protein by 5 or 10 g a week. At the same time, our planned daily macros will be increasing by 5, 10 or even 15 g a week. Eventually, the daily macros will equal the refeed macros, and the planned refeed day will be absorbed into the standard day.

When we implemented refeeds before the show, we tested which specific sodium and macronutrient distribution yielded the best results for our body composition and conditioning. Since that is no longer necessary, I suggest using the reverse refeeds to do just the opposite. Depending on how strictly you've taken prep, you've likely gone without restaurant food for months since it's so hard to track. In doing so, you've sacrificed a smorgasbord of flavors, textures, experiences and social settings. I encourage you to make your weekly refeeds during the reverse an opportunity to bring some of that back into your life. Stay relatively close to your daily macros throughout the week, just grant yourself the grace to try something new and different on refeed days.

I love to make the reverse refeed days my planned date night of the week. My wife and I give up restaurants and food prepared by others during the prep, so our "date night meter" is often in the red by the time reverse kicks in. By letting myself go out to eat on my refeed days, I can get some quality time with my wife, experience new flavors and enjoy myself for a change. Structuring the reverse refeeds this way also forces you to appreciate the experience much more. I assure you, a gourmet burger and wedge salad never tastes as good as it does after spending four to six months in competition prep.

If you do go out to eat for the refeeds, recognize that you'll have much less control over exact macros and sodium in your food. I recommend keeping your food selections ketogenic; no sense in deviating from that. Simply try and get as close to your macros as you can. There will be some fluctuations with water retention and digestion since you're increasing your food variety, but this is an instance where mental and emotional benefits can outweigh physical ones.

Eating out and having less control over everything is certainly not physically optimal, *but that's okay!* Prep is over. Grant yourself that flexibility and embrace the relaxation from a mental and emotional perspective. If you're nailing your weekly macros, a slight deviation in accuracy during the reverse diet refeeds should be tolerated reasonably well.

Of course, if you prefer to continue preparing all your foods during the reverse diet, that is fine as well—you can't ever go wrong with meal preparation.

Whether you choose to enjoy your refeed day at a restaurant or prep the meal yourself, the main thing is to enjoy this phase. By relaxing a little, you'll shed some of the anxiety and rigidity you forced upon yourself earlier.

RATE OF INCREASE

The whole goal of the reverse diet is to increase your caloric intake back to a healthy, sustainable level. As mentioned, this means you can be pretty aggressive with your initial bump in protein—but what next?

After that initial protein increase, your ratio of fat to protein will likely be near 1:1, but your dietary calories will still be far too low. Thus, you want to steadily and gradually increase your fat and protein macros by 5, 10 or even 15 g a week.

After increasing protein grams to a 1:1 ratio to my lean mass in pounds, I like to bump my fat macros to a 2:1 ratio relative to protein. For every 5 g I increase dietary protein, I raise my dietary fat by 10 g. This is reasonably conservative and allows my fat ratio to increase as well. Throughout this reverse phase, my body is hungry for additional fuel. I can tolerate the extra fat calories very well and use them throughout my daily energy expenditure. This provides enough protein to recover from more intense training sessions and enough dietary fat for energy to keep going.

The above recommendation is my personal preference and one I respond well to. You may tweak your numbers and find that your body can tolerate a much faster or slower pace of caloric increase. It is all dependent on how your body responds to manipulations. For this reason, it's imperative to continue tracking your metrics and monitor your body composition.

Hopefully, you've been taking bi-weekly progress pictures throughout this entire prep, so that habit should be ingrained at this point. I recommend continuing that practice throughout the reverse. By doing so (along with body circumference measurements and body fat scans), you'll be able to track how your body responds to food increases. You should expect to see an increase in body fat and a gradual decrease in muscular definition and vascularity.

Don't get depressed when it happens; it's supposed to! However, it's important that it occurs at a slow and sensible rate. You don't want to go from 5% to 25% body fat in a month or two. The specifics will vary, but body weight increases between 0.5 and 1.5 lb a week are pretty standard. If your rate shoots up at any point, tap the brakes on the rate you increase your weekly macronutrient intake.

METABOLIC SET POINT

Remember: your maintenance intake at this stage of the journey has been down-regulated from what it was at the onset of prep. With that said, understand that you won't be able to simply jump back to your initial maintenance intake and expect your body to respond well. If your maintenance was 2,800 calories when you started prep and you immediately jump back up to 2,800 post-show, you will put on unnecessary body fat.

Some coaches recommend recalculating your maintenance intake based on your current body stats and jumping to that intake. That may sound appealing and is certainly better than the first option, but it leaves a lot of room for error. Metabolism is such a tricky thing, and no calculator will give you a truly accurate value for your current maintenance intake.

Your training intensity, NEAT activity and average cardiovascular frequency have likely shifted tremendously since the beginning of the prep, which are all variables that are in play. After the initial jump in protein, I recommend a gradual increase in weekly calories. By gradually increasing both dietary protein and dietary fat by 5-15 g per week, you can determine your best macronutrient ratio distribution without exceeding your actual maintenance intake prematurely.

Every person has a homeostatic set point for body fat and composition. It is the point at which the body feels most comfortable, and it tends to fight to stay there. If you have a healthy set point, you're likely able to maintain healthy body weight and fat percentage during the off-season and throughout your typical day-to-day in a relatively effortless manner. When you transition into competition prep, you must push your body outside its normal range and force it to adapt to various stimuli such as a reduction in calories and increased cardio.

Your body wants to return to that same homeostatic set point as quickly as possible since that's where it's most comfortable. However, by maintaining a different composition or stressing your body for long enough, it's possible to reset that homeostatic set point at a new or different tier. If you were to lose a significant amount of body fat and then immediately return to eating a ton of food, you would likely return to your original body fat levels or worse! If you stay more disciplined post-show and intentionally stay leaner for a bit longer, you increase the chances that your body will reset its set point at a slightly leaner composition.

This is the primary reason I advocate for slowly reversing out of a massive deficit. Doing so allows your body to stabilize at a leaner composition than you started, which improves your homeostatic set point for the next time you compete. There is one other factor that dictates how much fuel you can consume and how your body responds: your training.

REVERSE DIET TRAINING

One of two things are likely to happen during the first phase of the reverse diet related to your training. On one end of the spectrum, you could experience a massive surge in energy and intensity brought on by an increase in calories. Your increased protein intake should help your recovery, and the increase in calories should boost your energy, both of which will lead to noticeable improvements in the gym.

On the other end of the spectrum is a delayed dip in performance. Sometimes a "lag effect," so to speak, is brought on by the weeks of decreased caloric intake and mental strain later in prep. I've seen competitors so high-strung toward the end of prep who finally relaxed when the show was over and their bodies dumped all the anxiety and stress they had been carrying for so long. Inevitably, this results in a week or two of decreased gym performance. This lag is only temporary and shouldn't last long. Once your body has had ample recovery time, both mentally and physically, your performance should bounce back quickly.

While all of this directly impacts physical performance, much of it depends on your mentality going into and coming out of the show. If you are at peace with the outcome and feel invigorated, you'll likely experience the aforementioned surge in energy and performance. If you feel incredibly taxed, you'll likely experience a dip. Either way, have the self-awareness to capitalize on a style of training that is best suited to your needs.

If you feel invincible and on top of the world, train hard and heavy and experience all the fulfillment that brings. If you feel mentally and physically exhausted, grant yourself a "de-load" week to train at a slightly reduced intensity. Regardless of where you fall on that spectrum, realize that there isn't a right or wrong approach. Do what is best for you until your body, mind and emotions stabilize. At that point, you can begin to take a more standardized approach to your training and cardio.

In general, I don't recommend deviating too far from the prep training split and protocol you're used to. Keep your current split constant and see how increased caloric intake impacts your performance. You'll likely have more intensity and be able to lift more weight.

Toward the end of prep, our primary goal was to keep lifting the same weight and volume you had been lifting to that point. Now that you are eating more, I encourage you to push the envelope a bit and see if you can increase weight resistance and total volume. Go for the PR you've been holding off on for several weeks. Don't get foolish and risk injury, but do capitalize on the extra energy that comes with the reverse diet.

You should notice a tangible difference in your recovery time as well. As your protein intake increases, you'll have more amino acids circulating to help your muscle recovery and growth. This should also aid your ability to train with more intensity and at a greater frequency. Rather than walking into the gym tired and beaten down, you should notice an enhanced zeal for lifting and appreciate training again!

So, what about cardio? Remember the inverse relationship cardio had to calories throughout prep? As calories got lower, cardio increased. That principle is still true, but in reverse. As calories increase in the reverse diet, cardio can gradually taper down. I don't recommend cutting cardio completely post-show, since that can have negative effects for maintaining a healthy composition and managing your increased food intake. Instead, I would slowly strip away cardio by either scaling back the intensity, duration or frequency (or a weekly combination of all three).

We want to create a sustainable environment in the reverse diet. Nobody wants to spend all their time on cardio! If you followed a cardio regiment like the protocol I described, you likely used the Stairmaster throughout prep. Toward the end, you may have been doing 20-minute sessions at an intense level four or six times a week. Going into the reverse, start dialing back, slowly but surely, week after week. Begin with dropping one day of cardio the first week.

Then, drop two minutes off each cardio session the second week. Decrease the intensity by a level or two the third week. Cycle back through and drop another session the fourth week and keep going through that rotation.

Even after several weeks of reverse dieting, I don't recommend removing cardio entirely. I encourage you to have a healthy baseline of cardiovascular activity to protect your cardiovascular health. Zero cardio conditioning spills over into your weight training and prevents you from reaching the volume necessary for optimal strength and hypertrophic growth. The goal should be to reduce your cardio training to a sustainable and even enjoyable level. Prioritize weight training and set yourself up for success, with the primary goal of building as much lean muscle tissue as possible throughout the reverse and building phases.

PHASE SIX MINDSET

Truth be told, this is probably the most challenging phase of the entire prep. The show is over, and the protocol is much looser. Free of distraction and discipline and with a newfound freedom of choice, how will you behave? The human mind is fascinating in that it can become incredibly obsessive over things it's been deprived of. If you feel you've sacrificed too much, you're more likely to want to replenish your tank. This outlook transcends food itself and spills over into your daily habits and training.

Post-show can be a time where the pendulum swings so far to the other end of the spectrum that you are left off worse than you started. Know this at the onset and plan accordingly. As I said, have a plan or plan to fail. Your body simply can't be left to its own devices at this point because it's simply not on stable footing. As such, intuitive eating is not a wise move immediately post-show. Competition day is not the "finish line." That mentality is what makes the pendulum swing so far in the first place.

That said, recognize that the show is, in fact, over. You can afford to take a deep breath and take your foot off the gas—though that's not the same as slamming the brakes. Coast out of prep, but don't drive off a cliff. Take this time to keep building on the healthy habits you've been following for so long.

Keep meal prepping, training regularly and hitting your cardio—heck, you could even keep posing for a bit. You'll learn a tremendous amount about your body and how it responds to increased food throughout this phase. Take advantage of that opportunity! Enjoy the fact that you're well-conditioned and in fantastic shape. Hold on to it for a bit and be proud of it.

Make this phase fun and sustainable. Grant yourself a weekly "date night" on your planned refeed day. Eat a bit more variety and give yourself some grace for your macros not being 100% accurate at all times. Stay within a healthy window and keep a weekly average instead of a daily requirement if it works well for you.

Take a trip and remove yourself from the bubble you've been trapped in for the past several months. Be okay with missing the occasional workout if it means spending some time with your family or loved ones. Set yourself up for success in a sustainable, healthy way that aligns with your lifestyle and fitness endeavors. Make this phase fun and enjoyable. Learn to look forward to the training sessions, meals and the day-to-day.

Another critical shift in mindset you should prepare for is your attitude toward gaining body fat. You will absolutely gain body fat during this phase—it is supposed to happen! We all intuitively know this to be true, but even so, it always seems to sneak up on us. Preparing in advance with the right mindset is crucial.

It's challenging to transition from waking up every morning and seeing a lower number on the scale and a new vein popping out to seeing that number trend upward and the seatbelt get tighter around your midsection. You've measured your success by one set of metrics up to this point; now, you have to shift those metrics. It can be a tough pill for most people to swallow.

Rather than measuring your success by a lower scale weight and increased definition, get excited about the weight you're pushing in the gym. Embrace the fact that your performance is improving and your recovery time has shortened. Get excited to see your training volume increase week after week.

Dig and ask yourself what matters long term. How can you make this a genuinely healthy sport, one that you can sustain for a lifetime? The answer is simple: work to get better every single year. The only way to do that is to have a productive building phase to counteract the extreme cutting phase. When you wrap your mind around that simple fact, you'll be in a better position to accept the reality of the fat gain that comes with the reverse diet rather than seeing it as a negative.

[7]
PHASE SEVEN: REVERSE DIET BASELINE AND BEYOND

This phase brings us to the end of the competition prep cycle. Does that mean it's all over? Not hardly! This entire journey should be viewed through a circular lens. As you cycle through the phases, you get better and better, improving your starting and ending composition and baseline with each full cycle. By viewing this process in a circular motion, you'll see that there is no "end." There is no point that you discontinue your aspirations to be the best you can be.

Phase Seven is designed to catapult you into a healthy, sustainable building phase that sets you up for long-term success. In this phase, we'll be able to phase out the ketogenic refeeds, establish your new caloric and metabolic baseline and bump you up into a healthy surplus to optimize your lean mass gaining potential—all to balance out the extremes of being in a caloric deficit for months.

It takes a significant amount of time to build substantial lean mass, especially as a natural competitor. Ensuring that you are in a surplus and prioritizing your training for gaining muscle is incredibly important. It's crucial to ensure that this phase is sustainable and enjoyable, and most of your time should be spent building rather than being in a deficit. As such, an entire book could and should be written on optimizing this phase in its entirety, though I'll save that for another day. Still, I want this section to provide enough actionable direction that you can step out of the competition prep cycle and into a healthy building phase in the most productive manner possible.

Remember that bodybuilding is a lifestyle, and it should be viewed as such; the same can be said about the ketogenic diet. Rather than viewing short-term challenges as just brief moments in time, I encourage you to take a more holistic view. Done correctly, the sport of bodybuilding coupled with a well-formulated ketogenic diet can provide you with a seemingly endless supply of growth potential, both physically and mentally. Capitalize on it!

Push your limits and see what your body and mind are truly capable of. Structure your day-to-day so you can move the needle forward over time. This phase is all about establishing your new baseline and beyond. Don't forget about the beyond! Leverage the lessons learned in this book and your desire for self-improvement to craft the best version of yourself possible. Do so in a manner you can sustain and appreciate so that your life transforms for the better. By doing so, others will take notice. You'll become an inspiration to others simply by being your best self.

We live in an era of quick fixes and short-lived hacks. By adopting a mindset of playing and winning the long game, we can get better and better. The better we are, the more stable we become. This stability creates a better foundation for ourselves and those that we regularly interact with: our family, our friends and the community at large.

The clearer we paint our picture of health, the likelier we are to inspire others to achieve similar results. True health and vibrancy are contagious and can't be ignored. By adopting a healthy lifestyle and living it every single day, we can positively impact the health of our fellow human beings. That is a cause worth living for.

PHASE SEVEN GUIDELINES

Phase Six should have primed your thinking toward shifting goals between the competition prep and the reverse diet. By this point, you've likely lost a bit of your definition and put on a few extra pounds. Good!

Hopefully, by now, you've embraced those extra pounds and experienced the benefits that come with ramping up calories. These benefits include increased satiety, greater mental focus, better sleep, more libido, increased strength and less obsession with food.

We often second guess ourselves when noticing a dip in our definition, and it makes it easy to seem like we're doing something wrong. Don't let that happen. Rest assured, you're on the right track. If you keep your food consumption in check and don't go off the rails on weekly food benders, you're doing everything right! Stay the course and make sure your goals around building muscle and sustaining a healthy lifestyle are top of mind.

It's tempting to look at your calendar to see what other competition dates are on the horizon, but I highly advise against doing so. If you spend most of your time in a deficit, it is nearly impossible to improve year after year. By now, you've been in a reverse diet for at least a month or two. You're starting to feel better and perform at a higher level. Why reverse that now that as things are just beginning to pick up? It doesn't make any sense.

If the temptation of another show on the horizon is gnawing at you, take a moment and reflect. Refocus your goals and ask yourself why you're doing this reverse in the first place. The answer is simple: to ramp up your metabolism, improve your baseline and catapult yourself into a building phase to put on more lean muscle tissue. None of that is possible if you transition into another cut—even just a "mini cut." Play the long game and appreciate what you're doing for your health and wellbeing at this point in the journey.

PHASE OUT REFEEDS

If you've been steadily increasing your fat and protein throughout the past several weeks while dropping your refeed intake, you are likely noticing little to no benefit from your refeed days. At this point, your average daily intake is likely not far from your planned refeed intake. When that becomes the case, the refeed days become redundant and can be absorbed into your average weekly macros.

Hopefully, you leveraged the increased flexibility of the weekly refeed meals provided in Phase Six and experienced some different flavors and textures. You can certainly still treat yourself to weekly date nights and explore that variety, but I would recommend keeping your macros and caloric intake more in line with an average day from here on out. Doing so will keep your weekly average intake a bit tighter, and you won't have to fall into the trap of having incredibly low intake days to balance out the high ones. In all, your average daily intake should be in a comfortable range that you can easily sustain and at which you can perform.

When you phase out refeeds altogether and are averaging the same daily intake throughout the week, it becomes much easier to standardize that fuel intake. If you're keeping your daily calories and macros within a reasonably tight window, you'll be able to fine-tune it to determine what your body responds to best. This leads us to the second objective of this phase: increasing overall intake to find your personal threshold.

INCREASE TOTAL CALORIC INTAKE

As mentioned previously, now that we can remove refeeds, we can determine what caloric intake and macro distribution you respond best to. As mentioned, I like a 1:1 ratio of fat to protein grams in a maintenance/surplus phase. There are times when I get a bit more aggressive with fat intake and I bump that ratio up to about 1.5:1 (during building phases). Everyone has their own personal "sweet spot," but generally, a 1:1 fat-to-protein ratio with minimal carbohydrate intake should yield around 68-70% of total calories coming from dietary fat. A 1.5:1 will be closer to a 75% intake of calories from fat.

The whole point of this reverse diet and maintenance phase is to increase overall caloric intake. Even with a higher fat ratio, you should still consume enough calories to have no trouble getting an optimal level of dietary protein. There is seldom any benefit to dipping below 1 g of protein per pound of lean body mass during the maintenance or building phase. Depending on how aggressive you are and how your body responds to various macronutrient ratios, you may even be able to get away with bumping your protein intake up to about 1.5 g of protein per pound of lean body mass (or more). If you are consuming ample calories, you'll likely still be able to maintain a higher fat ratio along with higher protein consumption.

Some people seem to respond pretty well to higher protein-to-fat ratios. While there is absolutely nothing wrong with that approach, it's likely not optimal from a ketogenic perspective. Keep in mind that protein is not an excellent substrate for energy. If you are genuinely trying to build lean muscle, it stands to reason that your training will be intense and your energy demands significant. It is better to give your body the fuel it needs to perform at a high level than to expect it to create energy inefficiently through excess protein consumption in the absence of enough fat.

With all that said, staying somewhere within the 1:1 to 1.5:1 ratio of fat-to-protein throughout this reverse phase while gradually increasing weekly or bi-weekly total calories is usually best—no need to be super aggressive. Simply ramping up your fat and protein grams by 5-15 g per week should be adequate to give your body the ability to ease into greater caloric intake with fewer adverse effects.

Keep in mind that everyone will be a bit different and only you will know precisely what macronutrient ratio you respond to best. The best way to figure that out is to standardize as much as you can and change only one variable at a time whenever possible. Pay close attention to your digestion, energy levels, sleep and recovery.

If you operate better outside the window I described, that's totally fine! The only way to determine your ideal ratio is to experiment and be gradual enough that you can determine your tipping point relatively precisely. By limiting yourself to 5-15 g manipulations and allowing a week between each one, you're sure to find when too much of a good thing becomes a bad thing.

The same is true with the increase in calories. There will be a slight increase in body fat as you increase your macros coming out of competition prep, which is normal and to be expected. The rise in fuel should equate to a tangible increase in energy and improvement in recovery. At some point, you'll cross a threshold where continuing to increase calories results in disproportionate increases in body fat relative to muscle gains. Once there seems to be a higher percentage of adverse outcomes from caloric increases than there are positive outcomes, you'll know you've hit that tipping point.

Ideally, you won't reach that point until you are well past your reverse diet and into a surplus intake. At that point, it's best to halt the caloric increase and give your body ample time to acclimate at a sustainable maintenance intake and build more lean tissue before increasing even further. It takes time to build muscle, and you can't rush the process. The more lean mass you have, the more fuel your metabolism will demand and the more calories you can consume.

There's no need to go too far beyond your equilibrium and risk putting on any unnecessary body fat. The most accurate and reliable way to gauge that tipping point is through consistent monitoring of your body composition and training stats.

MONITOR BODY COMPOSITION AND STRENGTH PROGRESSION

What gets measured gets managed. That age-old adage rings true during the reverse diet phase as well. Just as we monitored our body composition throughout prep with bi-weekly pictures, measurements and body-fat tests, I encourage you to do the same throughout your reverse diet. You likely won't need to continue tracking these stats as closely once you establish your maintenance intake, but I advocate for detailed monitoring up to that point. After months of dieting down for the show, the habit is already ingrained, so it makes sense to keep it up until you establish a new baseline.

By this stage, you'll likely have put on some body fat and won't be quite as vascular as you were during the last few weeks of prep and the first few of Phase Six. As such, the changes in composition—as shown through bi-weekly pictures—will be a little less pronounced. The photos, measurements and body-fat scans are used so you don't allow yourself to get sloppy and put on unnecessary adipose tissue. The goal is to maintain a slight surplus for muscle building and recovery. You won't be insanely shredded, but you also shouldn't look like the Michelin man!

As in prep, try taking bi-weekly progress pictures in the same place with the same lighting each time. You'll likely lose a good deal of your definition throughout the reverse and building phase, but there's no need to lose it all. I still like to see separation in my quads and a relatively detailed outline of my abdominals deep in my off-season. That will be a bit different for everybody, but it's important to be proud of and comfortable with your physique. You won't be as lean in the off-season, but you should still feel confident in your skin.

Taking detailed circumference measurements is also incredibly important. Once you reach your homeostatic set point, these measurements will likely hold steady. It takes a good deal of time to put on lean tissue and increase your measurements through muscle mass alone, so you likely won't see any drastic shifts once you've returned to a baseline; however, by tracking your measurements throughout the reverse diet, you can ensure that you're not jumping up too quickly on any area of your body. For example, if you add a few inches to your waistline in a matter of a week or two, it's clear that you would likely benefit from reining your rate of caloric increase.

Keep checking your body fat and lean mass throughout the reverse diet also. You'll hold more fluid with more calories, so your lean mass will likely increase from where it was in the depths of prep. That said, take the DEXA, InBody and 3D scans with a grain of salt. Fluctuations in fluid retention can have a massive impact on measured estimations of fat mass and lean mass. It's nice to have the data, but don't assume that it's entirely accurate—and certainly don't allow it to paint the reverse diet in a negative light. You are much better off putting your faith in the pictures you consistently take and your performance markers while training.

Track your training output and use this data as your primary proxy for progress. To stay motivated as your scale weight increases, the solution is to focus on performance in the gym as a success marker. You should witness an uptick in training output and performance with increased fuel intake and improved recovery time. That way, you can know with confidence that things are moving in the right direction.

If you can monitor your strength and volume gains in the gym and see your lifts increasing as you steadily implement progressive overload principles, you can rest assured that you're doing things correctly. This is a great way to provide peace of mind that a good deal of that increased scale weight is coming from muscle mass. After all, it's not body fat that's helping you hit those new PRs!

TRAINING ADJUSTMENTS

As you transition into a building phase late in the reverse diet, you'll be at a slight caloric surplus and your body will be primed to add more tissue. The best way to ensure that added tissue is lean muscle instead of body fat is to stimulate your body in a way that fosters muscle growth. Distilled to its essence, our goal is to subject our muscles to ever-increasing stress so that we are forced to adapt by building additional muscle fibers, accomplished by training with progressive overload principles. Progressive overload training means exactly what it says: we want to overload our muscles progressively.

This is most often thought of in terms of increased repetitions or increased weight load. While those are obvious ways to implement progressive overload, there are many options beyond those two including increased time under tension, drop sets, negative repetitions, burn-out sets, supersets and static holds. All of these are options to increase the training overload and intensity.

If you're reading this book while coming out of competition prep, you likely have a solid understanding of basic training principles and how to implement proper form and technique. Rather than focus so much on building muscle, I'd like this book to focus on competition prep itself with some simple guidelines towards the training and diet after the show.

As calories dip lower and lower during prep, your ability to implement progressive overload principles in your training has likely waned, which makes total sense. With less fuel, you have less ability to recover and grow more lean tissue. At that point, the primary goal was not to build more muscle; it was simply to hold on to as much lean tissue as you possibly could while in a deficit. The best way to do that was to continue subjecting your body to the rigorous training volume and load you'd worked up to by that point.

Now that we're entering a caloric surplus with adequate nutrition to build more tissue, you should be able to increase the training volume and workload beyond what you were previously capable of. The building phase is about adding as much lean tissue as possible while maintaining a healthy body composition and improving your metabolic and hormonal state. Take full advantage of this time to hit new PRs in the gym, experiment with new training splits and techniques, exhaust your muscles in new ways and subject yourself to different training stimuli to see what you respond best to.

(For the sake of transparency, I've included my personal training split and overload techniques in the appendix of this book. Feel free to try that split yourself and see how you respond to it.)

There is no one-size-fits-all when it comes to training splits. As with diet and nutrition, sustainability is key. Find something that pushes you but is sustainable enough that you can adhere to it and improve over time. Play around with training frequency; later, try less frequency but more intensity. You can experiment with drop-setting everything—and then supersetting everything.

Mix it up to see what you prefer but give your body ample time in each "experiment" so you can truly gain an accurate representation of how you respond to each style of training. Like your diet, remove as many variables as possible when conducting new training experiments so you can control for unknowns and confounding factors. Have fun with it, because that's what this is all about!

CARDIO ADJUSTMENTS

In Phase Six, we described the inverse relationship cardio has with calories in the reverse diet. That same concept holds here in Phase Seven and into the building phase. As calories return to a healthy baseline and enter a slight surplus, we can slowly taper our cardiovascular training down to a more sustainable level. Phase Seven is all about re-establishing our healthy baseline with food and putting ourselves in a slight surplus to build muscle.

Just as we want to establish a sustainable baseline with our caloric intake, we also want to establish a baseline for our cardio output. This generally means tapering our cardiovascular training down to a minimum viable dose. The minimum viable dose can be described as enough cardio to maintain cardiovascular health and conditioning but not so much that it inhibits our ability to perform or recover from resistance training.

Keep in mind that by having a minimum viable dose approach to cardio in the off-season, we're able to benefit more from slight increases in cardio activity during our next competition prep. If you do seven days a week of cardio in the off-season, you'll have less "cardio runway" in your next prep. However, suppose you reset your baseline in such a way that you're able to sustain a healthy minimum dose of cardio a week in the off-season. In that case, any slight increase in cardio should elicit a favorable response, and we can be more strategic about scaling that up throughout the next competition prep.

At the risk of sounding repetitive, remember that the primary goal of Phase Seven and the building phase is to put your body in a slight caloric surplus. That will be much harder to do if your energy output is amplified by tons and tons of excessive cardio training. It's far better to taper that training down so that you can enter a healthy energy surplus more effectively with a realistic increase in food.

I find a simple day or two a week of intentional cardio is all that's necessary to maintain a healthy baseline. This could take the form of a session or two on the Stairmaster at a moderate intensity, a brisk run a few times a week, HIIT training with a focus on cardiovascular endurance, sprint work, cycling or even some relatively intense hiking.

Make your cardio activities in the off-season enjoyable so you look forward to doing them. Standardizing and controlling cardio variables is best in competition prep, but that's not necessarily the case in the off-season. Instead, hop on the Stairmaster one day and go stand-up paddle boarding the next. Don't stress over the estimated caloric expenditure and take the fun out of the activity. Simply implement cardiovascular training to improve your overall health and quality of life. You're not trying to get lean in the off-season. You're trying to build as much muscle as possible and do it in a healthy manner! Prioritize strength training over cardiovascular activities and ensure that your cardio isn't a distraction—remember, it should serve your strength training!

DON'T JUMP RIGHT INTO ANOTHER PREP

It happens every time without fail. Whenever I'm working with a client through their first competition, they walk offstage in a euphoric state, go through a few weeks of reverse dieting and then start looking for future shows to jump into. Many federations have competitive seasons in both spring and fall. As a result, many first-time competitors start to imagine themselves doing a quick "mini cut" prior to the second season and jump back onstage in the same 12-month span as their first show.

I don't blame them. I totally understand where they are coming from. They've just subjected their body and mind to something new and exhilarating and, like a drug, they want to experience that euphoric high again sooner rather than later. For them, it's easy to rationalize jumping into another show in a short time because:

1. They are already pretty lean, and it wouldn't take much time or effort to dial things back in and be show-ready, and...
2. Why not?

The problem with that mentality is that it leads to a downward spiral of over-competing, chronic dieting and insufficient time for growth and improvement. As a bodybuilder or figure competitor, your goal is simple: be better than last time, every single time you step onstage. Come in with more muscle, more shape, better symmetry, more definition, improved conditioning and more polished posing.

This is nearly impossible if you don't give your body ample time to grow and improve in between shows. We introduced this topic at the beginning of this reverse diet section, but it bears repeating.

Remember, it takes time to build lean mass—a lot of time. It also takes a long time to diet down and minimize the loss of that hard-earned muscle.

Suppose you budget four to six months for prep itself, then another three months or so to return to a healthy baseline intake of calories. By that time, the year is almost over. You're spending nine months of the year in a deficit or in maintenance. That scenario isn't optimal for adding more muscle to your physique, and you may very well lose muscle during that period depending on your training and how low you take your calories.

As such, if you were to act on your euphoric emotions and jump straight into another prep, you might actually look worse onstage the second time, which should be avoided at all costs. Play the long game and make bodybuilding a sustainable lifestyle. Spend significantly more time at maintenance and in a surplus than you do in a deficit. Focus on your training and prioritize your building phase with the same intentional focus as your prep, and I guarantee you'll be better with each passing season. This way, you'll only get better and better.

You don't have to compete every single year. In fact, I highly encourage you *not* to (this is even more critical if you are a natural competitor). The hormonal fluctuations that happen in competition prep are not to be taken lightly. If you are competing as a natural, your diet and lifestyle factors will be your greatest antidote to correcting these hormonal dips. You won't lean on drugs to help keep things stable as you take your calories lower and lower. The only way to ensure your hormones are upregulated and functioning properly is to give yourself ample time at a healthy caloric intake and higher baseline body fat percentage. I take at least two or three years off between competitions. There is a method to this madness. You can't get better if you don't build on your foundational baseline. You can't build that baseline if you're constantly dieting down.

A good rule of thumb is to operate on at least a 3:1 ratio between time spent at a maintenance and surplus and time spent in a deficit. Using the earlier example of six months in a deficit and three months reversing up would be 27:9—27 months in maintenance or surplus and nine months in a deficit or reverse. With all this said, a 3:1 approach is on the aggressive side of the spectrum. I would personally recommend a 4:1 or 5:1 split. As always, what is optimal will vary by individual.

A younger competitor who is still experiencing some "newbie gains" will be able to put on much more muscle in a shorter time than a seasoned competitor. For that reason, they will likely be able to look significantly better between shows with less time separating the competitions than someone who has been lifting for 10+ years. Thus, they may be a bit more aggressive in their competitive timeline and spend less time building. Even so, I would argue that they would benefit even more by leveraging that time as a newbie to capitalize on their muscle-building potential and not squander it by dieting down too frequently.

While the importance of spending adequate time in a building phase can't be discounted, you don't want to be lazy and stay in a perpetual state of "bulking." There is much to be gained from cycling into a deficit, such as metabolic health, compositional improvement, cardiovascular conditioning and psychological perspective. The "yin and yang" philosophy of building and cutting phases goes both ways. Rather than chronically doing one or the other, strive to have a healthy blend of both—just recognize that you'll want to spend more of your time building than cutting. By following a simple template of keeping a 3:1 to 5:1 ratio, you should be able to plan your transition phases appropriately.

PHASE SEVEN MINDSET

How should one prepare themselves mentally for what lies ahead? After experiencing the rigors of competition prep and all that it involves, how can one possibly settle for anything less intense or invigorating? After the show is over and you've gone through the reverse diet, you must turn your attention toward the horizon and look ahead. Play the long game with this sport and with life in general. A common theme in this book is sustainability—in nutrition, training and life.

Phase Seven and beyond is all about exercising discipline and consistency around actions you can sustain for a lifetime. So many competitors are only on top of their nutrition in the months leading up to a show. So many athletes only push their bodies in the gym when it's crunch time in prep. The problem with being short-sighted in that way is that you leave so much potential on the table.

How much could you benefit if you trained with intention throughout the entire year, year after year? How much healthier would you be if you focused on the quality of the foods you consumed every single day of your life? The beauty of living a healthy life is that it has an exponential effect on the quality of your life for years to come. Your daily choices dictate your long-term outcomes. The habits you build now will be the same factors that define you later. At the root of all of that, sustainability is the key.

What can you sustain forever? You certainly can't maintain a competition level of conditioning indefinitely. You likely can't sustain detailed macronutrient tracking every single day for the rest of your life, either. That's fine; there is no need to. It's better to operate at 90% of your potential sustainably than to achieve 100% of your potential but flame out immediately after. Sustainability is the defining factor when it comes to discovering true health and success in life. The sustainability factor is why some people find great success with various diets, sports and career paths. It simply works for them. You must find and establish what works for you and is sustainable for the long haul.

For me and so many others, a quality ketogenic diet is sustainable. Simply removing all processed carbohydrates, sugars and hyper-palatable junk food can strip away foods that provide little and take much. By returning to a diet more in line with our evolutionary past and eating foods comprising high-quality proteins, fats and vegetables, we can set ourselves up for nutritional success.

Many would argue that sacrificing all carbohydrates is not a worthwhile price to pay. Maybe that stems from a dependency on treats, or perhaps from a lack of knowledge around how much impact the food you eat genuinely has on your health. Regardless, I wholeheartedly disagree.

The quality of my life and the life of so many others I know who adopted a ketogenic lifestyle has improved tenfold. Our relationship with food has improved along with our health markers, hormones and body composition. All those factors have led to a higher quality of life, one that I'm excited to sustain for the long haul.

All of this holds true for resistance training as well. Truth be told, we are all bodybuilders. Whether you step onstage and compete or not is irrelevant. We are all building our bodies in some form or fashion. We are either living a life conducive to building more lean muscle tissue, stronger joints and ligaments, more flexibility and better health, or we're "building" in a way that adds unnecessary fat, disease and inflammation that will eventually tear us down.

You hold the key to your outcome. Our bodies are designed to move. We should constantly be experimenting to see what we can handle and how we can test our capabilities. This is the case whether you're going for a new PR on squats or taking your grandkids to the park and climbing on the monkey bars with them.

Movement is fun! Exercise is liberating! Training your body is what leads to the formation and preservation of lean muscle tissue and operable joints. By staying active, you build the foundation necessary to carry your health into your later years. By building training habits early in your life, you ensure your body will perform well as you age. By adopting a resistance training protocol or sport that yields sustainable muscle growth and activation, you set yourself up for long-term success.

In my humble opinion, a well-formulated ketogenic diet paired with structured resistance training is both sustainable and the closest thing I have found to the fountain of youth. It checks all boxes from a nutritional and physical standpoint and sets you up for success now and in the future.

If you're reading this book, I assume you are interested in competing. The act of competing is not a vain endeavor. It's a catalyst and outlet for creating intentionality around your training and nutrition. Competing provides a tangible reason to transition through intentional periods of caloric surplus, build more lean muscle and dip into deficits focused on fat loss.

Transitioning through these phases is the very essence of what makes this sport and this lifestyle sustainable. Countless benefits come with putting your body in an energy surplus, just as they do from structured deficits. Competing provides the strategy for how to transition through these phases with a plan and a purpose. Doing so in a fat-adapted, ketogenic state ensures that you capitalize on all the benefits quality nutrition has to offer.

CHART OF MY 2020 COMPETITION PREP THROUGH THE 7 PHASES

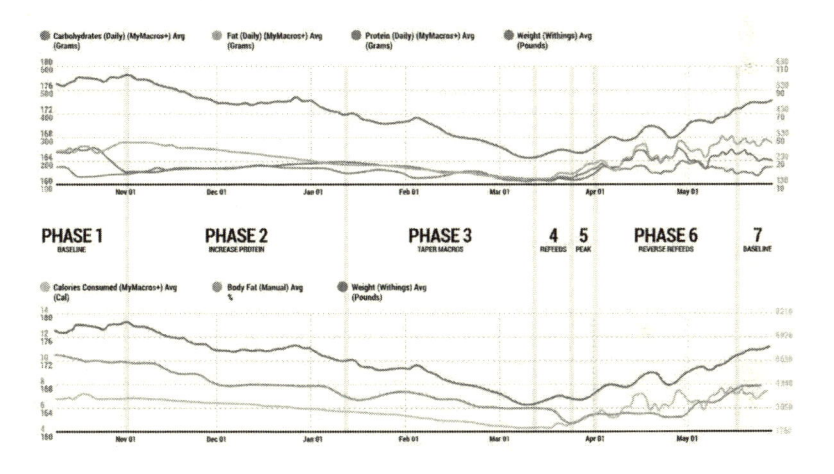

AFTERWORD

Discovering this proverbial fountain of youth and taking advantage of all the benefits it has to offer has been my greatest life's work. The ketogenic diet and natural bodybuilding have turned my health around and have given my life purpose. It has done the same for my wife Crystal, who struggled with countless gastric issues before adopting a ketogenic diet.

This lifestyle led to my creation of my Keto Savage and Keto Brick business empire, giving me a vehicle to create and share the knowledge I've gained through years of experimentation. This business employs many people who have since adopted a ketogenic diet and shared these principles with their families and loved ones.

The content I put out in my weekly newsletter, podcast, YouTube videos and social media content has garnered millions of views, downloads and interactions. The emails, DMs and messages I get from audience members who have implemented my protocol in their own lives have made my work and my life worthwhile. The letters I get about 87-year-old grandmothers who adopt a ketogenic lifestyle and get a few more quality years with their loved ones, or from 24-year-old kids who start bodybuilding and discover confidence and a calling that they didn't realize they had, all make my day.

I receive emails like these daily, and they are truly the reason I do what I do. Seeing how people's lives are genuinely transformed for the better by adopting these principles is what brings me true fulfillment and satisfaction in life. They illustrate beyond a shadow of a doubt that I am doing what I was put on this earth to do.

I am incredibly passionate about this lifestyle, and I commit to it freely and forever. Putting out information around the topic of ketogenic bodybuilding and all its benefits will be something I do forever. This is sustainable for me, and I am excited to do it until the day I can't. On that day, know that I'll have died with a smile on my face and a ribeye in my belly.

[PART 3]
APPENDICES

OVERVIEW

My goal with this appendix is to deliver a ton of actionable takeaways in the form of nutritional choices, training methods, posing techniques, supplement recommendations and miscellaneous bodybuilding information.

The book itself is a step-by-step guide in how to manipulate your macros and training to arrive at the destination in show-level conditioning. This appendix provides lists, graphs and templates you can easily leverage with your prep if you don't currently have something in place.

This appendix is not designed to be read in novel form. Feel free to skip around and use these resources as needed.

[1]
NUTRITIONAL OVERVIEW AND OBJECTIVES APPENDIX

The point of this section is to provide actionable takeaways as it relates to your nutritional manipulations. I'll give a few sample meal plans so you can gain perspective. I have no intention or desire to "paint you into a corner" and create an exhaustive list of meal plans you feel enslaved to.

Truth be told, one of my biggest frustrations as a nutrition coach is clients who expect weekly meal plans. In my experience, rigid meal plans and black and white guidelines around food choices do much more harm than good. They are rarely followed, so rather than wasting energy with a list of detailed meals, I'd rather teach you how to prioritize nutrient density and manipulate macros.

Equipped with that knowledge, you become much more flexible and adaptable—two attributes that contribute significantly to sustainability.

MEAL PREP BASICS

Meal prepping is often viewed as a massive inconvenience, but there is a certain art to prepping your meals in advance. The truth is that the process can be streamlined. When done correctly, it will save you a tremendous amount of time.

Because your macros change weekly in this ketogenic prep protocol, I highly encourage you to meal prep for the week at a given set of macros in advance. As your macros change, you can simply adjust your meal plan to target new macros and provide some flavor variety. By keeping your meals consistent throughout an entire seven-day period, you'll be able to control for more variables and dial in your nutrition with greater precision.

As mentioned in the manual, having your base macros come from quality fat and protein sources and using smaller items to supplement in adjustable 5-10 g increments will make this process much more manageable.

Whole eggs can easily help with these fluctuations because each whole egg contains about 6 g of protein and 5 g of dietary fat.

Ground beef is a great base to build from as it's so versatile. Since the contest prep protocol starts at a relatively high dietary fat ratio, start with a 75/25 ground beef as the base of your nutrition. As your protein intake increases and your dietary fat decreases, slowly transition to 80/20 ground beef, then to 85/15 and eventually 90/10 or even 96/4, depending on how high your protein ratio becomes. By swapping out your ground beef percentage as macros change, you can easily hold many other variables in your meal plan constant. As your protein intake drops throughout Phases Three, Four and Five of this protocol, simply return to a fattier ratio of ground beef. This simple hack is the most accessible and efficient means of adjusting to changing macro ratios.

If you are not a fan of ground beef, feel free to incorporate other cuts and other types of **red meat, white meat, fish and shellfish**. Many people love steak, and I'm one of them! Still, recognize that steak varies quite a bit from one cut to the next. One day's ribeye may include a ton of marbling, while another could have very little. This disparity results in significant deviations in macros and total calories. The best way to mitigate this is to source meat from a consistent supplier if at all possible. In general, I avoid cuts that are incredibly inconsistent whenever I'm in competition prep. Instead, I opt for choices that are easily tracked and manipulated. For this reason, ground meat is easier than steak or steak cuts.

Bulk cooking preparation is a bit tricky. How can you possibly account for all the fat drippings that get cooked out of food? When I'm in prep, I avoid using cooking methods that result in a loss of macros. When I'm in a deficit, I want to ensure I'm consuming everything I'm tracking. As such, I avoid grilling my foods when I'm prepping my meals and focusing on macronutrient accuracy.

The fattier the cut, the more you lose to drippings that cook out of the meat and fall to the flames of a charcoal or gas grill. Since we follow a ketogenic diet and so many of our meats are relatively fatty, I prepare my meats in the oven or a cast-iron skillet on the stove. After the meat is cooked, I make sure to pour any of the remaining fat drippings left in the skillet back onto my food so it can reabsorb those nutrients.

Realize that it will be impossible to get everything precisely perfect from one meal to the following, but close enough counts. Things will average out over a week. This is another reason why keeping your meals consistent over an entire week is a wise move. When meal prepping, I cook several servings of meat in a cast-iron skillet, portion out each day's allotment into a separate Tupperware dish and then pour the remaining meat drippings evenly into each container before sealing them back up and placing them in the refrigerator.

GROCERY LIST

The following is a comprehensive list of various sources of dietary protein, fat, and carbohydrates. Feel free to incorporate these into your meals as long as they add up to hit your desired macronutrient targets.

> *Note: The carbohydrates are characterized by their net carb count, but I highly encourage you to track your total carbs, not net carbs.*

FAT SOURCES:

- Avocado
- Avocado oil
- Almond oil
- Bacon grease
- Beef suet, preferably from grass-fed cattle
- Beef tallow, preferably from grass-fed cattle
- Butter, preferably grass-fed and unsalted
- Broth
- Chicken fat, organic
- Cheese (hard)
- Cream (heavy or whipping)
- Duck fat, organic
- Eggs (whole)
- Ghee (butter with milk solids removed)
- Keto Brick
- Macadamia nuts

- Macadamia oil
- Mayonnaise (made with an avocado oil base)
- Olives
- Organic olive oil
- Organic coconut oil, coconut butter and coconut cream concentrate
- Peanut butter: make sure to use unsweetened products and limit due to omega-6 content.
- 85-100% dark chocolate can be used in small amounts

PROTEIN SOURCES:

- Red meat/ruminants (variety of cuts and options), including beef, lamb, venison and goat
- Pork products, such as pork loin, Boston butt, pork chops, ham, bacon and sausage
- Poultry (free range is better if it's available), such as chicken, turkey, quail, duck, goose and pheasant
- Fish, including anchovies, calamari, catfish, cod, flounder, halibut, herring, mackerel, mahi-mahi, salmon, sardines, sole, snapper, trout and tuna
- Shellfish (an exception is imitation crab meat, as it contains sugar, gluten and other additives), such as clams, crab, lobster, scallops, shrimp, squid, mussels and oysters
- Whole eggs, whether fried, hard-boiled, poached, scrambled or eaten as omelettes

Note: When applicable, grass-fed meat is generally preferred, as it has a better fatty acid profile.

VEGETABLES:

All of these have fewer than 5 net carbs, but for best results, I still recommend tracking total carbs.

- 1 cup of alfalfa sprouts (1 net carb)
- 1 cup raw broccoli (2 net carbs)
- 1 cup bok choy (< 1 net carb)
- 1 cup cooked broccoli (4 net carbs)
- 1 cup raw shredded cabbage (2 net carbs)
- 1 cup boiled cabbage (4 net carbs)
- 1 medium raw carrot (4 net carbs)
- 1 cup cauliflower (2 carbs)
- 1 stalk raw celery (1 net carb)
- 1/2 medium cucumber (3 net carbs)
- 1/2 cup cooked eggplant (3 net carbs)
- 1 clove raw garlic (1 net carb)
- 1 cup lettuce (< 1 net carb)
- 1 cup of mixed greens (< 1 net carb)
- 1 cup raw mushrooms (2 net carbs)
- 1 cup mustard greens (3 net carbs)
- 5 green olives (< 1 net carb)
- 1/4 cup raw onions (3 net carbs)
- 1 cup raw green bell peppers (4 net carbs)
- 1 cup raw red bell peppers (5 net carbs)
- 1/2 cup raw radishes (< 1 net carb)
- 1 ounce raw shallots (3 net carbs)
- 1 cup raw spinach (1 net carb)
- 1 cup raw summer squash (4 net carbs)
- 1 medium red tomato (4 net carbs)
- 5 cherry tomatoes (2 net carbs)
- 1 cup turnip greens, cooked (3 net carbs)

RECIPES

The following recipes are all options that can easily be added into your competition prep. I've included a few of my favorites here, but feel free to experiment and swap out foods as you see fit. There's no need to feel trapped in a rigid meal plan. As long as you're accurately hitting your target macros, controlling for as many variables as possible and sourcing your food from quality sources, you're setting yourself up for success!

* * *

ZERO CARB MEAT PANCAKE

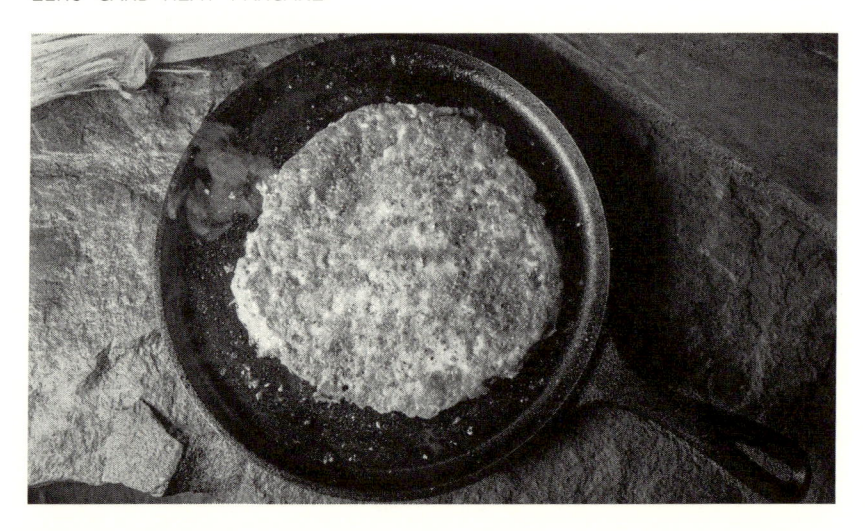

Yield:
1 Serving

Prep Time:
5 minutes

Cook Time:
5 minutes

Macros:
84F | 68P | 0C

Ingredients:

- 2 whole eggs
- 4 oz ground beef (80/20)
- 1/2 cup of cheese
- 2 tbsp oil (we use beef tallow and duck fat)
- 1 tbsp beef gelatin

- Desired seasonings

Directions:

1. Cook your 4 oz of ground beef and place in a mixing bowl.
2. Pour the 2 tbsp of oil into the cooked ground beef and mix together.
3. Mix the remaining ingredients (eggs, cheese and gelatin).
4. Spray your cooking pan with quality oil and warm the surface.
5. Pour mixture into the pan and cook one side.
6. Flip the "pancake" over and cook throughout until both sides are nice and crispy.
7. Enjoy pure deliciousness!

* * *

"FATHEAD" PIZZA

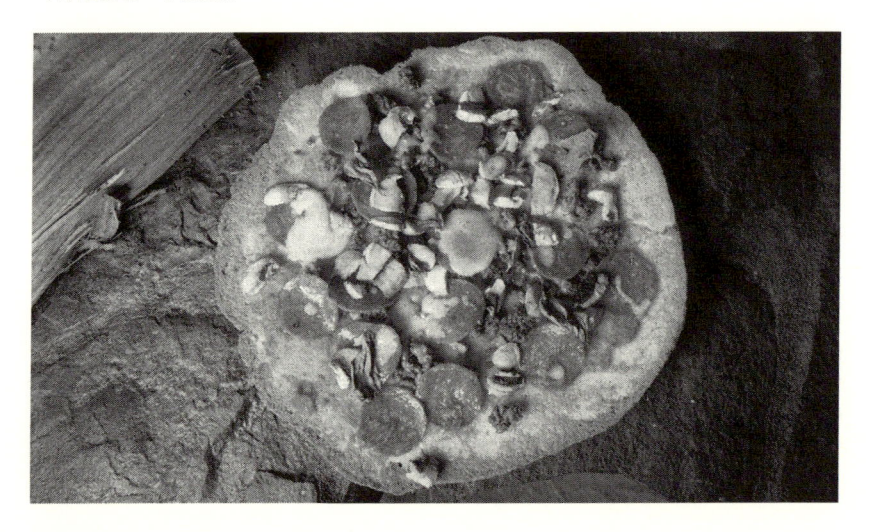

Yield:
1 serving

Prep Time:
5 minutes

Cook Time:
20 minutes

Macros:
96F | 68P | 20C

Ingredients:

- 6 oz shredded mozzarella cheese
- 3 oz almond flour
- 1 oz cream cheese
- 1 whole egg
- Desired toppings

- Desired seasonings (we use Redmond Real Salt)

Directions:

1. Place the 6 oz of cheese and 1 oz of cream cheese in a medium microwave-safe bowl.
2. Microwave for 1 minute, stir and warm longer until fully melted.
3. Add the 3 oz of almond flour to the melted cheese and stir.
4. Once blended, add one egg to the mixture and mix until it makes a dough.
5. Add in your desired seasonings and knead well.
6. Take the dough and place it on a stone pizza pan or baking sheet with parchment paper.
7. Flatten the dough to the size of the pizza you would like using parchment paper. At this point, you can form it into whatever shape you like and however thick or thin you desire.
8. Bake at 400 degrees for 12 minutes and then flip over the dough.
9. Bake on the opposite side for an additional 5 minutes.
10. Add desired toppings and broil in the oven until toppings are crisp and the cheese toppings are melted.
11. Dig in!

* * *

FRITTATA

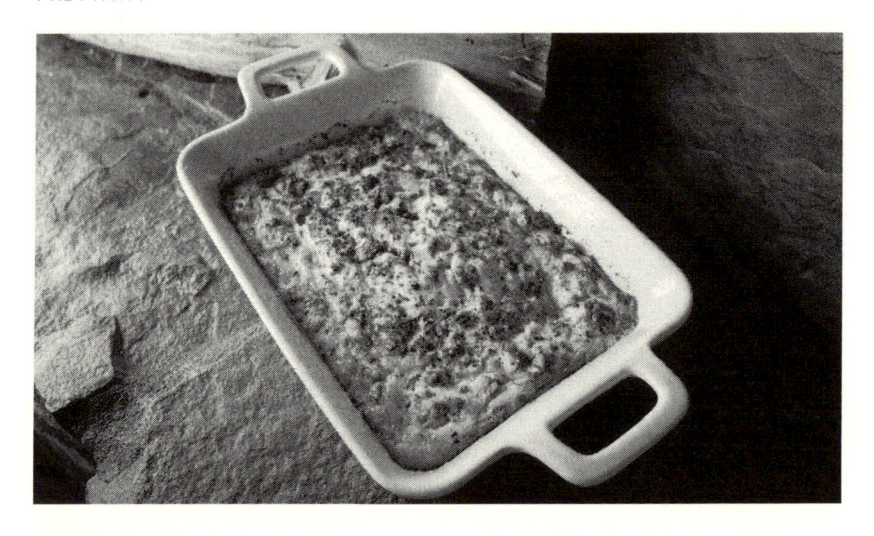

Yield:
1 serving

Prep Time:
10 minutes

Cook Time:
25-30 minutes

Macros:
68F | 55P | 2C

Ingredients:

- 4 whole eggs
- 2 oz cheese
- 2 tbsp heavy cream
- 4 oz ground beef (80/20)
- Veggies of your choosing

- Desired seasonings

Directions:

1. In a small/medium bowl, scramble together the eggs and whisk in the heavy cream.
2. Mix in the seasoning of your choice.
3. Mix in the remaining ingredients, cheese, desired veggies and pre-cooked ground beef.
4. Spray cooking spray into baking dish and ensure even coating.
5. Pour the mixture into the baking dish.
6. Bake at 350 degrees for 25-30 minutes.

* * *

ORGAN MEAT BURGER

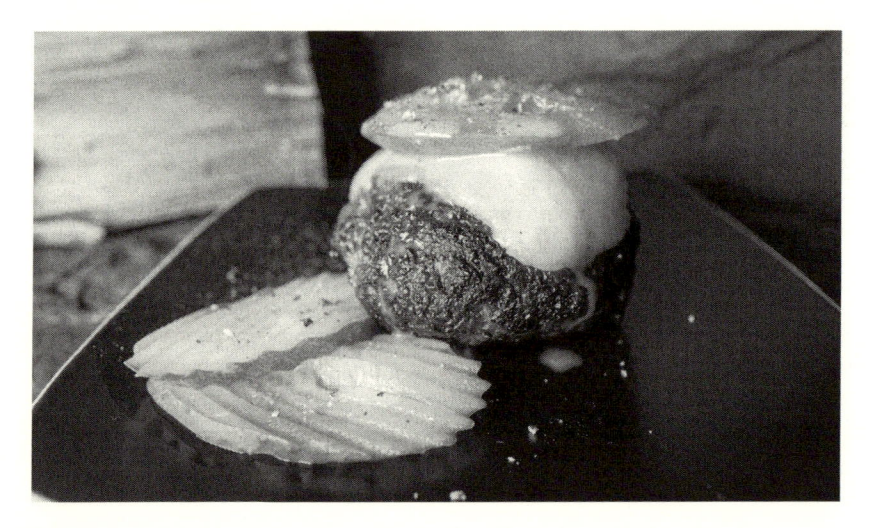

Yield:
10 servings

Prep Time:
15 minutes

Cook Time:
16 minutes

Macros:
23F | 32P | 2C

Ingredients:

- 8 oz heart
- 8 oz liver
- 1 lb venison
- 2 lb bacon
- 1 lb ground beef

- Desired seasonings

Directions:

1. Cut up all of your meat into chunks small enough to pass through the grinder.
2. Run all cuts through a meat grinder and ensure a consistent blend.
3. Season the meat and get your hands dirty. The better the mixture, the better the burger!
4. Pack the meat into patty portions; we went with an 8 oz patty size.
5. If using an air fryer, set to 390 degrees and cook for 7-8 minutes per side.
6. Add toppings and dig in!

* * *

BAKED SALMON

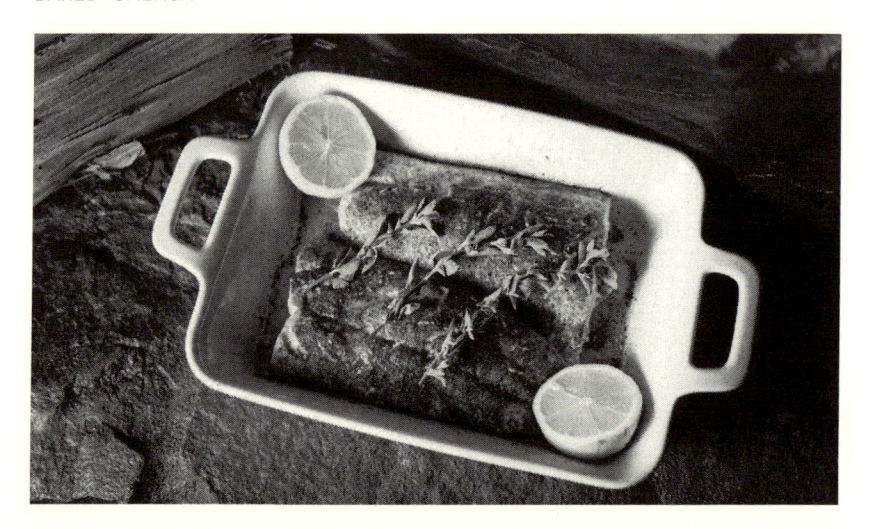

Yield:
4 servings

Prep Time:
5 minutes

Cook Time:
15 minutes

Macros:
17F | 46P | 3C

Ingredients:

- 1.5 lb salmon (preferably wild-caught)
- Lemon slices (enough to cover the baking sheet)
- 2 tbsp olive oil
- Smoked paprika
- Chili lime seasoning

Directions:

1. Preheat oven to 400 degrees.
2. Grab your baking dish and spray the bottom with oil.
3. Lay lemon slices to cover the bottom of the baking dish.
4. Pat dry salmon with paper towels.
5. Pour the 2 tbsp olive oil over the top of the salmon and spread evenly.
6. Sprinkle on seasonings as desired.
7. Place in the oven and bake for 10 minutes at 400 degrees.
8. Once cooked, place on broil for another 5 minutes.
9. Squeeze fresh lemon on top for added flavor.

* * *

BUFFALO BACON BURGER-BITES

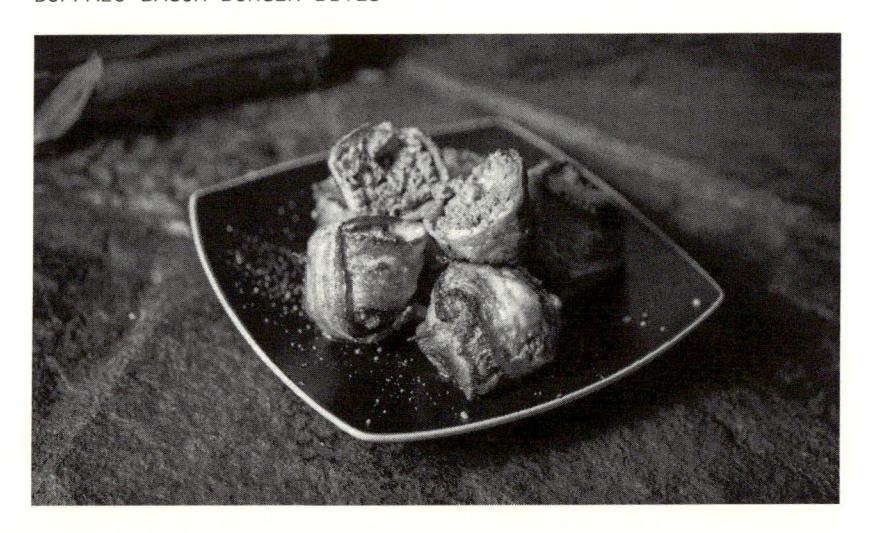

Yield:
12 burger bites

Prep Time:
10 minutes

Cook Time:
30-35 minutes

Macros:
19F | 16P | 1C

Ingredients:

- 1 lb ground beef (80/20)
- 3 oz cheese
- 1 pack of bacon (about 12 slices)
- Desired seasonings (we use buffalo and salt)

Directions:

1. Cut cheese into 12 even squares.
2. Place ground beef in a bowl and add seasonings.
3. Once the meat and seasoning have been well mixed, separate and roll the beef into 12 even-sized balls.
4. Wrap the ground beef ball around one of the cheese squares (make sure cheese is covered).
5. Then wrap that ball with bacon, poke with a toothpick and get it ready for the oven.
6. Place in oven for 30 minutes at 350 degrees.
7. If you enjoy your bacon a little crisper, then place the range on broil and cook for another 5 minutes.
8. Let them cool slightly and enjoy!

* * *

SWEET AND SIMPLE CHAFFLE

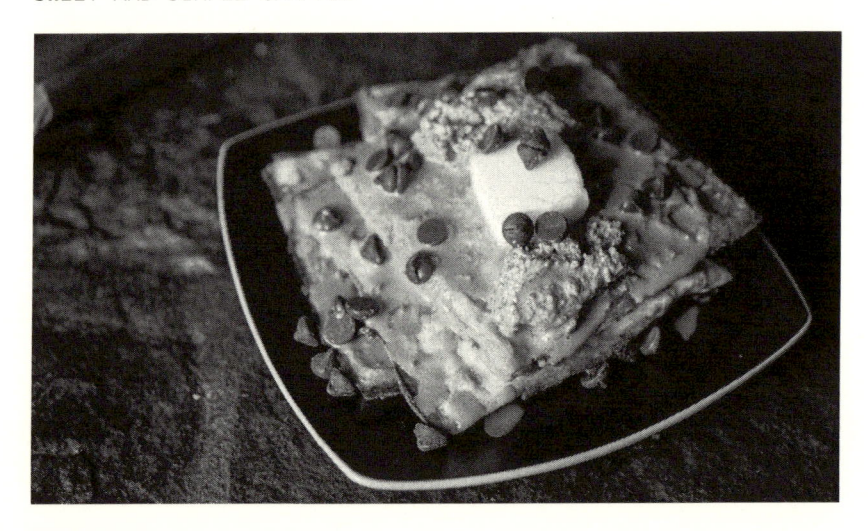

Yield:
1 serving

Prep Time:
2 minutes

Cook Time:
5 minutes

Macros:
39F | 46P | 3C

Ingredients:

- 1 cup mozzarella cheese
- 3 eggs
- Seasonings (if you want it savory)
- Sweetener or extract (if you want it sweet)

Directions:

1. Turn on the waffle maker and spray with cooking spray.
2. Mix the cheese and eggs.
3. If you want it savory or sweet, add in your seasonings, sweetener or extracts.
4. Pour the mixture onto the waffle maker and spread evenly.
5. Leave the waffle maker on until desired crispness.
6. Remove the waffle and add toppings you like.
7. Let them cool slightly and enjoy!

* * *

CHICKEN PICCATA

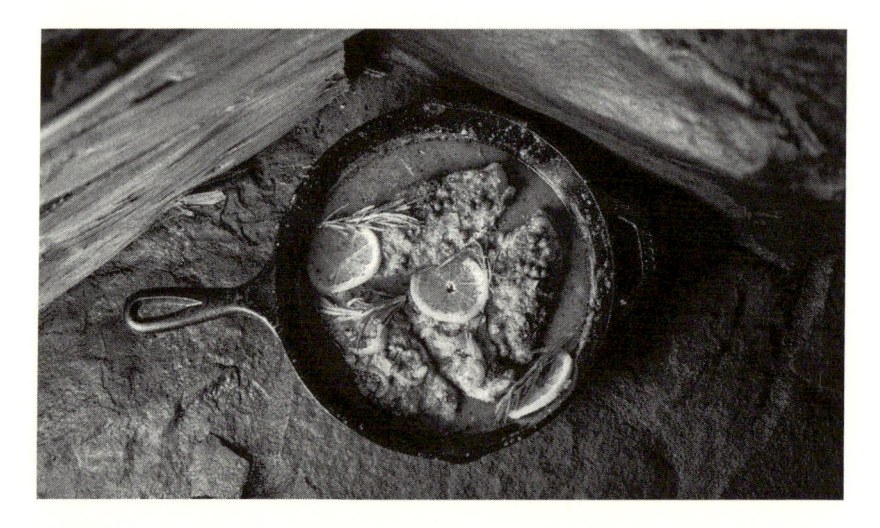

Yield:
2 servings

Prep Time:
5 minutes

Cook Time:
10-15 minutes

Macros:
122F | 160P | 12C

Ingredients:

- 1 lb chicken
- 1 cup bone broth
- 2 tbsp olive oil
- 5 tbsp butter
- 3 tbsp capers

- 1 shallot
- 1 squeezed lemon
- 1/2 cup almond flour
- Desired seasonings

Directions:

1. Fillet the chicken breast.
2. Place oil and butter in the pan and allow to melt completely.
3. While that is warming in the pan, cover the chicken breasts entirely with almond flour.
4. Place chicken in the pan of oil and butter. Cook until internal temperature reaches 165 degrees.
5. Remove the chicken from the pan and set it aside, keeping the stovetop on.
6. Add the diced shallots to the remaining oil and sauté.
7. Add bone broth to the shallots and allow it to simmer and reduce.
8. Once the broth has reached the desired consistency, add in the lemon juice and capers.
9. Remove from heat.
10. Place chicken back into broth mix or pour broth mixture over the top of the chicken.
11. Serve and enjoy!

* * *

DRINK RECIPES

As far as your drink options go, try to keep things clean and simple. I always avoid drinking my calories unless I'm implementing a fat fast and being strategic with consuming a bolus of dietary fat in my morning coffee.

KETO COFFEE

Add heavy cream, MCT oil, butter, ghee or another clean fat source into your coffee drink. If you desire an added sweetener, try liquid stevia (as it will typically be your cleanest option).

KETO TEA

Same as above, except use tea instead of coffee. Many people have a sensitivity to caffeine or coffee and prefer tea. One of my personal favorites is a London Fog Tea. This is simply Earl Grey tea, heavy cream and sugar-free vanilla liquid stevia.

BROTH DRINKS

Many people enjoy drinking plain bone broth. This is fine, but I encourage you to pair it with a fat source to avoid drinking a pure protein without any dietary fat. It's always a good rule of thumb to pair your protein with fat to slow the absorption of the protein and reduce a blood glucose response.

ELECTROLYTE DRINKS

A straightforward way to give you some flavor variety is to mix up the electrolyte drinks you use. I typically recommend sticking with Redmond Re-Lyte because it has a perfect 2:1 ratio of sodium to potassium built in. Each scoop of Re-Lyte contains 1,000 mg of sodium and 500 mg of potassium. They offer unflavored blends, but they also have a vast array of flavors that all taste great! All are sweetened with stevia and provide a welcome change in flavor from plain water. I'll often mix my day's worth of electrolytes, creatine and water into a large gallon jug and sip from that throughout the day.

CARBONATED DRINKS

A little bit of pop and fizz goes a long way when your calories are low. Something about the carbonation seems to fill you up a tad more and take the edge off. I'm all for incorporating an occasional Zevia carbonated beverage or carbonated mineral water, but I encourage you to consume these in moderation. You never want the majority of your fluid to come from carbonated sources.

HUNGER HACKS

What are "hunger hacks?" These are food options and fillers that provide a relatively high degree of fullness and satiety with a minimal caloric load. As I mentioned in the book, I tend to avoid leveraging high-volume, low-nutrient filler foods when possible. Not only do they provide little benefit from a nutritional standpoint, but the filler fibers can also reduce some of the nutrient absorption from the primary foods you consume.

I included many more hunger hacks when I was following a bro diet and consumed a much higher percentage of my calories from lean sources. My underlying satiety level was significantly improved by simply increasing my dietary fat intake with this ketogenic prep protocol. There is a stark contrast between merely being full of high-volume foods and experiencing true satiety.

A bowl full of lean meat and watercress contains much more volume than a fatty ground beef and egg blend, and it's easy to assume that increased volume directly correlates to increased satiety. This simply is not the case. The body craves nutrients, and the hormones crave a certain baseline of dietary fat. By swapping out the leaner cuts for more nutrient-dense, fattier options, you can likely improve your satiety level significantly with less overall volume. Taking all this into consideration, why would I bother including a section on hunger hacks?

It's simple: sometimes you simply need to satisfy that urge to chew and consume. When you are deep into a competition prep deficit and have transitioned to only one or two meals a day, your mind starts playing tricks on you. Your body is physically hungry; there is no doubt about it. However, finding some way to convince your mind that you "should" be satisfied is a valuable tool to have at your disposal.

I highly encourage you *not* to become overly dependent on these hunger hacks as they offer little physical benefit; the main benefit they add is mental. In all, these are more of a crutch than an actual benefit. Have these tools at your disposal, but don't lean on them too heavily.

SHIRATAKI NOODLES AND RICE

Shirataki noodles are long, white noodles. They are often called miracle noodles or konjac noodles. They are made from glucomannan, a fiber that comes from the root of the konjac plant. Konjac grows in Japan, China and Southeast Asia and contains very few digestible carbs. These noodles typically come prepackaged and are made by mixing glucomannan flour with water. The mixture is boiled and then shaped into noodles or rice-like pieces.

Shirataki noodles are about 97% water and 3% glucomannan fiber. As a result, they are incredibly low in calories and are often used by individuals trying to consume more food bulk without any additional caloric load. Glucomannan is a highly soluble fiber that moves through your digestive system very slowly. This slow transit can temporarily create a sensation of fullness but delays nutrient absorption into your bloodstream.

If you've never prepared these noodles before, you'll likely be put off by how smelly they are when you first open the package. They are packaged in water to prevent them from drying out, so simply strain out the water and boil them to remove the smell. Then, I recommend drying them out in a warm skillet so that they can lose a bit of their moisture and take on the texture of actual rice or noodles more closely. The noodles themselves lack any real flavor, so feel free to season or sauce them heavily to make them palatable.

In my IIFYM days, I would prepare a massive bowl of miracle rice and then drench it with zero-calorie Walden Farms syrup and a few spoonfuls of peanut butter to create a tasty dessert. While delicious, this dish was utterly void of nutrients and filled with chemicals and artificial sweeteners. Since then, I've transitioned to using the miracle rice and noodles as a savory dish. I'll prepare my ground beef and then dry the noodles off in the same cast-iron skillet so that they can absorb more of the fat left from the meat. After that, I'll mix everything to create a higher volume stir fry or casserole.

KELP NOODLES

Another alternative comes in the form of kelp. Kelp noodles are a sea vegetable made of only kelp, sodium alginate and water. They are fat-free and very low in carbohydrates and calories. Like konjac noodles, kelp noodles have a neutral taste that allows for various uses. One significant benefit of kelp noodles is that they contain a considerable dose of iodine, a trace mineral that most of us are deficient in.

No cooking is required—just rinse and add the noodles to any dish and they are ready to eat! These noodles are incredibly crunchy, so I like to mix them with my ground beef to simply provide a change in texture.

EGGS

Eggs are a fantastic source of nutrition! Not only does a whole egg provide a healthy dose of quality fat and protein, but it also is a culinary miracle for its uses in cooking. You can blend eggs with other foods and bake them in the oven to create different textures. Due to the unique rising nature of eggs, it is possible to create a variety of recipes that are easily absorbed, nutrient-dense and surprisingly high in volume. A simple Google search for "keto mug cake" will yield tons of options that you can factor into your daily macros.

ZERO CALORIE "SNOW CONES"

This is straight out of the bro bodybuilding playbook, but it is surprisingly effective! Simply purchase a cup of crushed ice from Sonic or a snow cone dealer and drench it with a zero-calorie water enhancer. I'll sometimes use Mio as my flavoring agent, but Mio is full of Sucralose and Ace-K as a sweetening agent, so I prefer to use something a bit more keto-friendly.

Sweet Leaf makes a water enhancer that avoids coloring agents and only uses stevia as the sweetener. Chowing down on a cup full of crushed ice and zero-calorie sweetener will garner some strange looks, but it keeps the hunger at bay. I'll often incorporate this snow cone when my macro allotment is depleted at the end of the day but I'm still hungry because it satisfies the desire to chew things (even if it's only frozen water).

My one word of caution is to consume this as your final meal before going to bed. The sweetener can elicit a cephalic phase of insulin response that incites more hunger. If you consume this and go to bed shortly thereafter, you can usually fall asleep before any increase in hunger has you rummaging through the cupboard looking for something else.

READY-TO-EAT FOODS

Recipes are great, but sometimes you are in a time crunch and need something that nails your macros in a quick and easy, grab-and-go manner. Ideally, you have meals prepped for the week, but what about when the stars don't align? What do you do when you need something in a time crunch? I like to keep a stash of simple grab-and-go options that are easy to fit within my macros. The following is a list of my preferred ready-to-eat options.

KETO BRICK

I may be a bit biased, but a shelf-stable, 1,000 calorie ketogenic meal replacement brick with perfect macros is hard to beat. I eat one of these every single day, and I have for the past several years. The ingredients are all top-notch and easily absorbed. These bricks were literally made for the very purpose of optimizing a ketogenic competition prep: high-quality nutrition with zero gastric bloat or digestive issues. The cacao butter in the bricks is an excellent source of stearic acid, which has been shown to provide a ton of benefits.

CANNED SARDINES/OYSTERS

Canned sardines, oysters, clams, mussels, mackerel, trout and salmon are all fantastic options! Seafood provides a ton of micronutrients and minerals. Always try to get canned fish and seafood packaged in pure olive oil and not a processed, hydrogenated blend. Also, if the macros include the oil in which the fish is canned, try to consume all of it with the fish. If the macros are based on the can being drained, make sure the can is drained!

PARM CRISPS

If you don't have any food sensitivities to dairy, I highly encourage you to try baked parmesan cheese crisps. These are easy to make at home, but many brands are popping up that offer these as a quick and easy prepackaged option. Many gas stations are starting to carry these baked cheese crisps as well.

As with all prepackaged foods, check the entire ingredients list! Many companies are getting lazy and trying to capitalize on the popularity of keto at the expense of quality ingredients. With something as simple as parmesan crisps, the only ingredient should be cheese and seasonings. Nothing else is necessary!

MEAT STICKS

Meat sticks are a good option for keto-friendly grab-and-go snacks. Unfortunately, most mainstream brands contain a ton of added sugars and preservatives, so you'll likely have to pay a bit more for one with quality ingredients. Duke's brand, Fire Creek Snacks, Epic and Chomps are a few popular brands that contain quality ingredients.

Many prepackaged meat options have a ton of added sodium, so keep that in mind when you factor these into your macros. A significant bolus of sodium above your normal baseline will likely result in a temporary increase in water weight and fluid retention. If you have a day that you consume significantly more prepackaged foods, anticipate this temporary increase in fluid retention and plan accordingly.

PILI NUTS

Many nuts are incredibly healthy and acceptable from a macro standpoint. Macadamia nuts are often touted as the best "keto nut," but the true victor is the pili nut! Pili nuts are high-fat, low-carb and provide an excellent source of magnesium, manganese, vitamin B1 and phosphorous.

A 1/3 cup serving of pili nuts contains a whopping 40 g of dietary fat and only 3 g of total carbs! I'm a massive fan of the Pili Hunters brand, as I know the owner, Jason, personally and trust his product. Jason sources these nuts from local gatherers in the Philippines and does a ton to pay it forward to the individuals gathering these nuts by hand.

PORK RINDS

People's minds automatically go to pork rinds when they hear the word "keto." Pork rinds aren't an excellent source of protein or dietary fat, so I would never encourage making them a staple; however, sometimes you must have a quality crunch. Nothing compares to the crunch of a tasty bag of pork rinds!

I like to snack on these when I'm on a road trip or as a substitute for chips whenever I'm preparing keto nachos. Many pork rind brands use subpar ingredients and fillers, so avoid that whenever possible. I'm a huge fan of the Epic and 4505 brands, as they typically use clean ingredients. Like other preserved meat snacks, pork rinds contain quite a bit of additional sodium, so keep that in mind when planning out your electrolyte intake for the day.

POST-SHOW CELEBRATORY MEAL

I wrote about the best tactics to adopt post-show at length in the book itself. I highly suggest you reread that chapter before letting your desire for overindulgence get the best of you.

No good comes from deviating too far off the path that led to your success with this journey in the first place. By all means, eat a hearty meal after the show and take pleasure in knowing you've accomplished something extraordinary. Just don't let that meal turn into a week and that week morph into a month.

Don't deviate from the habits and practices that you've built your foundation upon. If you've followed a quality, ketogenic dietary protocol up until this point, don't stray from it in the final hour. Feel free to grant yourself a meal of additional intake but keep the food selections ketogenic and relatively high quality. Otherwise, you'll most certainly suffer from some significant gastrointestinal issues. If you've suffered from disordered eating habits in the past and have a hard time moderating certain foods, avoid them entirely. No good comes from opening Pandora's box after a show when your willpower and discipline are all but used up.

My preferred indulgence after a show is to join my family and friends for a celebratory meal at an all-you-can-eat Brazilian steakhouse. This provides an impressive spectrum of flavors and textures, and nearly everything on the menu is well within the realm of a ketogenic diet. I'm able to eat until I'm stuffed and not ever feel guilty about the foods I'm consuming.

Even with a massive bolus in calories from this celebratory meal, it's rare to suffer any adverse effects from a digestive standpoint if all of those calories are coming from quality sources I know my body responds well to. Prepare a keto-friendly dessert in advance and enjoy it after the primary meal if you're craving something sweet.

There is no need to sacrifice your nutritional integrity after a show. Focus on the experience and the relationships with the people there supporting you. Enjoy the food but don't let it have a hold over you. Feel free to deviate from the target macros on show day with the celebratory meal and even allow yourself plenty of grace the following day. Just be sure and get back on target the next week as you transition into a structured reverse diet.

[2]
POSING AND JUDGING APPENDIX

POSING AND JUDGING CRITERIA OVERVIEW

What follows are the exact posing and judging requirements presented by the INBF and WNBF federations. Each federation will be slightly different, so I highly encourage you to dive into their unique needs and specifications. The INBF/WNBF federations are the ones I'm most familiar with, which is why I've included them below.

Their posing and judging criteria will showcase posing requirements mirrored by most federations within these divisions. There are a few divisions that I've not included below, such as Women's Fit Body, Women's Physique and Women's Bodybuilding. If you plan to compete in those divisions, be sure to read up on their specific requirements.

I've tried to present these criteria in easy-to-read, bulleted lists. I've also included illustrations whenever possible. You already have a million things on your mind during this phase of the show prep, so the easier this information is to absorb, the less likely you'll be to stress about it.

***

WOMEN'S BIKINI

The Bikini Division is designed to find athletes with a fit and shapely body that is not heavily muscled or overly defined. In the bikini division, athletes wear a two-piece bikini posing suit. The top ties straight across and the bottom is a bikini cut that flatters the athlete's physique. Thongs, micro-cut, scoop cut or suits that do not provide moderate coverage are not allowed. Brazilian cut suits are preferred in the INBF/WNBF.

COMPETITION ATTIRE

- Multi-colored or solid color
- Two-piece bikinis

Fabric may be decorated and jewelry is permitted. Studs, rhinestones, beads or appliques are allowed. Designs may include connectors, straps and hip connectors. Moderate coverage in the back of the suit is required. Shoes are required, but the height of the heels is optional.

ROUNDS SCORED

ROUND 1: FITNESS AND BALANCE

Round shoulders, defined abs, soft lines in legs and tight glutes. Overly lean, muscular, hard or vascular physiques will be scored down.

ROUND 2: PHYSICAL APPEARANCE

The overall appearance of the athlete. Stage presentation, suit choice, tanning, hair and makeup are all encompassed by this round. The information on the next page outlines competitors' poses for the Fitness and Physical Appearance rounds.

FACE FRONT

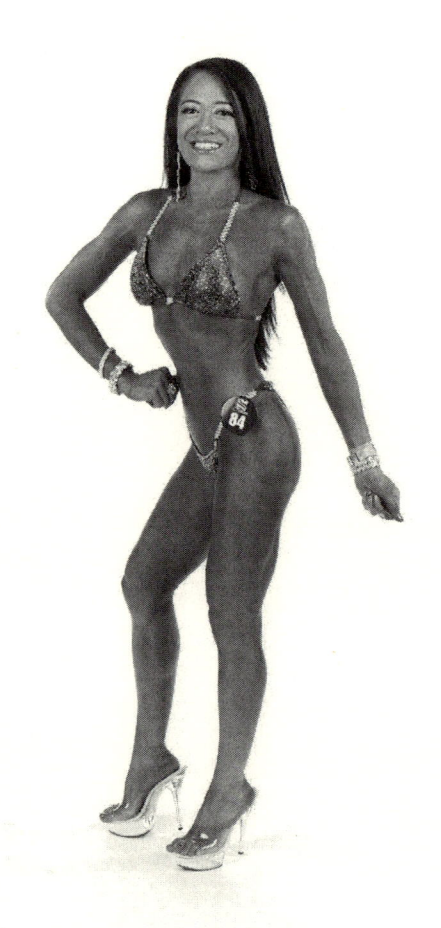

- Hips and toes shall be positioned forward.
- One leg is extended to the side. Either leg is acceptable.
- One hand must be on the hip and the other arm should hang below the hips (not extended to the side).
- Arms should not be raised or spread wide, impeding another competitor's space next to you.
- Lats should be open but not overly flared as in the figure division.

- A slight twist is allowed as long as both hips and shoulders are visible from the front.

QUARTER TURN TO THE RIGHT

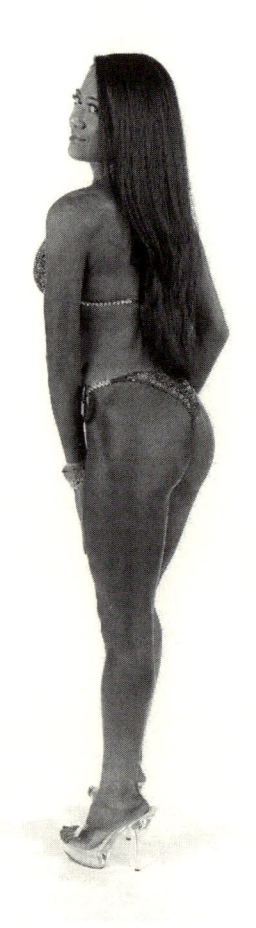

- From the front, competitors execute a quarter turn to the right and adjust stance.
- Upper body turned 35 degrees toward judges to see the rear shoulder.
- The hips face the side of the stage; you may twist your shoulders toward the judges.
- Turn your head and look directly at the audience and judges.

- The front foot may be offset. A slight lift of the heel onto the toe is permitted.
- Long hair should be pushed back behind the shoulder.
- The rear hand is placed on the hip, the other hanging freely.

330 / ROBERT ORION SIKES

FACE BACK OF THE STAGE

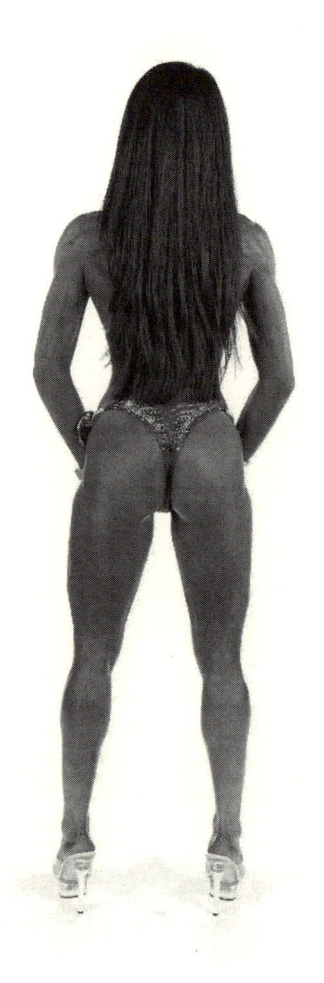

- From the side pose, competitors execute a quarter turn to the right and face the rear of the stage.
- Heels can either be together or spaced less than shoulder-width apart.
- Weight can be centered or shifted to either side.
- Other options for leg positions include legs crossed over and feet in a staggered T-position.

- Arm position is optional and can include arms down or placed at the top of thighs.
- One hand on the hip does not apply in the back pose.
- Lats will be open but not over-flared to show upper body shape.
- Hair should be pushed to the front (apologies for not being pushed forward in the picture above)
- At no time during the rear stance is a competitor permitted to turn their head to look at the judges.
- Standing in a wide straddle or bending over excessively is not allowed and will be scored down.
- At any time, if a competitor's posing does not meet the criteria, the head judge will give a general warning. If the pose is not corrected, they may call the specific athlete number to fix an issue. If the competitor still does not correct course, the competitor may be scored down.

QUARTER TURN TO THE TIGHT

- Same as the first side pose, but from the opposite side.

FRONT AND BACK STAGE WALK

This optional walk is called by the head judge. Bikini competitors walk from the front of the stage to the back of the stage as a group. Competitors are asked to execute a back pose at the back of the stage. They transition by turning back around, facing the judges and walking to the front of the stage. This walk may be performed multiple times.

A normal T-walk can be included in prejudging and used at finals. The stage walk or T-walk is the competitor's opportunity to show grace, poise and confidence. Competitors should execute the T-walk in a tasteful, confident manner. Overexaggerated posing or performance outside bikini division (bodybuilding poses and gymnastic moves) will be scored down.

This stage walk is the same as Figure and Men's Physique, usually executing three points onstage. The stage walk will be conducted according to the promoter's site restrictions, and competitors will perform the T-walk in the pattern designated by the promoter. Competitors who fail to follow the designated walking pattern may be scored down.

SCORING EACH ROUND

Judges will score each round and give competitors a final placement before the head judge moves to the next round.

For example, in a class of eight competitors, judges will rank competitors 1-8 in each round. When the judges have completed scoring for both rounds, they will add the scores together to determine the final placement for each competitor.

* * *

WOMEN'S FIGURE

Figure is a class of physique competition judged equally on symmetry and muscle tone. Stage presence (to include posing and the stage walk) shall be a tie-breaker. Judges use two rounds to assess competitors in each of these physique-based areas.

COMPETITION ATTIRE

- The two-piece posing suit must be in good taste; thongs are not allowed.

- The posing suit may be adorned with rhinestones, sparkles or sequins for added effect.
- High-heeled shoes are required.
- Jewelry is permitted; body jewelry (piercing) is allowed if it is not offensive.
- Other jewelry (earrings, necklace, bracelets) may be worn but should not obscure the physique or be in poor taste.

ROUNDS SCORED

ROUND 1: SYMMETRY

Competitors will perform mandatory quarter turns; judges will compare competitors against each other. Judges will be looking at balance and proportion (e.g., between upper and lower body and sides). Figure athletes should be symmetrically balanced; the upper or lower body should not overpower the other; no one body part should overpower the rest of the physique.

ROUND 2: MUSCLE TONE

Competitors must show good muscle tone. Leanness and muscle development are expected; however, competitors should *not* exhibit as much conditioning and muscle mass/size or present an over-conditioned physique as in the bodybuilding division.

POSING EXECUTION

Mandatory quarter turns for symmetry and muscle tone include the following:

FACE FRONT

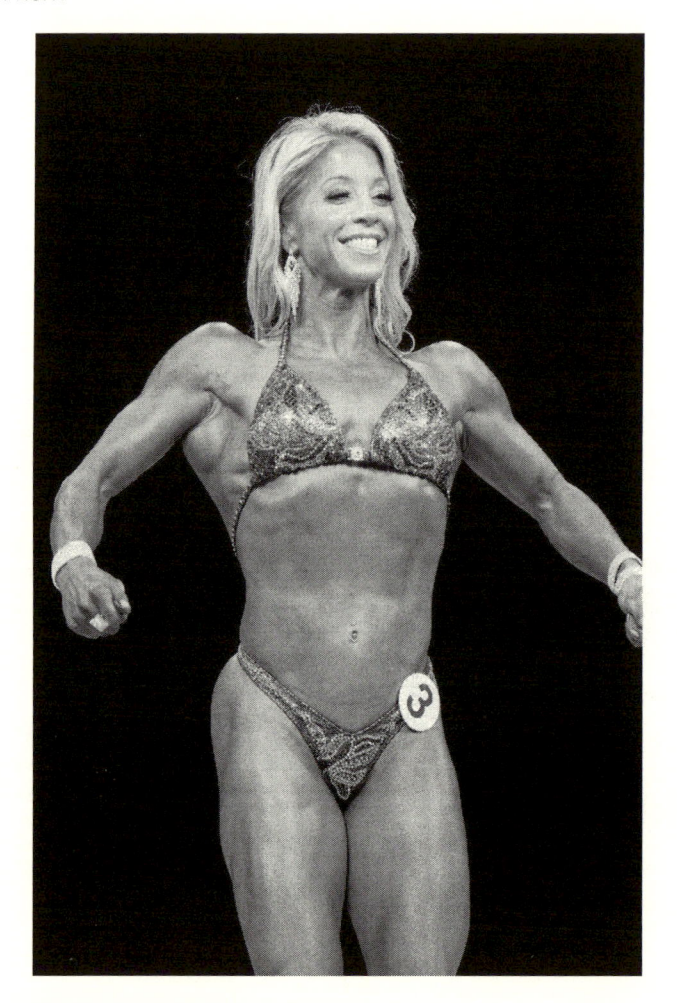

- Heels must be together and in line, without either foot ahead of the other.
- Hips must face the judges, and arms must remain to the sides (although they shouldn't touch the sides or spread overly broad).
- Lats should be open/flared to show a nice V-taper.
- Toes must face the judges, but competitors can angle

their toes out slightly if it helps to accentuate their quad presentation.

336 / ROBERT ORION SIKES

SIDE POSE

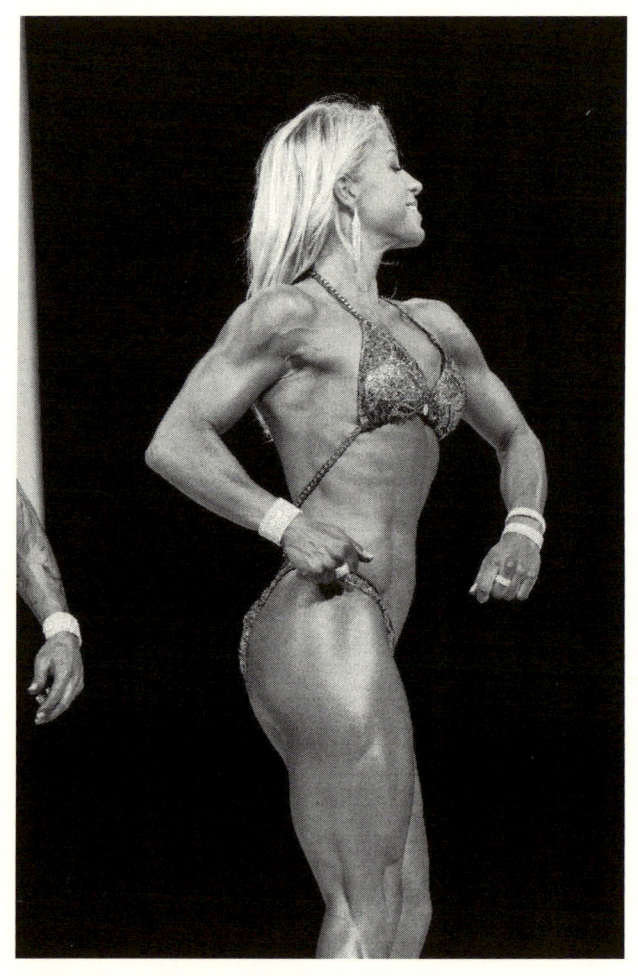

*This photo reflects the opposite side pose.

- Competitors execute a quarter turn to the right and adjust stance from the front pose.
- Upper body turned 35 degrees toward judges so the rear shoulder can be seen.
- Hips must face the side of the stage.
- Eyes must face the side of the stage.
- Toes must face the side of the stage with both feet flat.

The feet can be offset only half the foot's distance (front or back foot offset).
- Long hair should be pushed back behind the front shoulder to avoid obscuring the view.
- Front and rear hands should hang freely with palms toward the body.

REAR POSE

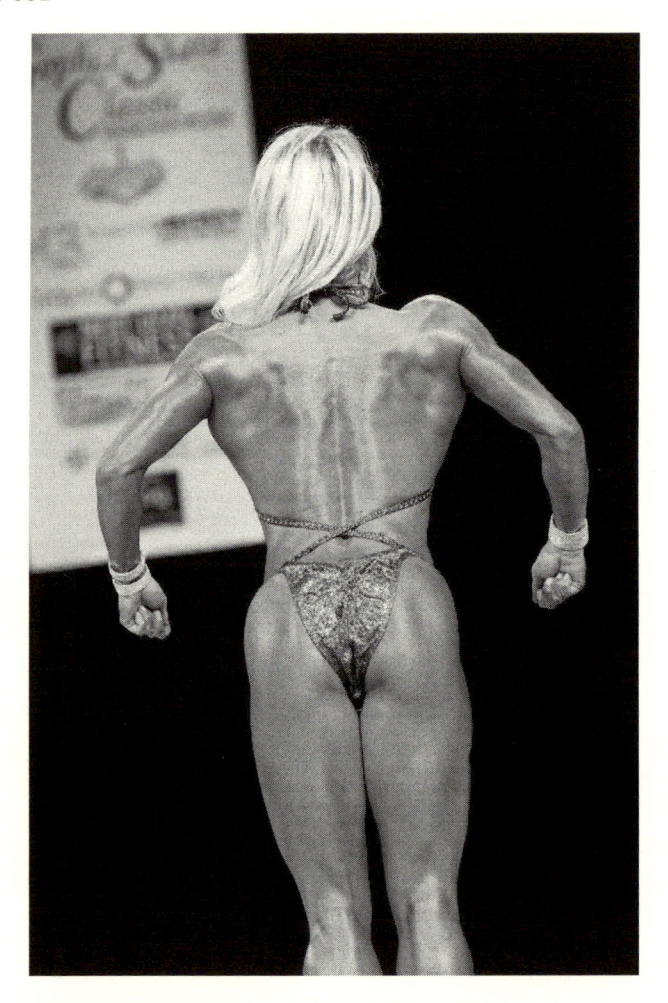

- From the side pose, competitors execute a quarter turn to the right and face the curtain or rear of the stage.
- Both feet must be together or very close.
- Toes cannot be spread wide apart.
- Feet cannot be offset to any degree (i.e., one in front of the other).
- Competitors should brush their hair to one side so their backs can be seen.

- Arms must be at the sides with the hands hanging freely, palms toward the body.
- Lats are spread wide to show upper body symmetry.

PRESENTATION AND STAGE WALK

This portion is to be used as a tiebreaker and is not given a score/ranking.

- Hair and makeup should complement your figure.
- Posing suit and shoes should complement your figure.
- Skin tone and tanning products/foundation color should complement the hair and suit and enhance the overall figure.

OVERALL STAGE PRESENCE

Judges will assess competitors' ability to execute quarter turns, present confidence and poise seamlessly and change places with other competitors.

During the stage walk, judges will consider the above elements and how well you walk and present yourself during the mandatory poses. Judges will be looking to see if all the above components work together as a whole to present a total package. Subtotal scores can be positively or negatively affected by the walk, moving a competitor up or down by breaking ties.

PREJUDGING WALK

- A normal T-walk should occur with all competitors remaining onstage at the back line.
- Competitors should execute a side pose facing toward the

middle of the stage when posing near the outside posing spots.
- In the middle area, competitors should perform a front pose, back pose and turn back to a front pose before walking to the following outside posing spot.
- Poses should not be held for more than three seconds each, and the entire individual presentation should be completed in 30 seconds (the head judge may allow more time depending on the size of the stage).

The stage walk or T-walk is the competitor's opportunity to show grace, poise and confidence. Competitors should execute the T-walk in a tasteful, confident manner. Exaggerated posing or performance outside the figure division (such as bodybuilding poses and gymnastic moves) are not allowed.

SCORING EACH ROUND

Judges will score each round and give competitors a final placement for that round.

For example, in a class of eight competitors, judges will rank competitors 1-8 in each round. When the judges have completed scoring for two rounds, they will add the two scores together to determine subtotals for each competitor. The stage walk shall break ties.

* * *

MEN'S PHYSIQUE

Physique Division competitors are lean, fit and muscular, yet do not have the muscle mass or extreme leanness required for the Bodybuilding Division. Athletes wear conventional board shorts cut above the knee.

COMPETITION ATTIRE

Men's Physique competition attire should be conventional board shorts with inseams no shorter than six inches and no longer than 11 inches. The waistband should fit no lower than three inches below the navel. The legs of the shorts should fit appropriately to accentuate the athlete's physique.

ROUNDS SCORED

ROUND 1: SYMMETRY AND MUSCLE TONE

ROUND 2: PRESENTATION

The physical criteria that judges are looking for is a lean, fit, muscular physique that is balanced and aesthetically pleasing. Athletes should be appropriately groomed, possess a small waist and have a good V-taper from the shoulders to the obliques. Judges are not looking for the level of muscle mass or extreme leanness that is necessary for success in bodybuilding.

POSING EXECUTION

Posing will be conducted in four-quarter turns to the right. The head judge will guide competitors through this process.

FRONT POSE

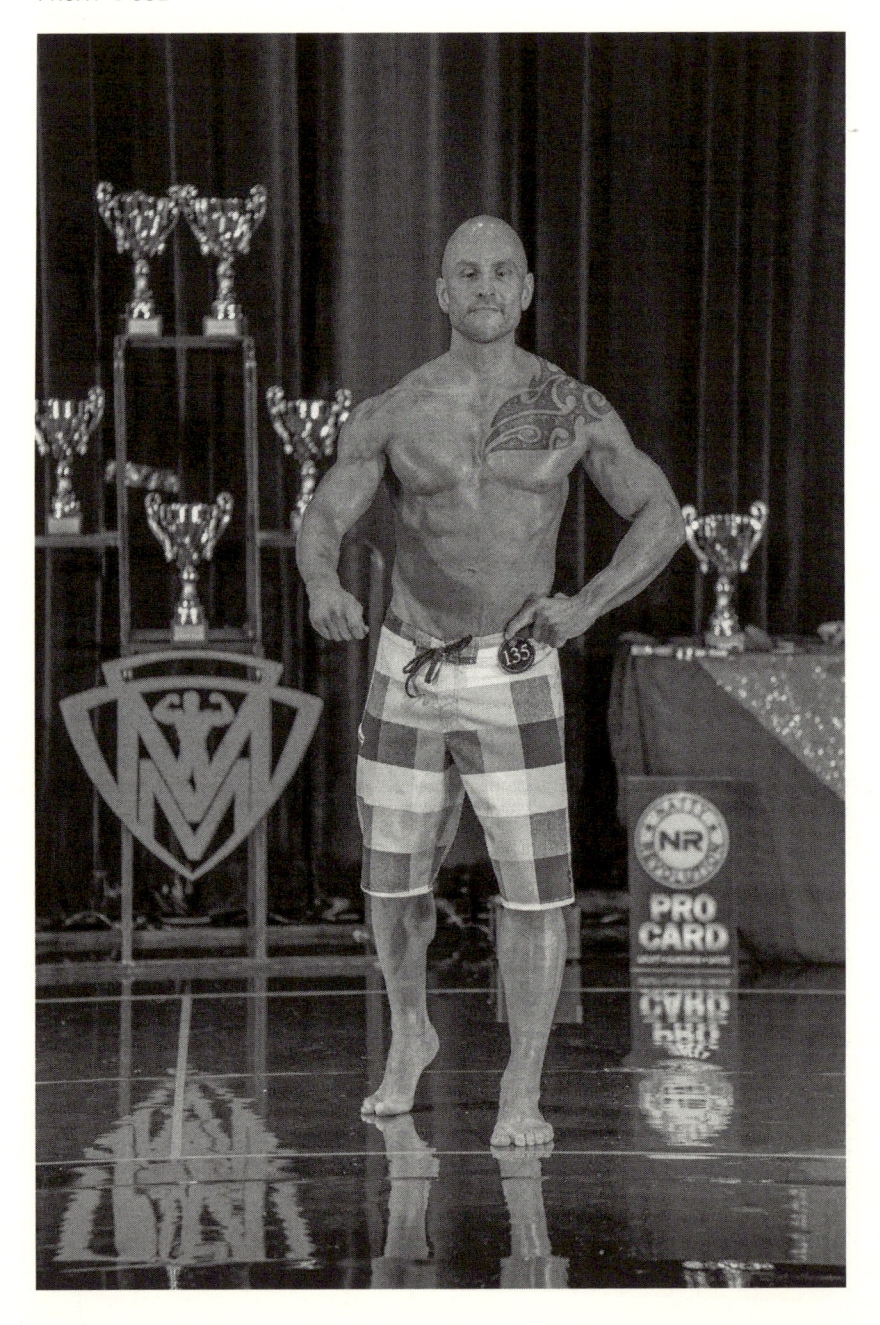

- Competitors will face the judges.
- The feet must remain parallel, but some lateral positioning of the toes is acceptable.
- Hands may be held at the sides momentarily to display symmetry, but this should not look like a bodybuilding front relaxed pose.
- Over-flexed posing and clenching of the fists is not preferred.
- Physique athletes shall have one hand on their hip on all quarter turns to differentiate men's physique from bodybuilding. The head judge will remind competitors to place one hand on the hip if needed.

344 / ROBERT ORION SIKES

SIDE POSES

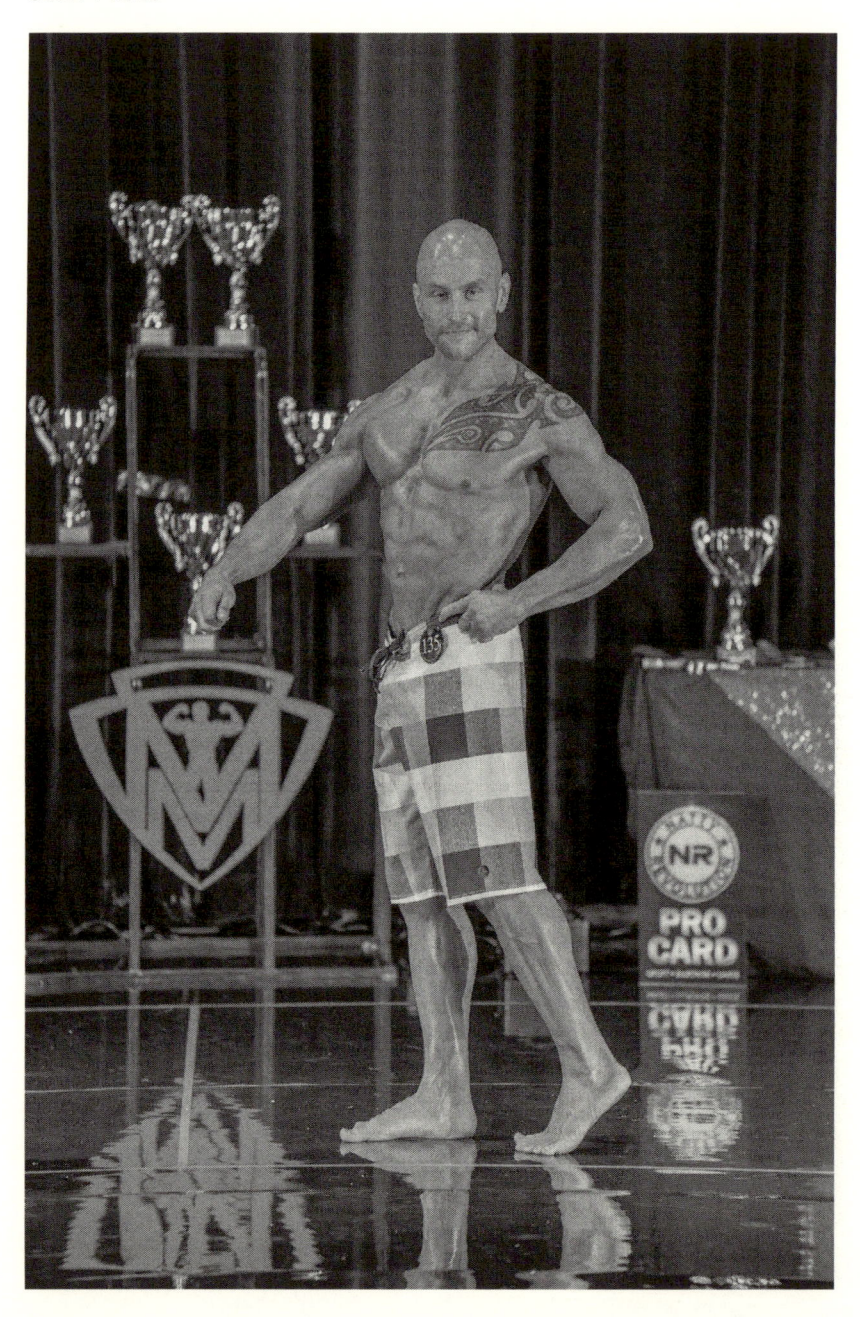

- Competitors' hips must face the side of the stage and heads should be turned toward the judges.
- Shoulders may be rotated as much as 35 degrees toward the judges to accentuate their V-taper.
- One arm shall hang down, and the other hand shall be placed on the hip.
- Feet shall be staggered and the back calf tightened.

BACK POSE

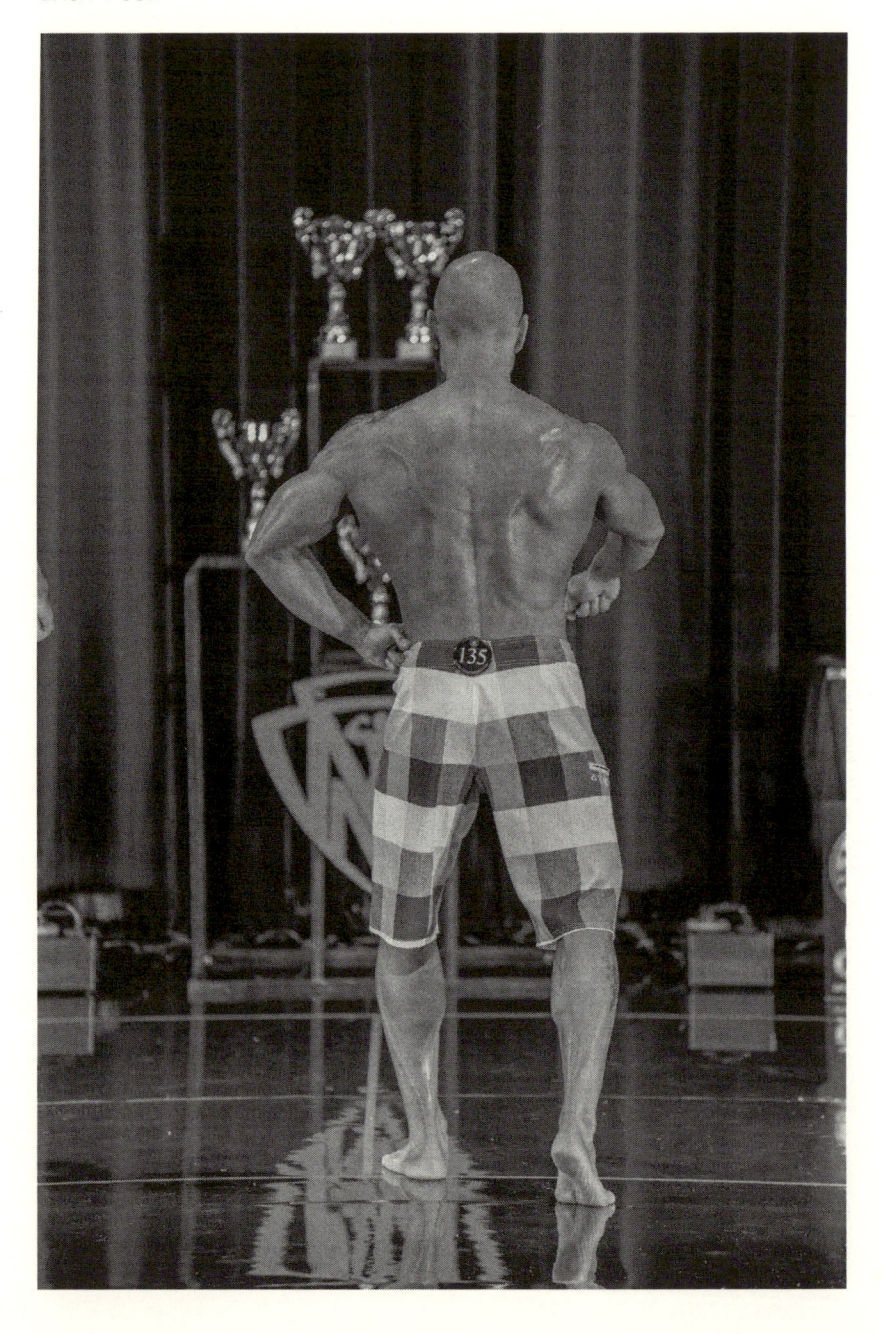

- Competitors will face the back of the stage.
- Feet must remain parallel.
- Lats should be spread to display V-taper.
- Hands may be held at the sides momentarily but then transition to one hand on the hip. The head judge will remind competitors to place one hand on a hip if needed.

INDIVIDUAL STAGE WALK

Conducted during prejudging, judges will evaluate poise and stage presence during the walk to determine the overall presentation score. If a T-walk is performed, competitors should execute a side pose facing the middle of the stage when posing on the outside posing location. At the center of the stage, competitors should perform a front pose, back pose and turn back to a front pose before walking to the following outside location.

Poses should not be held for more than three seconds each, and the entire individual presentation should be completed in 30 seconds (the head judge may allow more time depending on the size of the stage). For large shows, competitors will walk to the middle spot onstage and perform a front pose, side pose, back pose and finish with a front pose. In the large show format, competitors should complete their presentation in 15 seconds.

> *Note: Men's Physique competitors should execute no bodybuilding poses during competition.*

SCORING EACH ROUND

Judges will score each round and give competitors a final placement before moving on to the next round.

For example, if there are eight people in the class, the judging panel will place athletes 1-8 in each round. When judging is complete, both scores will be added together to develop the final placement for each competitor in that class.

* * *

MEN'S BODYBUILDING

The Bodybuilding Divisions will be judged through a series of poses that allow the judges to evaluate individual body parts and the "whole package." Athletes wear a bodybuilding posing suit.

COMPETITION ATTIRE

- Bodybuilding Posing Suit

ROUNDS JUDGED

ROUND 1: SYMMETRY

Symmetry encompasses overall balance and conditioning from top to bottom and side poses.

ROUND 2: MUSCULARITY AND CONDITIONING

Athletes will be judged on the size of muscles and conditioning/definition by executing a series of mandatory poses. Competitors must perform all mandatory poses in a timely manner. Judges are looking at the complete package from all parts of the physique, not just one body part at a time.

POSING EXECUTION

Note: At all INBF/WNBF events, the Head Judge reserves the right to penalize an athlete a ranking if the athlete refuses to perform the requested pose properly. The athlete will be given the warning to perform the pose correctly, and if the judge's request is ignored, a penalty may be imposed, affecting their final placement. Athletes will perform only the poses requested by the Head Judge.

SYMMETRY POSES

FRONT RELAXED

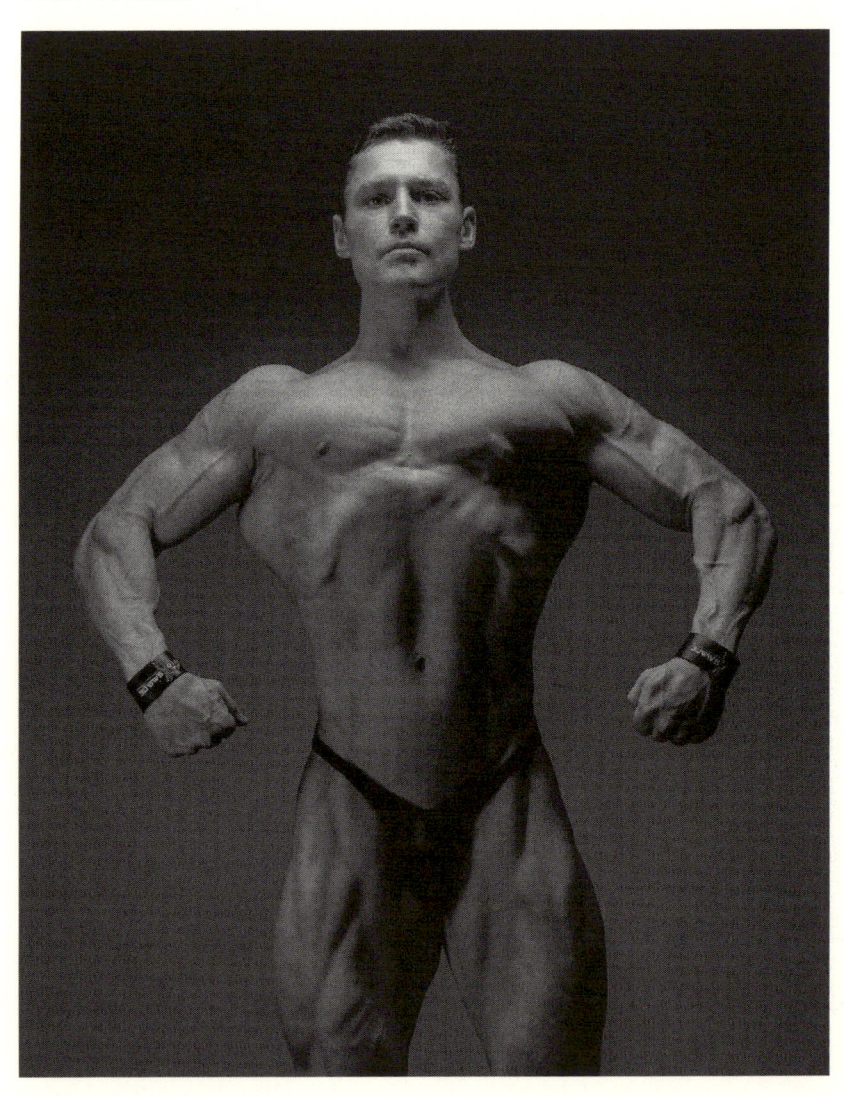

SIDE RELAXED

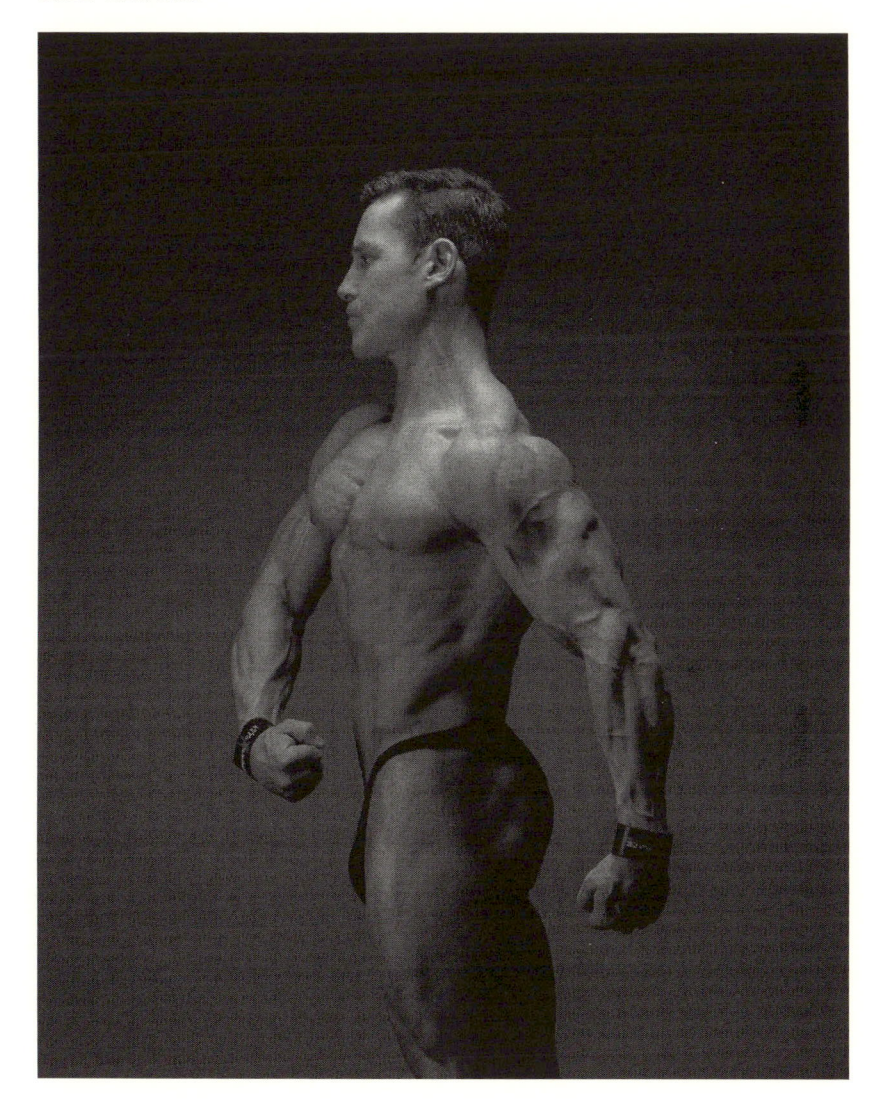

352 / ROBERT ORION SIKES

REAR RELAXED

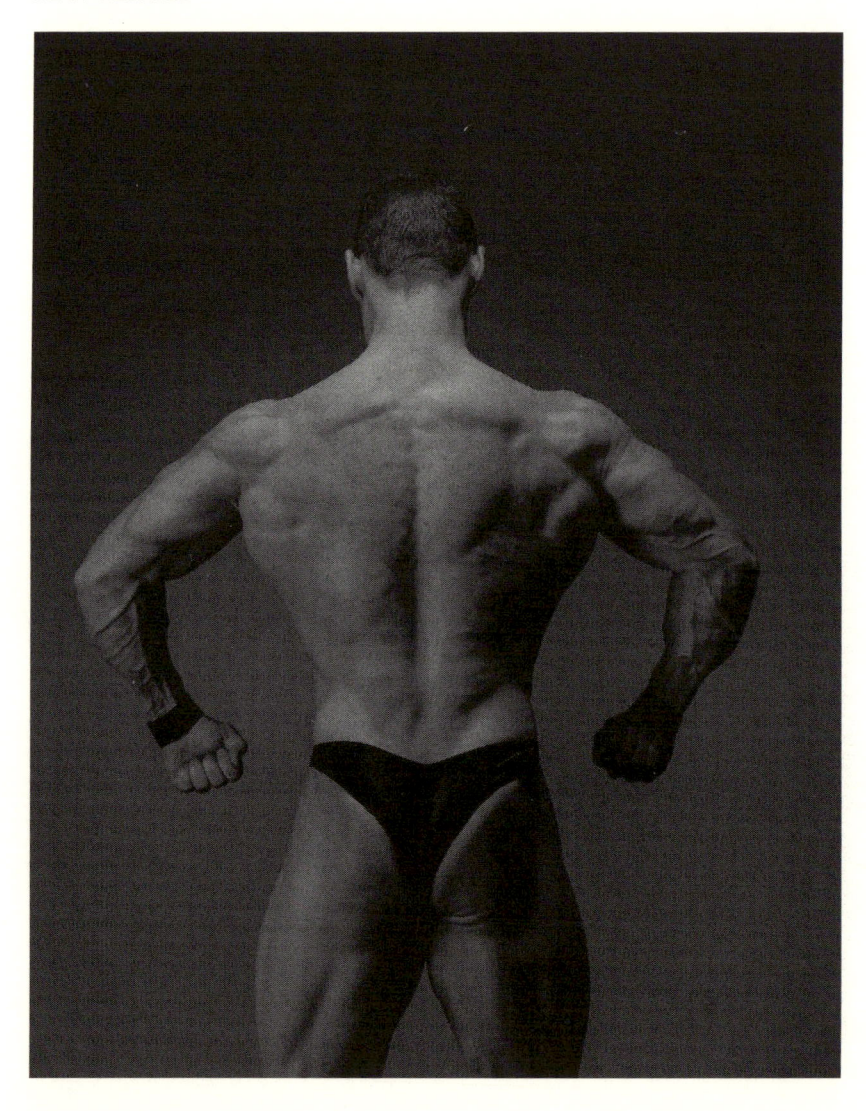

SIDE RELAXED, OPPOSITE SIDE

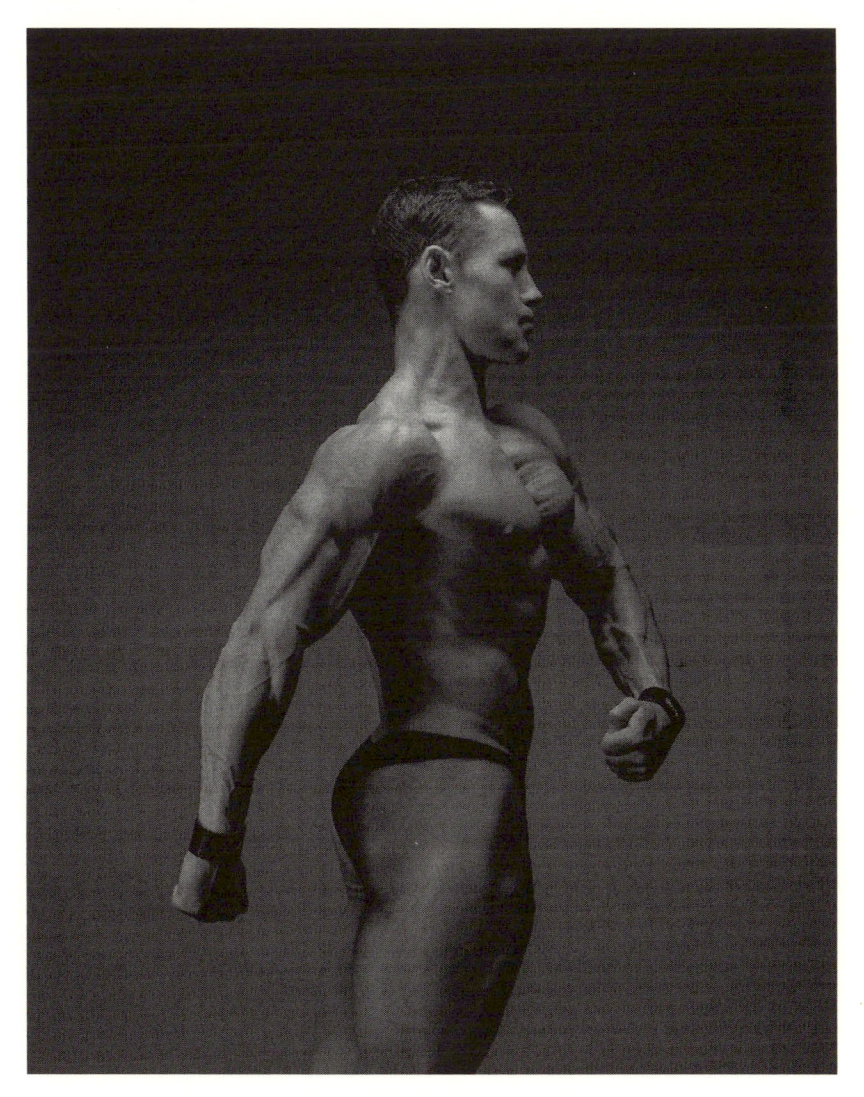

354 / ROBERT ORION SIKES

MANDATORY MUSCULAR POSES

FRONT DOUBLE BICEPS

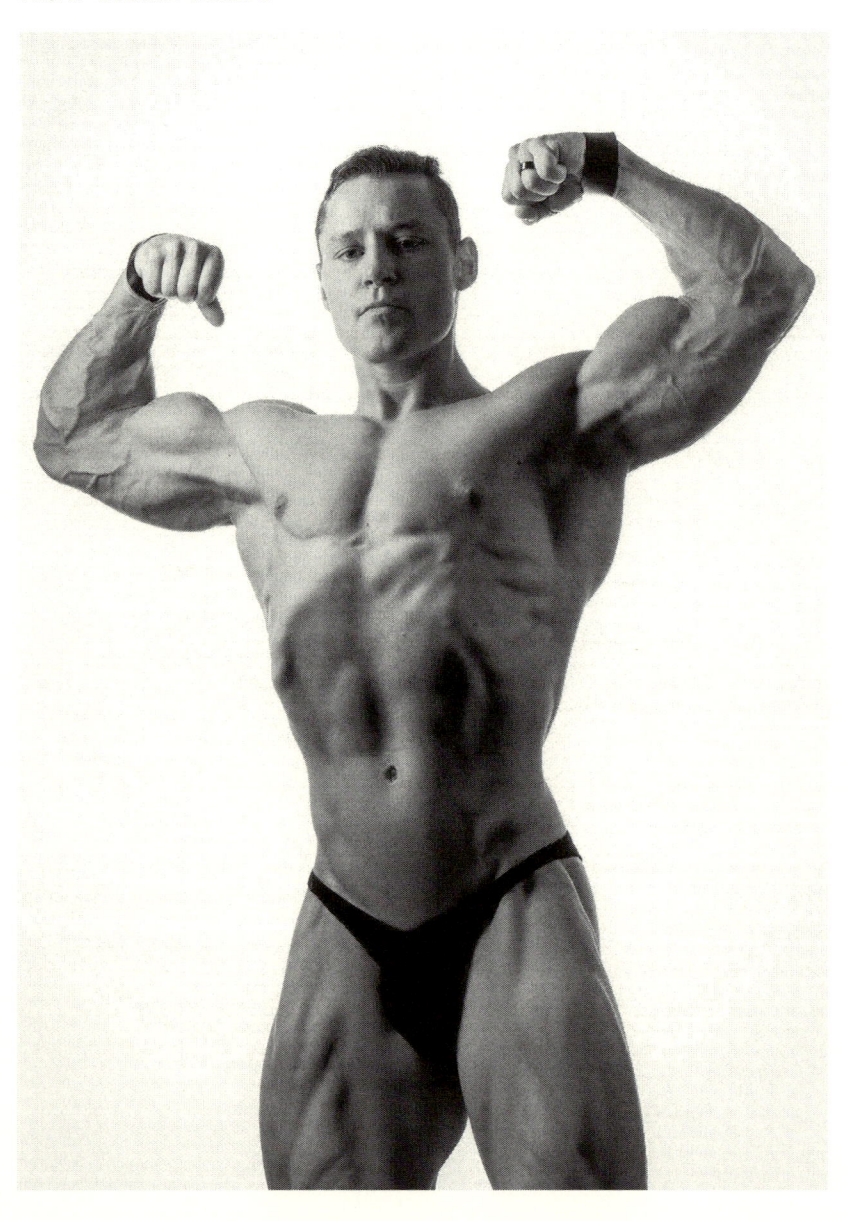

SIDE TRICEPS

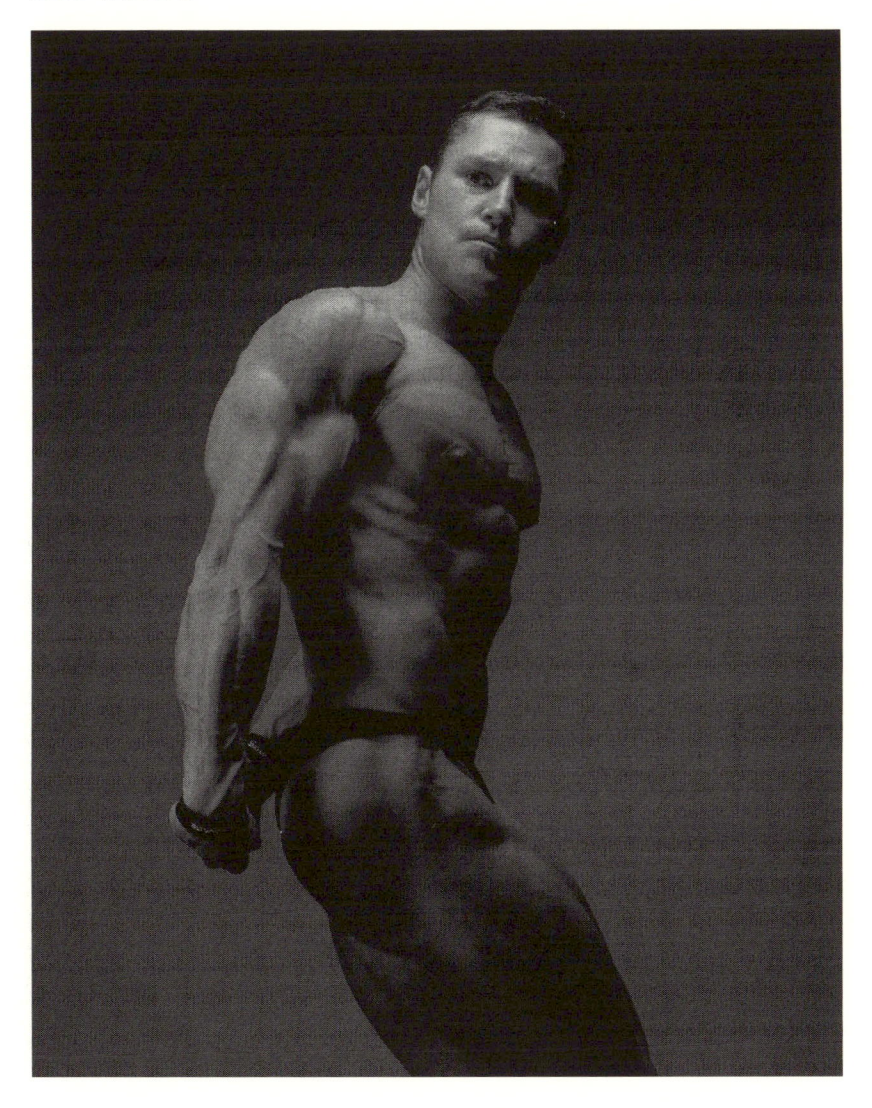

ABDOMINAL AND THIGHS

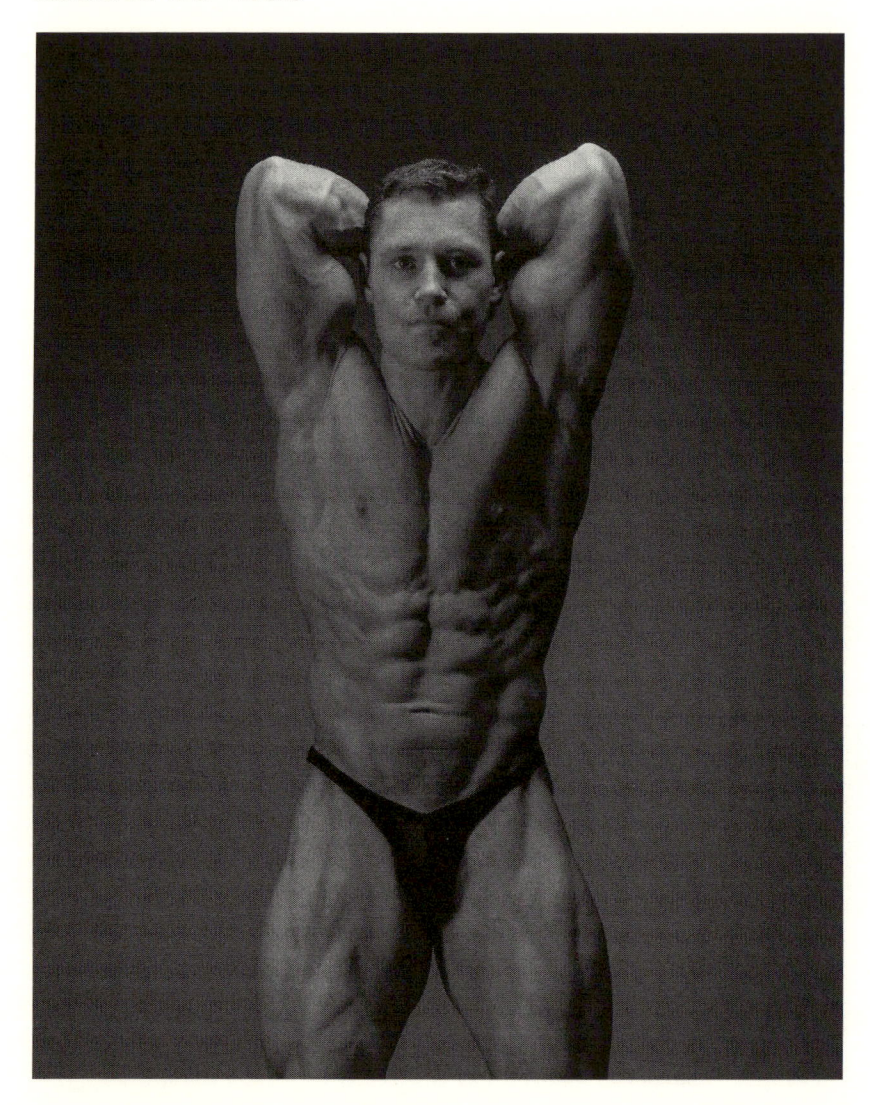

KETOGENIC BODYBUILDING / 357

FRONT LAT SPREAD

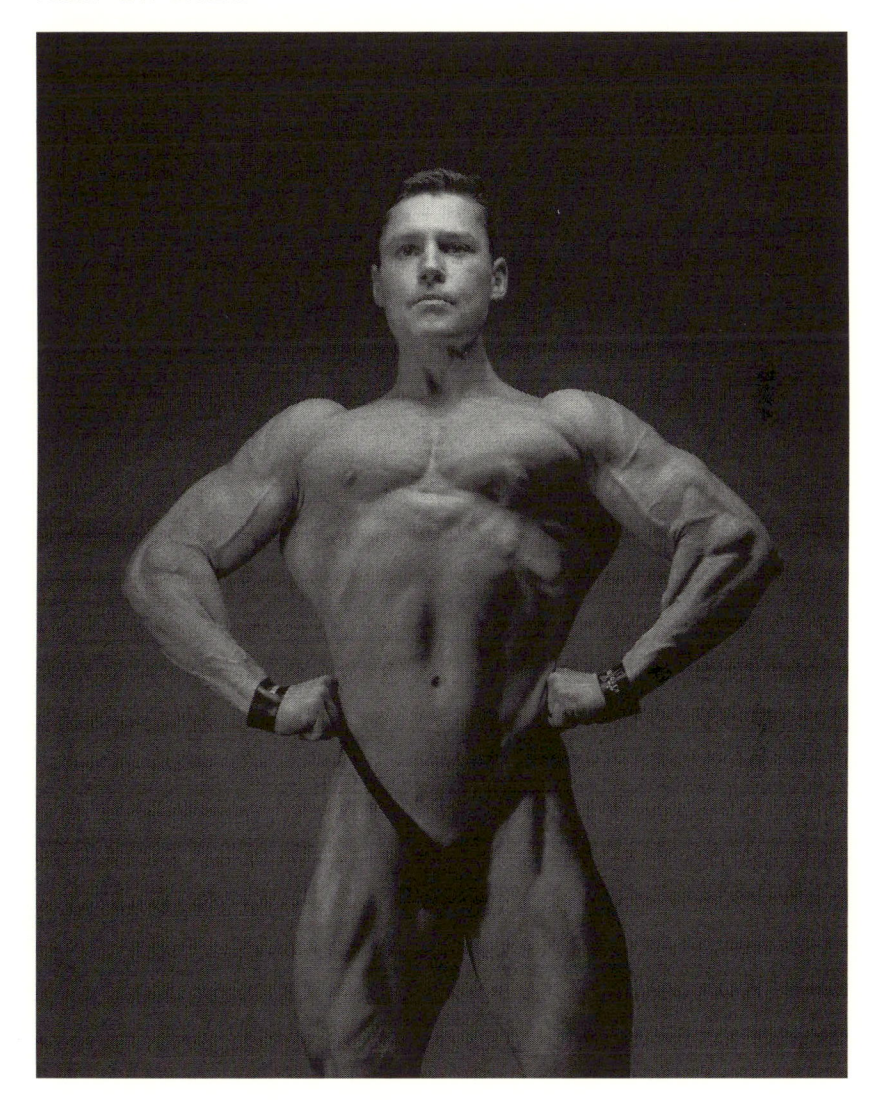

REAR DOUBLE BICEPS

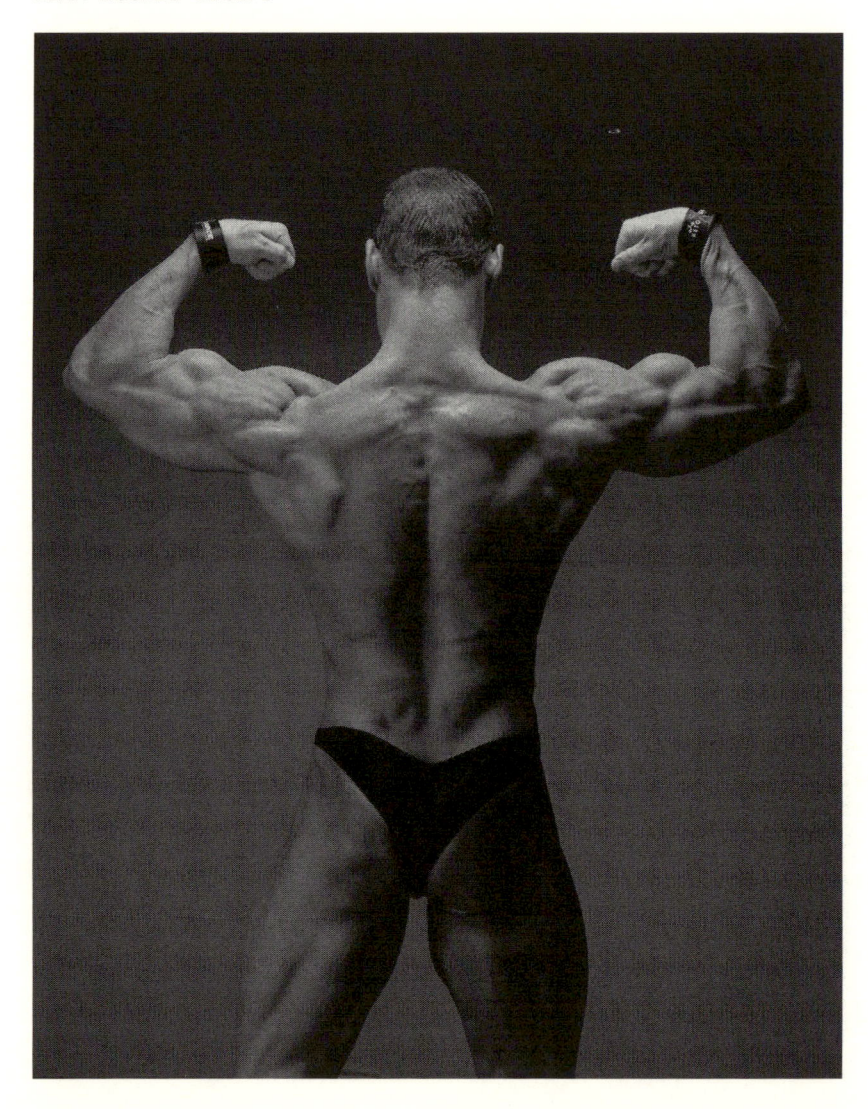

KETOGENIC BODYBUILDING / 359

HANDS-ON HIPS MOST MUSCULAR

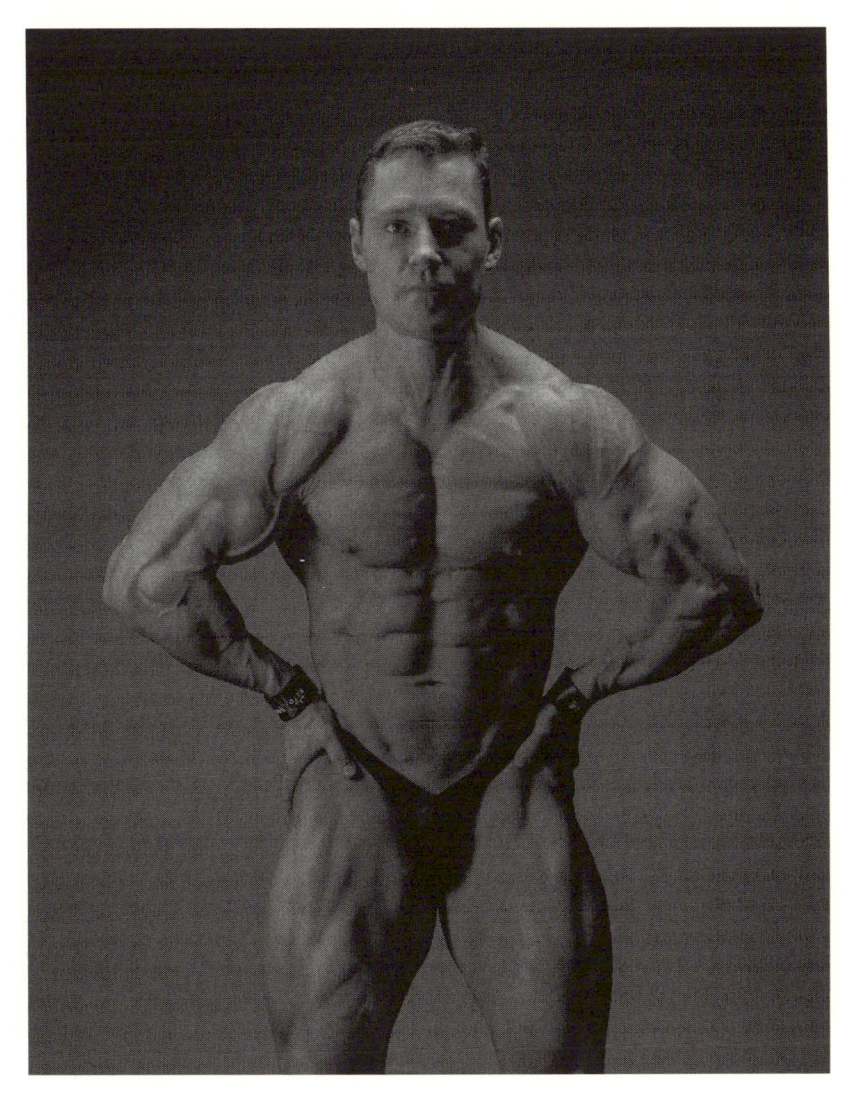

SIDE CHEST

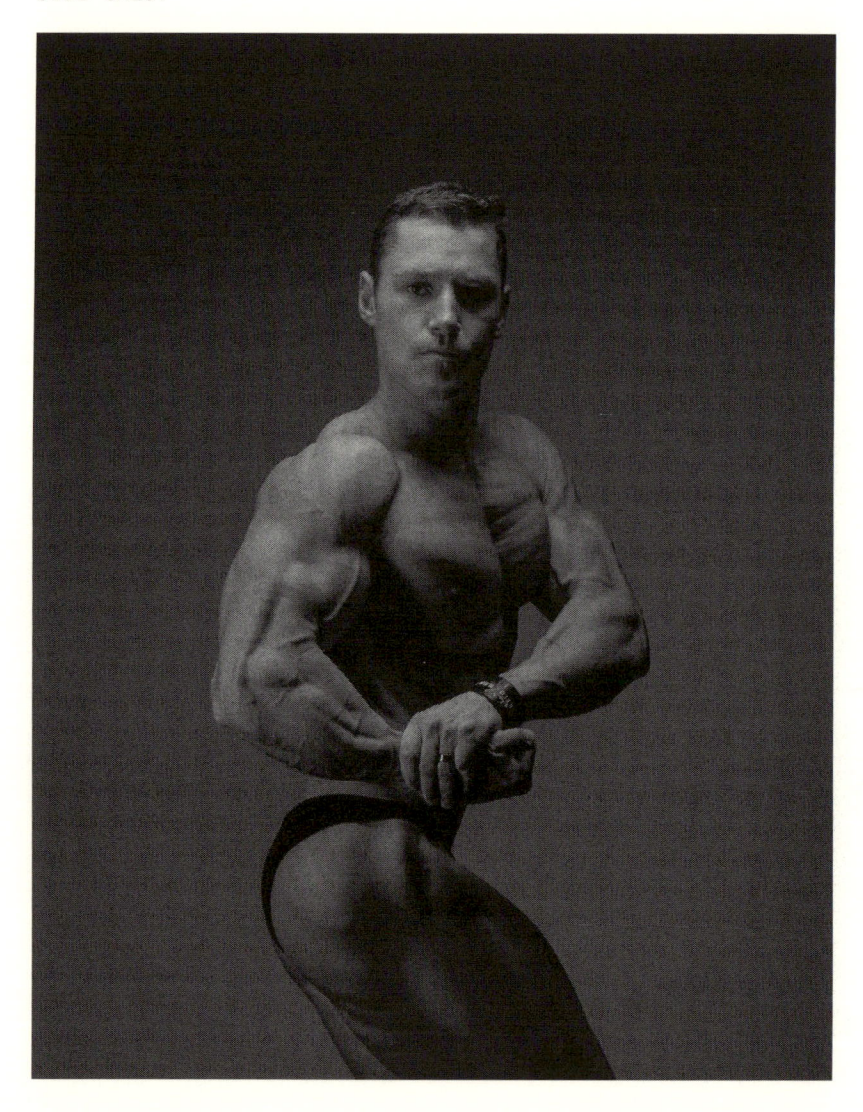

REAR LAT SPREAD

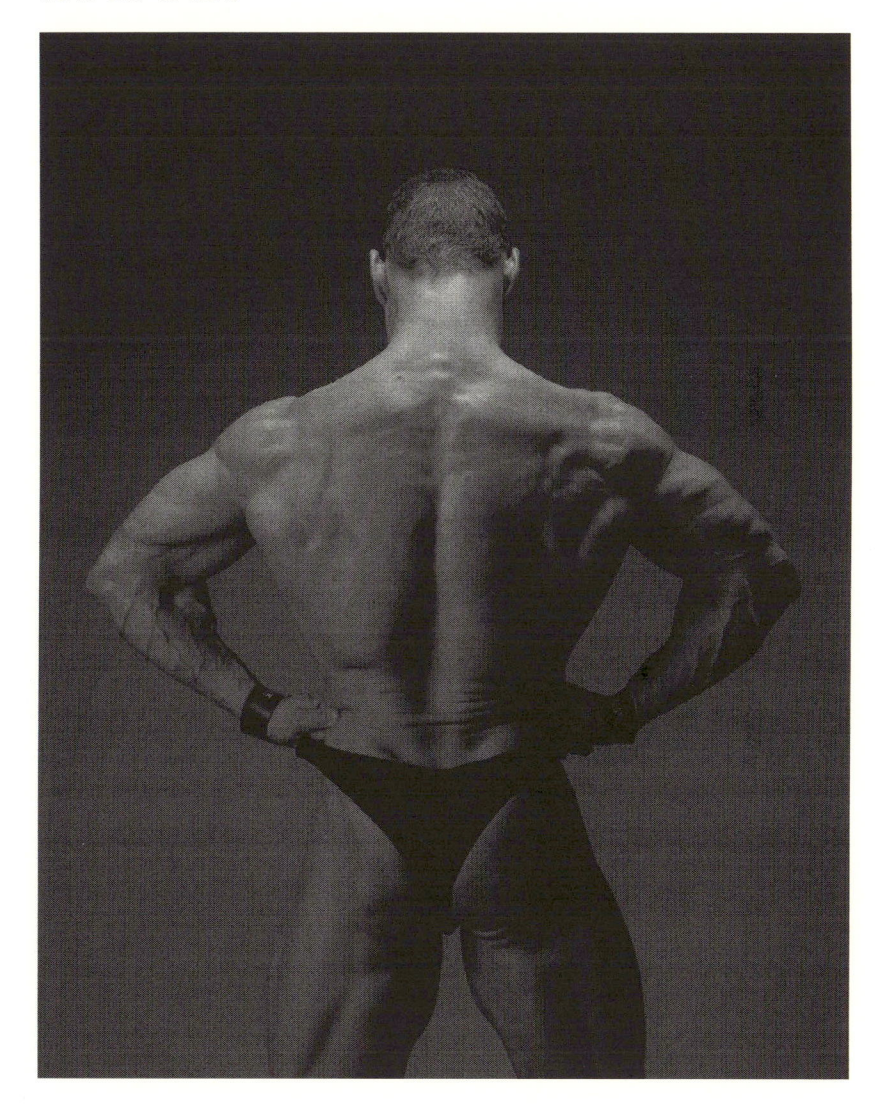

CRAB MOST MUSCULAR

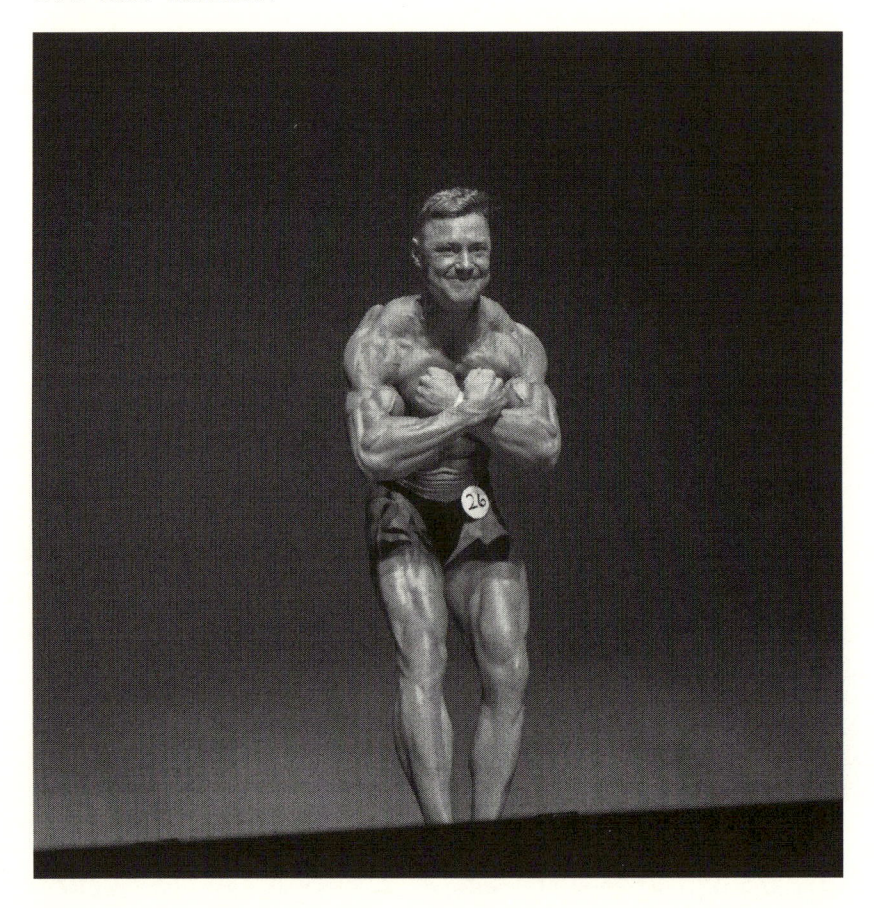

SCORING EACH ROUND

Rounds scoring differs by division, but the main guidelines for each division are described below.

INBF Amateur: Judges will score each round and give competitors a final placement for that round before moving on to the next round.

For example, if eight people are in the class, the judging panel will place athletes 1-8 in each round. When judging is complete, both scores will be added together to develop the final placement for each competitor in that class.

WNBF Professional: Judges will score each round and give competitors a final placement for that round before moving on to the next round.

For example, if there are eight people in the class, the judging panel will place athletes 1-8 in each round. When judging is complete, both scores will be added together to develop the final placement for each competitor in that class.

Pro-Posing Routines: Final placings for professionals will be determined after free posing routines are finished. Judges may break ties or move a competitor up or down one placing in this final judging process.

* * *

MEN'S CLASSIC PHYSIQUE

The Classic Physique Division is not currently offered by many of the natural bodybuilding federations. It is not an option within the INBF/WNBF federation at the time of this writing. However, I want to include a quick discussion of it here and present the posing requirements of the NPC federation.

It's been fantastic to see the popularity of the Classic Physique Division take off as many people have become less impressed with the mass monsters and more focused on building an aesthetic physique of shape and symmetry. Classic Physique was created as an outlet for returning to the traditional roots of bodybuilding, popularized in the golden era of Frank Zane, Arnold Schwarzenegger and Serge Nubret, when a tiny waist and proper proportions were the goals. I hope this new division continues to thrive and creates greater interest in developing a physique reminiscent of the foundation from which bodybuilding was built.

COMPETITION ATTIRE

Competitors are required to wear posing shorts. You are *not* to wear board shorts or bodybuilding posing trunks. Competitors must wear the same type of cut, and all shorts worn in competition must be black.

All suits will be inspected at the check-ins. Every competitor must wear their competition suit under their clothing to check-ins for inspection. If your suit is not inspected, you will not be permitted to compete. No exceptions.

MANDATORY POSES

The judging will consist of comparisons of the symmetry round quarter turns and the following five mandatory poses:

KETOGENIC BODYBUILDING / 365

FRONT DOUBLE BICEPS

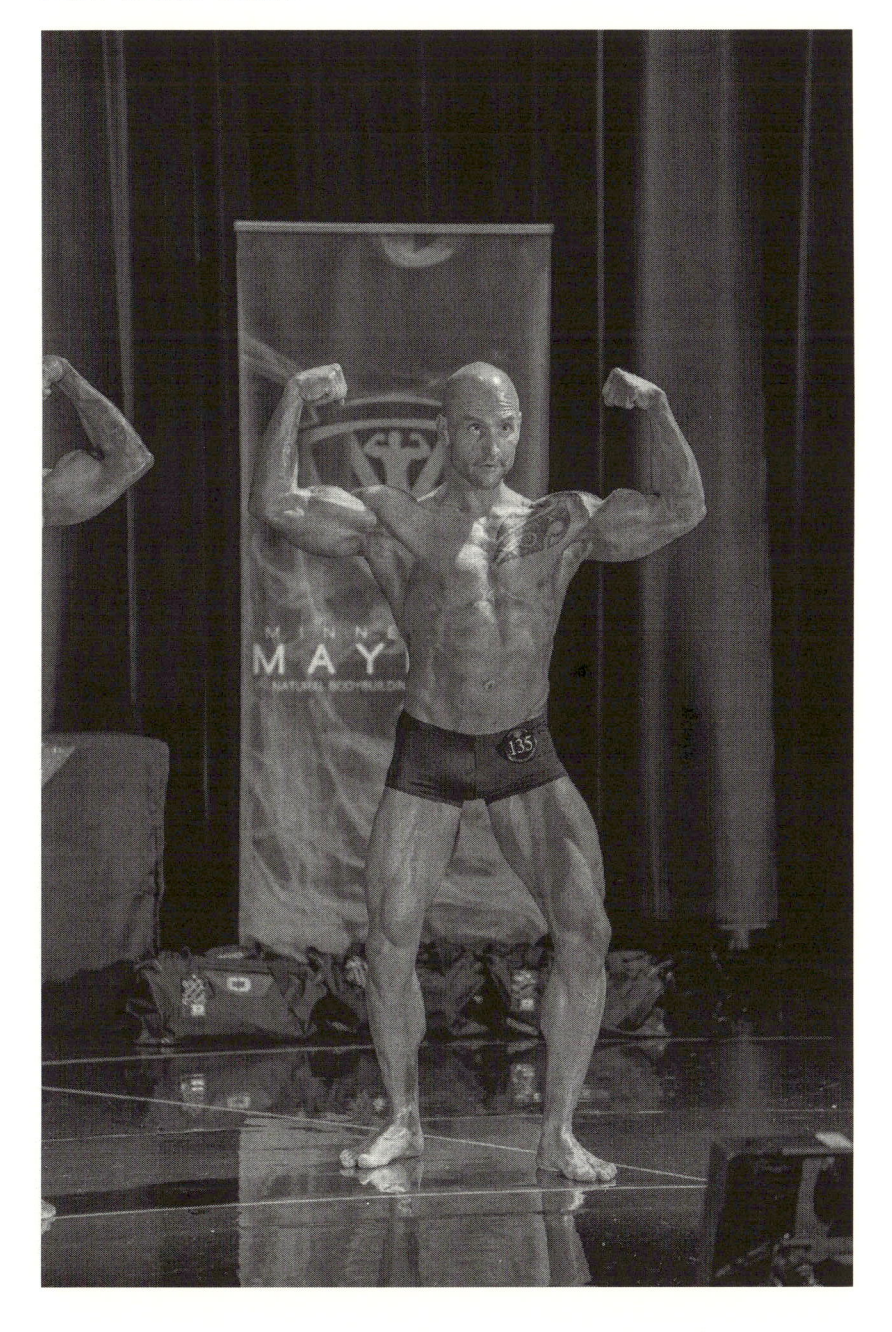

SIDE CHEST

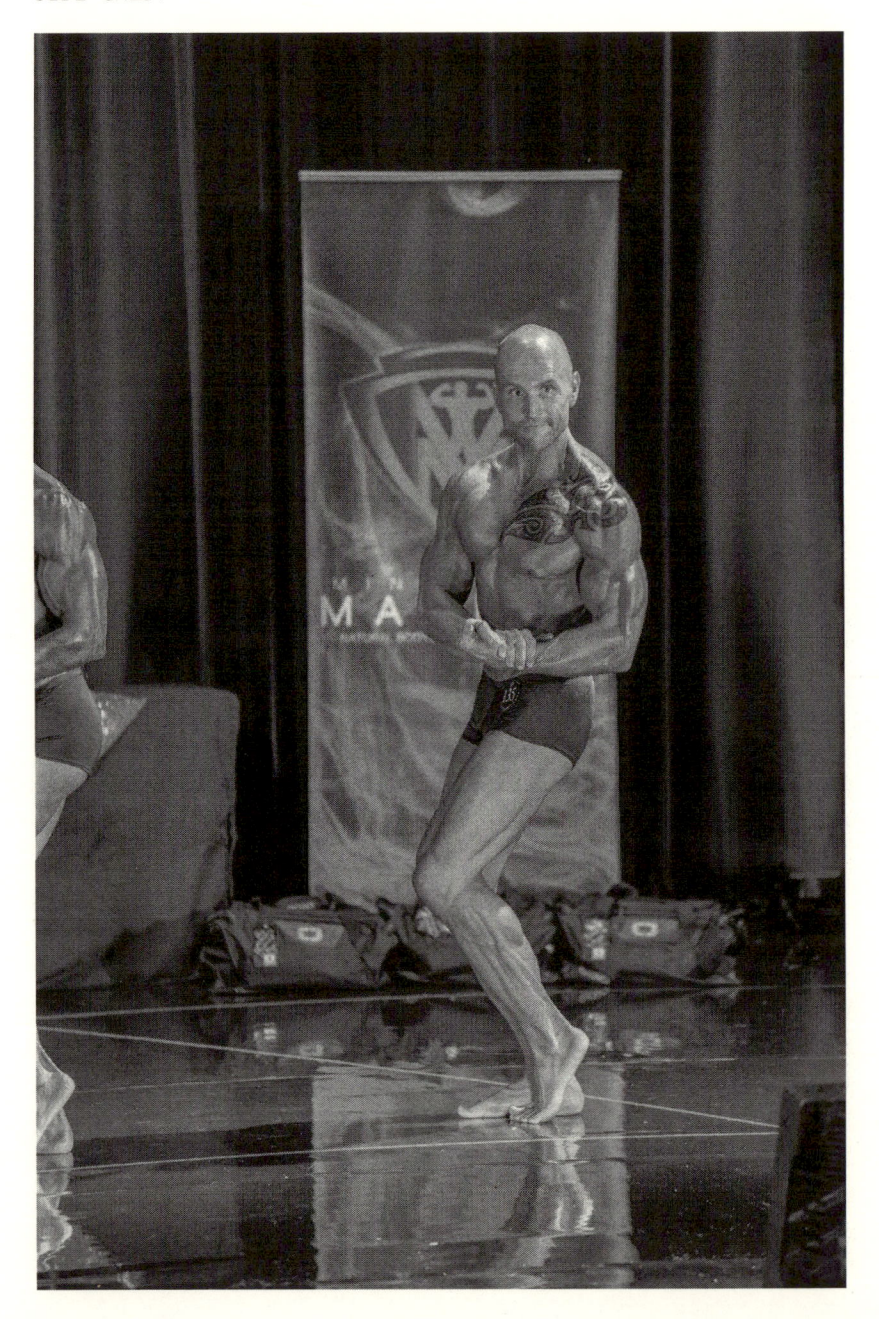

BACK DOUBLE BICEPS

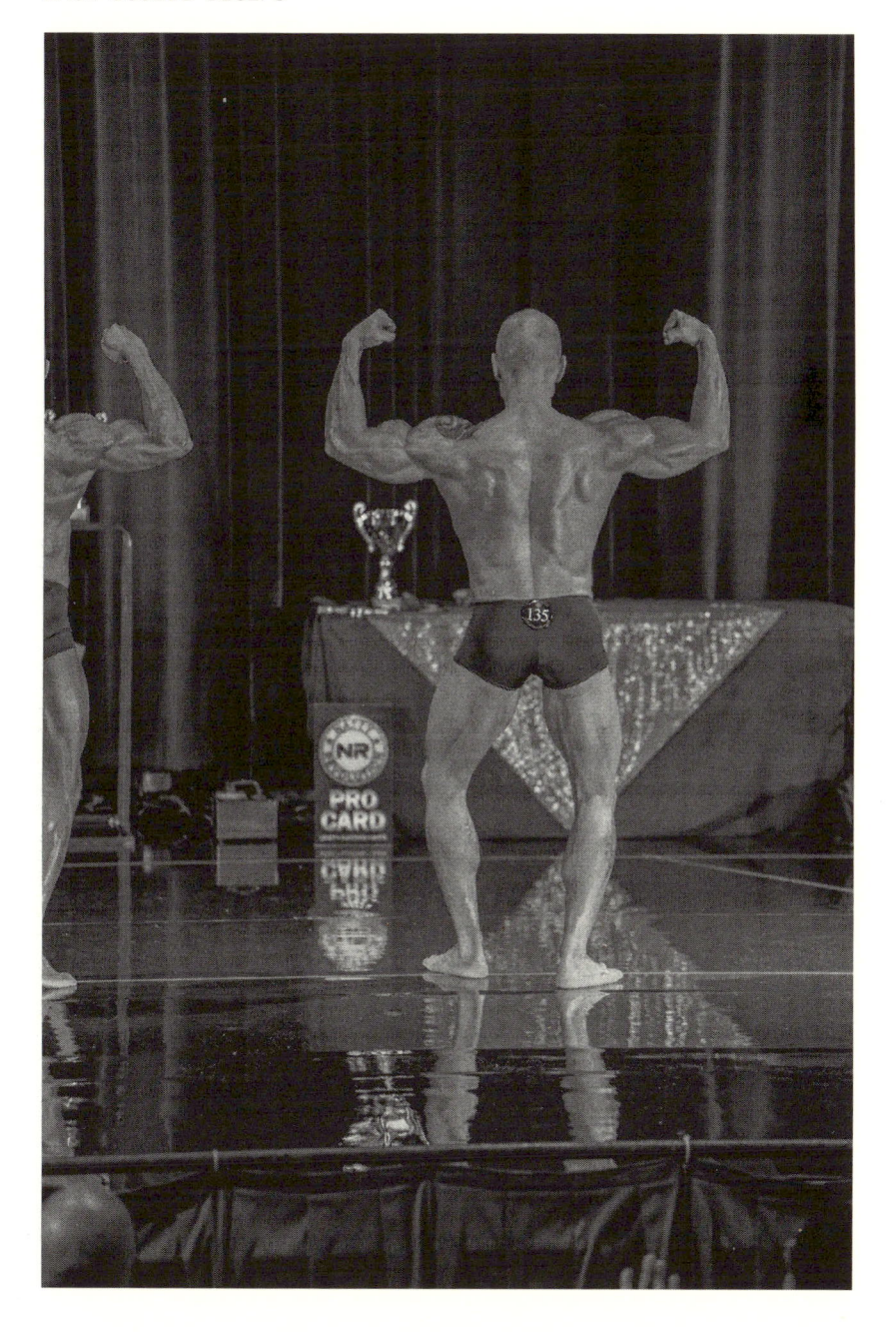

ABDOMINAL AND THIGHS

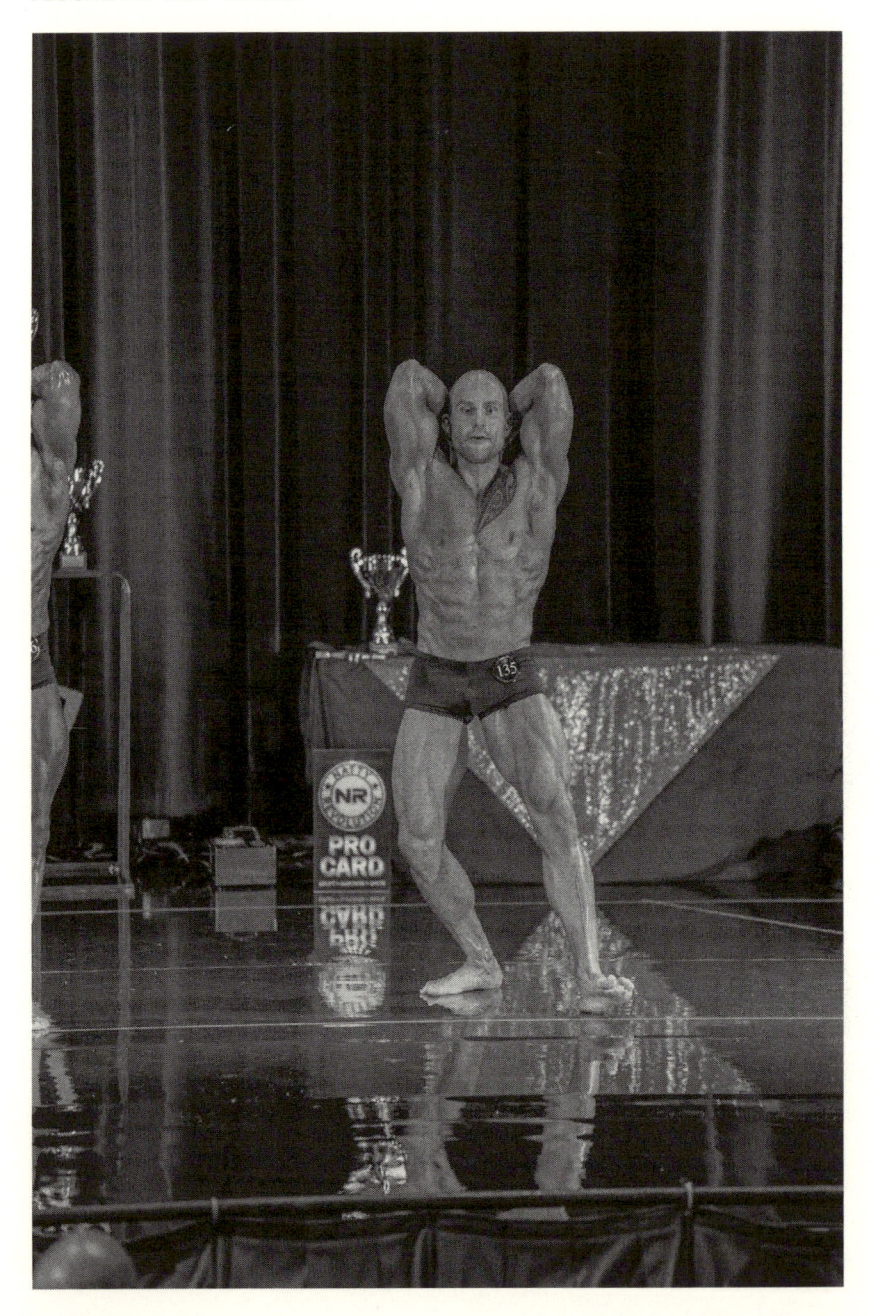

KETOGENIC BODYBUILDING / 369

FAVORITE CLASSIC POSE (NOT MOST MUSCULAR, VACUUM POSE PICTURED BELOW)

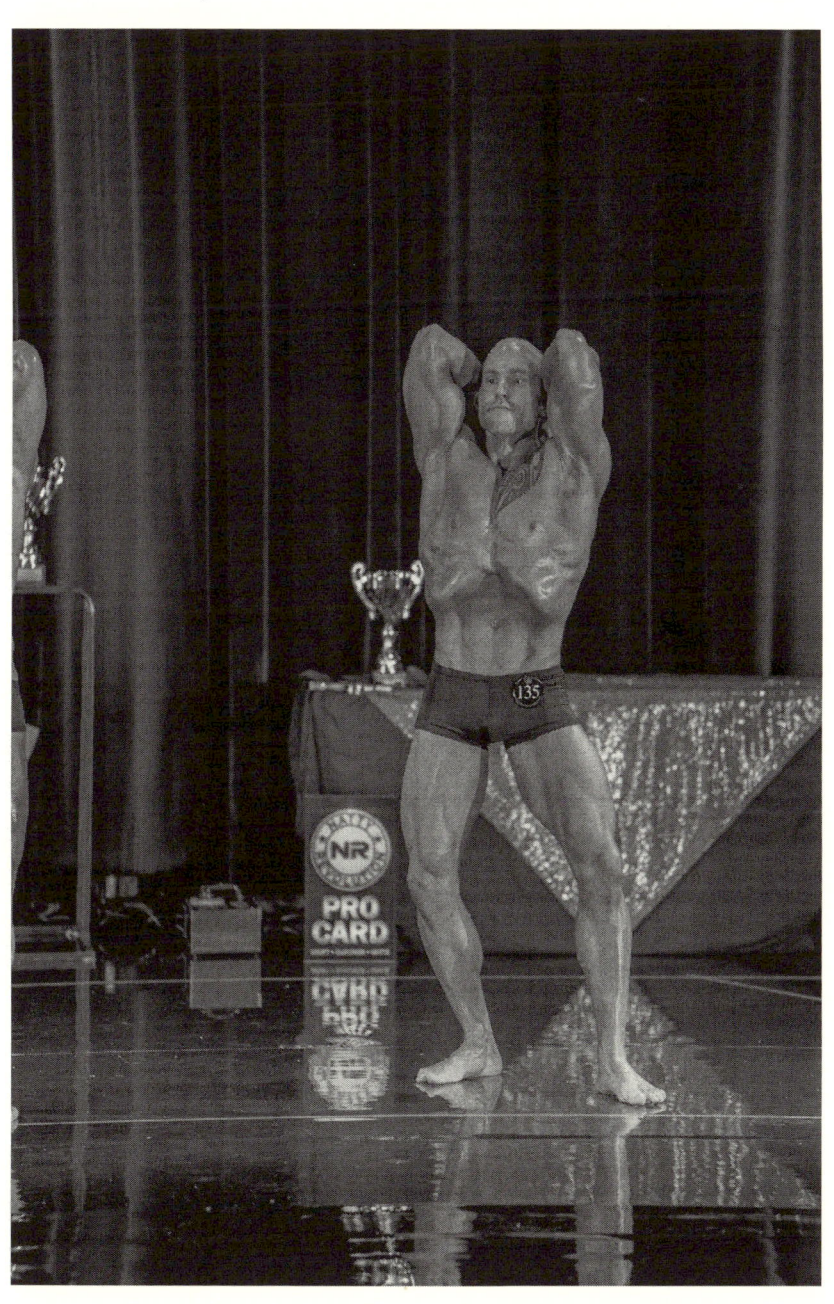

[3]
EXERCISE APPENDIX

EXERCISE APPENDIX OVERVIEW

As mentioned earlier, the purpose of this book is not to teach proper training form and function; I'll assume you are well versed if you're considering a competition prep. Still, there is just as much bio-individuality in the training department as there is within nutrition. What works wonderfully well for one individual may not be effective at all for another. Experiment with your training to see what works well and is sustainable for you. That said, I'd like to use this appendix as a repository for some high-level training principles and techniques that are generally accepted. I'd also like to provide you with a detailed template of the training protocol I've implemented throughout my last several years of competitive bodybuilding with a high degree of success.

RESISTANCE TRAINING

Resistance training is simply the act of physical exercises designed to improve strength and endurance.

Everyone would benefit from resistance training whether they intend to step onstage or not. Many people take up weight training to simply look good naked, and there is nothing wrong with that; however, strength training does more than increase lean muscle tissue. It also leads to better bone density, stronger tendons, joints, ligaments, better body composition, improved metabolic rate and a laundry list of other perks. I would encourage people to resistance train as a simple hedge against sickness and poor health span if nothing else. Incorporating a structured training protocol into your life is one of the single most effective means of improving your health and longevity.

CARDIO

Aerobic exercise or "cardio" training is designed to improve the strength and endurance of the body's cardiovascular system. This system relies on oxygen to adequately meet energy demands during exercise via aerobic metabolism. There are many different forms of cardio ranging from LISS (Low Intensity Steady State) cardio, which involves a consistent, steady stimulus like walking on a treadmill or using the Stairmaster, to HIIT (High Intensity Interval Training) like running hill sprints or cycling through battle ropes.

For the sake of accuracy, I prefer to implement more LISS cardio when my goal is centered explicitly on body composition. I'll incorporate more HIIT if I'm trying to focus on metabolic conditioning and improve my time at an obstacle course race or something of that nature. When trying to account for all variables and manipulate your training with a high degree of accuracy, I highly encourage you to stick with a form of cardio that can be standardized and tracked. LISS tends to work better in this regard and also makes it much less likely you'll pull a muscle or risk injury. You are much more susceptible to injury when in an extreme deficit and sleep-deprived, so it's generally better to play it safe in competition prep.

PROGRESSIVE OVERLOAD

Our bodies are incredibly adaptable. If we constantly provide a stimulus in increased resistance, our bodies adapt by creating more muscle fibers and stronger tissues to withstand that increased resistance. If that resistance holds steady, there is no demand on the body to adjust further. This explains the concept of progressive overload. Our goal as bodybuilders is to progressively overload our bodies to ensure increased stimulation and demand for further growth and adaptation. This adaptation leads to increased strength and muscle hypertrophy. The following pages demonstrate a variety of techniques you could implement to overload your training progressively.

INTENSITY

Training intensity refers to the difficulty of the actual exercises throughout a session. Usually, this corresponds directly to the total weight lifted and the Rate of Perceived Exertion (RPE). For example, say the RPE scale goes from 1-10. A 10 would indicate that you are going all out with maximum effort. You wouldn't be able to perform another rep if your life depended on it. A four or below would indicate that you aren't exerting yourself much at all, and it would be no trouble to pump out multiple reps with little issue. The higher your exertion on the scale, the more intense the workout. Numerous techniques can be leveraged to increase the intensity beyond weight alone, but weight is usually the most manipulated factor.

VOLUME

Volume refers to the summation of the total weight moved when the number of sets, reps and weight are all factored together. Simply multiply sets by reps by weight to calculate your total lifting volume for a given training session.

FREQUENCY

Frequency is simply the number of times you train throughout the week. If you divide your training into body part splits, frequency refers to the number of times you target a specific muscle throughout the week.

* * *

Training intensity, volume and frequency are the three primary levers you can manipulate to stimulate your body to adapt, strengthen and grow lean tissue, thus resulting in the ability to overload your training progressively.

HOW TO MANIPULATE THESE VARIABLES

A Google search for the best training split and style will yield more controversial and conflicting results than a simple query for nutrition. People have been arguing over the best ways of building muscle since the first caveman picked up a heavy rock. Scientific research on the subject is pretty daunting as well. Like nutrition research, one can find studies that support or deny anything they want.

Rather than get lost in the minutiae, I tend to experiment for myself to see what my body best responds to. Generally speaking, it isn't possible to go all out on all three variables. You can't sustain maximum intensity with a ton of volume on an incredibly frequent basis, as doing so doesn't give your body time to repair and grow. As such, it's usually best to think of these three levers using a "high, moderate, low" rubric.

For instance, you can train with high intensity, but you're better off implementing lower volume and moderate frequency if you go that route. Conversely, if you train with high volume, you should probably implement moderate intensity and lower frequency.

Periodization is the act of modulating through these three variables and having periods of higher intensity, periods of greater volume and periods of greater frequency to reach a desired goal. There are several variations of this, which is where you'll genuinely have to experiment to see which combination works best.

Some people perform wonderfully with incredibly high-volume training. It's not uncommon to see them crank out sets of 20 or 30 reps each and train the same muscle group multiple times throughout the week. On the opposite end of the spectrum, I've seen people have tremendous success with super short but incredibly intense workouts that only involve one or two working sets at a very heavy weight. These people often won't train the same muscle group for another six or seven days.

With such a broad spectrum, how could I possibly suggest a protocol that is best for *you*? I can't. It would be impossible. You'll have to try a variety of styles and see what resonates with you most. If you respond amazingly to high intensity but hate it and dread going to the gym, you're not going to be able to sustain it, and therefore it's not optimal for you. Like nutrition, the most crucial factor here is consistency. Anybody can go all out in the gym for a single training session; there's nothing too impressive about that. What *is* remarkable is witnessing somebody be consistent with their training every week, every month, every year, every decade and so on. Above all, determining which style is most sustainable for you is the most critical factor.

Another important training characteristic is the mind-muscle connection. The mind-muscle connection is a phrase that often gets tossed around in conversation, but what is it? Simple: having a connection between your mind and your muscle means training with intention and purpose.

Practice feeling the individual muscle fibers contract as you move weight throughout an entire range of motion. So many people walk into the gym and go through the motions. They pick up a heavy weight or bang out a ton of reps, but they lack the focus necessary to maximize their training potential. If you are distracted throughout your workout, you can't possibly learn everything your body is telling you. You can't know with any degree of certainty if you are feeling a full contraction. A distracted mind leads to a limited body. Be present and be aware. Walk into the gym with a sense of purpose and train accordingly. If you do this consistently, you cannot fail.

TRAINING FOR KETO

Rather than give you a long-winded answer, I'll keep things simple. You *do not* have to train any differently if you are following a ketogenic diet! That said, you will most likely experience a temporary dip in training performance as you first start a ketogenic lifestyle, and you should plan accordingly.

When you completely shift your body's primary source of fuel and energy from carbohydrates and glucose to fat and ketones, it makes sense that your ability to perform at a high rate temporarily takes a hit. Still, that temporary dip doesn't mean you should alter your training! Simply give your body the time it needs to adapt. If you need to go a tad lighter with the weights or reduce your volume slightly, so be it.

Don't feel like you have to alter your split structure or training techniques. Depending on your lifting style, resistance training can be an incredibly glycolytically demanding sport. If your body hasn't adapted to preserving and replenishing muscle glycogen without dietary carbohydrates, you'll likely feel more fatigued and have difficulty obtaining a great pump. That is temporary. Do what you are capable of, and your body will return to or exceed your previous best as soon as you are fully adapted. This is why I highly encourage individuals to be deeply keto-adapted before diving into a competition prep!

ADVANCED TRAINING TECHNIQUES

The following techniques can be leveraged to increase the intensity of a training session beyond simply increasing the resistance or the number of repetitions.

MUSCLE FAILURE

Before we dive into various techniques to go beyond our natural muscle failure, let's first explain what muscle failure is. Muscle failure is simply reaching a point in a session or set where you can no longer complete another repetition.

For instance, imagine you're training chest with the barbell bench press exercise. If you're able to knock out 10 reps at 225 lb and then reach a point where you lower the weight but can't get it back up if your life depended on it, you've reached muscle failure. Your chest muscles have "failed" the repetition. Many people advocate for training to failure regularly as a means of increasing overall training intensity. In general, I'm a fan of doing this on the last movement set to not drastically diminish my overall training volume. I do not advocate for failure training on every set, as you'll likely pre-exhaust yourself too early in the workout.

SUPERSETS

Supersetting my exercises is one of my favorite methods for increasing training intensity and reducing overall time spent in the gym. Suppose you have two exercises left to do. Rather than doing your set on one, taking a rest set and then jumping back into another, simply perform your set on the other exercise during your "rest set" from the first exercise.

I love supersetting opposed muscles within the same muscle group—for example, biceps and triceps. I can do four sets of bicep curls and four sets of tricep extensions in half the time by simply supersetting the two. I'll bang out a set of bicep curls, skip my rest set and go immediately to the cables to knock out my tricep extensions. Once those are done, I'll immediately repeat another set of bicep curls.

By super setting opposing muscle groups, I still allow each muscle adequate time to recover before targeting it again. My bicep muscle is "resting" as I'm doing the tricep extensions and vice versa. While it's not a true rest set, it's generally ample recovery to not inhibit either bicep or tricep training. The result is significantly more blood in the entire arm and an enhanced pump.

GIANT SETS

Giant sets are similar to supersets, but they contain additional movements. Supersets usually alternate between two different exercises, whereas giant sets generally consist of four or more. You would cycle through four or more exercises with minimal rest and then rest for a minute or two at the end of that "giant set." The entire circuit is only one set and is repeated several times to comprise the whole workout session.

PYRAMID SETS

Pyramid sets are an excellent hedge to include more volume and more intensity at once. Pyramid sets, as the name suggests, pyramid up in weight and down in reps.

For instance, imagine you are doing four sets of bench press. Rather than simply doing four sets of 10 reps at a constant weight, you would start with more reps in the beginning and pyramid up in weight while simultaneously reducing the number of repetitions. I'll often do this with a 15, 12, 10, 8 scheme. On bench press, I may do 135 lb for 15 reps, 155 lb for 12 reps, 185 for 10 and finish with 205 lb for eight reps. One of the main benefits of this structure is that it allows your muscles and joints to warm up with a lighter weight before going into heavier sets.

DROP SETS

Drop sets are a simple way to increase volume and intensity without a high risk of injury. A drop set is simply the act of dropping the weight after you've reached muscle failure at a given weight and continuing with more repetitions at the lighter weight. For instance, say I reach muscle failure on my last bench press set after several reps of 225 lb. I wouldn't be able to do another rep at 225 lb, but if I strip a 45 lb plate off each side of the bar and am left with 135 lb, I can crank out a few more reps.

Since I'm training with a lighter weight, I can hit a few more reps and increase the overall volume lifted. A general rule of thumb is to go into the drop set relatively quickly without a long rest set in between. I like to drop the weight and go immediately into the next set at a lighter weight. This drop set protocol can be repeated multiple times with each additional set using a lighter weight.

NEGATIVES

Doing negative reps is a slang word for eccentric training. The eccentric movement throughout a rep is the portion of the movement that lengthens the muscle. This is the opposite of the concentric movement, which involves the contraction of the muscle. We are stronger on the eccentric portion of the repetition than we are on the concentric. This provides a unique opportunity to train past our natural muscle failure.

Continuing with our bench press analogy, say you have reached muscle failure at 225 lb. You couldn't lift the 225 lb bar off your chest if you had to, but if you had a skilled spotter who could raise the bar for you, you could easily control the weight on the way back down throughout the eccentric or "negative" portion of the repetition. This is a spectacular method for pushing your body beyond its natural sticking point and increasing overall training intensity. It's crucial to have a skilled spotter when training negatives with free weights. If you're training solo, many of the machines make it easy to push the resistance beyond the "sticking point" and focus on the eccentric portion of the exercise.

FORCED REPS

Forced repetitions are like negatives in that they allow you to train past your natural muscle failure and generally require the help of a spotter. Unlike negatives that focus on the eccentric range of motion, forced reps also involve pushing through the concentric portion. This is where a spotter comes in.

A skilled spotter can support your elbows or the bar while doing a bench press and provide a little assistance—just enough to help you push through the entire repetition. While it's true that you aren't lifting the total weight, you are still increasing your overall training volume and intensity by squeezing out a few more reps, even with slight assistance. The key word is "slight"—if your spotter is the one doing most of the work and you just leave the extra weight on the bar to appeal to your ego, you're not doing yourself any favors. Drop the weight and do the work yourself.

TIME UNDER TENSION

Time under tension is, as it sounds, the amount of time your muscles are subjected to an exercise's resistance. More time under tension equates to more muscle stimulation and growth. Increased time under tension demands more muscle control and balance and forces you to work on all your complementary stability muscles.

As it relates to overall lifting volume, time under tension can be a bit tricky. Say you're doing bench press and lifting 135 lb for 4 sets of 10 reps. That would yield a total training volume of 5,400 lb. That holds whether you lift that weight as quickly as possible, letting it fall to your chest on the eccentric portion of the rep, or if you go incredibly slowly, controlling throughout the entire range of motion. One technique is more challenging than the other, but that isn't necessarily reflected in the total training volume. This is where measuring only volume as a proxy for training progress can be a bit iffy.

I am a huge advocate for training with quality form and function. Ideally, the last rep of your heaviest set will look just as flawless as your first rep on your lightest warmup set. I realize that this is often wishful thinking and much more easily said than done, but we should strive for it. As such, having control of the weight throughout the entire range of motion is of paramount importance. This control will most certainly increase the total time under tension, as you will likely be moving a bit more slowly throughout the repetition.

PARTIAL REPS

I'm going to use this section on partial reps to contradict myself. I stated earlier that the full range of motion and increased control is of paramount importance. That is true, but what happens when you simply can't muster another rep at the full range of motion? You can drop the weight, or you can knock out a few partial reps. Partial reps are simply another tactic to shorten the overall range of motion and eke out a few more reps to stimulate your muscles further. These often aren't as pretty as they should be, and you may get a few looks at the gym; however, a few partial reps are better than nothing, given the option between partials and simply calling it quits.

* * *

The tactics above only scratch the surface of what is possible in your training. There are countless ways of increasing training intensity to push your body a bit further than you previously thought possible. Still, these are the basics—and you can't ever go wrong with the basics! Feel free to sprinkle these intensity techniques throughout your training split to increase the overall training stimulation and keep things interesting. As with everything we've talked about, be sure to give your body time with each technique so you can genuinely gauge its effectiveness.

YEAH, YEAH—BUT WHAT SHOULD *I DO?*

Personally, I like intensity; it makes me feel alive. I like to push myself to the limit and feel like I'm accomplishing something when I step into the gym. For that reason, I'm a massive fan of going heavy, pushing the envelope, implementing a ton of drop sets and supersets and leaving the gym utterly exhausted.

In all honesty, I would probably still train this way even if definitive research came out that said high intensity was the least effective way to leverage the three variables. I just prefer training in this manner. That said, I also like doing enough repetitions of a given movement so that I can get an amazing rush of blood. Because of this tradeoff, I tend to find myself in the 8-12 rep range with most movements. I'll go a little lower than that and stick with 4-6 reps on some of my heavier compound lifts and will go a bit higher than that (around 15 reps) on some of my smaller muscle group auxiliary lifts.

Over my several years of training, I've improved my muscular endurance to a point where I can lift with a relatively significant degree of intensity at this 8-12 rep range. I'm not too fond of powerlifting-style training that involves incredibly long rest sets and very few repetitions. I also don't prefer a ton of lower-weight, higher-volume training because I love racking a ton of weight on the bar. Depending on the split I'm using, I train each muscle group once or twice a week. This frequency has proven effective at my intensity level and gives my body ample time to recover before targeting it again.

As stated earlier, I can't possibly give you an exact training protocol that will work best for you. Even so, I've included a few sample templates at the end of this training appendix that will give you a foundation to build from. Implement these into your routine to see how your body responds.

I preached the importance of tracking metrics and stats throughout the bulk of this book as it relates to the prep and our nutritional manipulations, and the same is true when experimenting with your training protocol. Stick with a given protocol for long enough to measure if it's working or not. I typically recommend at least three or four months on a given program.

Track as many relevant metrics as possible. Your weight, your body composition, lean mass, fat mass, strength and measurements as well as how you feel, your recovery, your sleep, your hunger and your satiety as a result of the training, how you look in the mirror, your new PRs and your ability to consistently increase your progressive overload: these are all factors that can provide great insights on the efficacy of your training routine.

TRACKING YOUR TRAINING

All this talk of training metrics and body stats begs the question: what can you use to track your training progress?

Just as there are dozens of apps to track macros and calories, there are dozens of apps to track your training. Many of these apps allow you to track the changes in total volume lifted over time, monitor new PRs and even log your RPE on a given set. The fancier apps also include plate weight calculations, rest timers and automatically generated training templates.

To be completely honest, I still haven't found a training app that I'm absolutely in love with. Fidgeting with my phone throughout a workout to enter data is quite distracting and can hinder my ability to train at a higher intensity. As such, I often train intuitively and keep a solid mental tab on what I lifted the prior week and what I need to try and best. The downside to this method is quite apparent: I don't have nearly as much data on my training over the years.

Throughout my last competition prep, I used a training app called RepCount to ensure that I didn't drop below my volume or training intensity as I got deeper into prep. That is the main priority and benefit of leveraging one of these monitoring apps. As calories drop, you want to fight the urge to decrease your training volume and intensity. It will be harder to maintain your lifts with fewer calories coming in, but it's crucial to try and do so. Maintaining training intensity and volume throughout your prep is the best way to ensure you don't lose much of your lean tissue while in a caloric deficit.

Many people ditch the apps altogether and go old school with a pen and paper. I'm entirely onboard with this philosophy if it works for you. I generally do not recommend untracked, intuitive training during a prep unless you have quite a bit of experience under your belt and are incredibly in tune with your body.

What about apps and wearables that track your caloric expenditure throughout the day? Oura Rings, watches, WHOOP straps and Fitbits have become very popular over the years to monitor step count, heart rate, sleep and recovery. I think these apps are great at providing a rough estimate of your NEAT activity. For example, you may start this journey at a healthy maintenance intake and be brimming with energy throughout the day. You probably skip to work, are on your feet all day and walk every evening after dinner to burn all your pent-up energy. However, as calories decline, you may find yourself dragging your feet and scanning the room for comfy chairs to rest in.

This energy shift often happens subconsciously and without warning. In those cases, step count calculations or estimated caloric expenditure can be helpful pieces of information. If you can see this trend moving downward, you can correct course and try to fight it with more intentional evening walks or by spending more time playing with your kids.

I do not put much stock in the accuracy of caloric expenditure calculations as they pertain to training. Wearables are not great at gauging intensity, and that variable will have a significant impact on actual caloric expenditure. I don't ever recommend using the estimated caloric expenditure from these apps as hard data. Certainly don't factor it into your meal planning, macro manipulations or refeeds. It's nice to have as a way of keeping track of your NEAT activity, but there is still no way of assuring its accuracy.

All your training and nutritional manipulations should be based on how you look and feel and what your body composition stats show you. I've seen many ill-informed individuals look puzzled after comparing their wearable's estimated caloric expenditure and the nutrition app's total caloric intake. Just because your wearable says you're burning more calories than you're consuming doesn't mean you actually are! Don't get caught up in misguided addition and subtraction. Focus on what your body is telling you daily, not on what your wearable suggests.

This concept holds true for your "recovery index" as well. Many apps consider your sleep time and quality, heart rate, HRV and other factors to generate a recovery or "readiness" score. This score is designed to show you if you are fit for duty that day or not. If the score is low, the app prompts you to take a rest day and recover. If it's high, you're permitted to train hard. I may be ruffling some feathers here, but I am not a fan of these readiness scores at all. More often than not, I see people use these low scores as an excuse to be lazy.

I can't tell you the number of PRs I've hit in a training session after my Oura Ring suggested I "take it easy" that day. Maybe I'm stubborn and just train harder to spite my wearable; that is certainly a possibility. I just don't think these readiness calculations are all that accurate. I am a huge fan of leveraging the data you have available to make informed decisions; however, I'm not a fan of leaning on readiness scores at the expense of learning to read your own body.

You know if you feel good or not. You know if you can train hard and kick ass. You also know if you're totally whupped and need to take a day to let your body recover. You shouldn't have to lean on a watch to grant you permission one way or the other.

DELOAD WEEKS

A "deload" week involves lifting at significantly reduced intensity and volume so your body can fully recover from the progressive overload you've been subjecting it to. The scheduled rest days sprinkled throughout your training protocol are great, but sometimes you need more than a day or two. This is where deloads come in.

There isn't a standardized method for implementing deload weeks, as it will be different for everyone. I'll often implement a deload week after six to eight weeks of consecutive training if my body seems to need it. Some indications could include lingering plateaus, the inability to go heavier, trouble recovering or nagging injuries. If you don't lift with much intensity, you'll likely be able to go longer in between deloads.

Just as there are no standards for how often you should do a deload, there aren't any standards for *how* to do them. Some people take the week off entirely and don't pick up a single weight; others find success in continuing to lift heavily but with a significantly reduced rep count and volume load. I prefer to train at about 40-60% of my usual training intensity and focus on increasing time under tension and muscle contractions. By going much lighter, I can have maximum control over the weight I'm moving. This increased control allows me to focus on perfecting my form and increasing the total time under tension.

Fixating on the contraction of every single muscle fiber throughout a range of motion is an effective use of my deload weeks. This generally results in a ton of blood flow despite the reduced intensity. My central nervous system gets a break by simply reducing the heavy loads throughout the deload week, and I often come back stronger than ever the week after. A structured deload protocol is one of the best ways to ensure your progressive overload training blocks are sustainable and that they improve over time.

Implement a deload week during your competition prep if necessary, but don't leverage them too frequently. Remember, your ability to implement more progressive overload principles will be hindered as your calories continually drop. The main priority is to maintain the muscle you've built. Deloads can be effective during competition prep, but they are generally used while in a building phase. Being tired in an extreme deficit is bound to happen, so don't use deloads simply because you want to shirk your training and binge Netflix while you should be pumping iron.

ADAPTATIONS TO TRAINING OVER TIME

Keep in mind that our bodies are adaptable. Just as we experience metabolic adaptations to increases and decreases in calories, we also experience adaptations to our training.

When you first start lifting, your body is shocked with all the new stimuli you're subjecting it to. As a result, many beginner lifters can put on significant lean mass seemingly against all odds. These "newbie gains" can come when in a caloric deficit—they can even come with poor training form and poor nutrition! It's almost as if a beginner lifter can do everything wrong and still put on a ton of muscle. This honeymoon phase of resistance training doesn't last forever, though.

As you become more and more experienced, your body matures and adapts to the constant training load. As such, it becomes much more difficult to continue seeing significant increases in lean mass. It's not uncommon for a new lifter to put on 20 lb in their first year of training, whereas a natural athlete who has been lifting for several years is happy to put on a few pounds of solid lean muscle tissue a year!

As you continue to train, you'll notice fewer changes in overall size but more significant changes in muscle maturity. How your muscles look and function will continue to improve. Your total weight may not change much from year to year, but your proportions, symmetry and overall condition will likely improve significantly. Through it all, remember that building lean muscle tissue takes a lot of time. If you're a natural athlete, recognize this and embrace it wholeheartedly. Don't get down on yourself if you don't add 10 lb to your frame year after year. Play the long game and fall in love with the lifestyle. Train regularly with intensity and purpose and the muscle will come. The compounding effect of this consistent training year after year is what leads to truly remarkable physiques.

CHANGES TO RESISTANCE TRAINING THROUGHOUT PREP

As I mentioned in the primary text of this book, your resistance training shouldn't change drastically throughout your competition prep. Many people make the mistake of thinking that their training should differ significantly between a building phase and cutting phase. This simply isn't the case.

The misguided belief that you need to lift heavier weights with fewer reps to build and less weight with more reps to cut needs to die. On the contrary, continuing to train hard and heavy is one of the single best things you can do to ensure you retain as much lean muscle tissue as possible during prep while in a caloric deficit.

When you're in an extreme deficit, your body looks for anything and everything it can to fuel its bodily functions. Muscle tissue is incredibly demanding from a metabolic standpoint, requiring a ton of calories to maintain. If you're not using that muscle tissue, your body sees no need to support it and will catabolize it to fill the gap created by fewer calories. However, if you continue to subject your muscles to the rigors of intense and strenuous training, your body will be less likely to tap them as a fuel supply. It's a simple case of "use it or lose it."

There is no need to train less intensely or with lighter weight. That said, it will become much more difficult to train hard and heavy as the calories continue to drop. Fight the urge to lighten the load—it's where the mindset component comes into play. Strive to continue training hard despite your waning energy and fuel supply. Don't beat yourself up if you aren't hitting any new PRs throughout the prep. If it does happen, great! Just don't expect it. Instead, keep training as hard as possible to preserve as much lean mass as possible. You've worked hard to get that muscle; now, work hard to keep it!

CHANGES TO CARDIO THROUGHOUT PREP

Cardio, on the other hand, should change quite drastically throughout your prep. As mentioned in the book, it's best to start with minimal cardio. Use it as a "trick up your sleeve," so to speak. As discussed above, our bodies adapt to whatever we subject them to. If you start with seven days of cardio a week, your body will quickly adapt and you'll have no room left to increase further.

Implement cardio with a minimum effective dose mentality—the least you can do to elicit a positive response, the better. Most compositional changes will result from dietary manipulations throughout this contest prep. Cardio will be one of the levers you can pull as changes from nutrition alone become less pronounced.

Generally speaking, cardio has an inverse relationship with calories; as your calories continue to drop, your cardio will likely increase. If your body reaches a plateau, pull the cardio lever a bit harder. If you start with minimal cardio, you'll have a ton of room to increase it sustainably as needed. The more opportunity you have for increasing cardio throughout the prep, the more variables you control.

Cardio is a tool, not the end-all-be-all to your success with this journey. Don't become a slave to hours of endless cardio a day, as that can suck the fun right out of this prep. Increase your cardiovascular work incrementally by increasing your cardio training sessions' intensity, duration or frequency. Feel free to leverage my cardio progression template below if you want something that easily integrates with this prep protocol.

MY TRAINING AND CARDIO ROUTINE

I implemented this eight-day rotational heavy/hypertrophy split throughout my last competitive season with much success. Since it follows an eight-day protocol, any given muscle group never falls on the same day of the week consecutively. I've found this to be advantageous for many reasons.

Traditional splits that parallel a standard seven-day week are often structured so that chest falls on Monday and legs always fall on Friday. As such, if you are having a wonderful Monday, you've just come back from a relaxing weekend and are feeling rejuvenated, you'll likely have an excellent chest workout. By Friday, however, you may be worn down from the rigors of the workweek, and that exhaustion will be reflected in your leg day.

By staggering what you train while following this eight-day cycle, each group gets its own day week after week, and you'll be more inclined to average your good days and bad days as they impact your training. This factor alone has improved my symmetry tremendously because no muscle group gets left behind.

Another unique factor of this eight-day split is that it blends heavy training intensity protocols and higher volume techniques. Most muscle groups get targeted twice throughout this eight-day rotation, one being a heavy day and the other focusing more on hypertrophy. This is an excellent way to hedge your bets when it comes to stimulating a muscle group. You can implement all the heavy intensity techniques we discussed earlier on the heavy day. You can also integrate more volume training and focus on increasing overall blood flow on the hypertrophy day.

As you'll notice, I set aside one day exclusively for barbell squats. Many people, myself included, have a love-hate relationship with barbell squats. They are heavy, they hurt and they are freaking intimidating! Many people get anxious at the thought of cranking out a few difficult sets of squats during their workout. Rather than try and hide a few of these difficult sets between other exercises, I wanted to remove all distractions and dedicate an entire day to this king of leg exercises! As such, I do a *ton* of squat work on a squat day. I'll often do a pyramid set that starts with 135 lb and increases to 405 lb throughout 13 or 14 total sets. That is a lot of intensity and a lot of volume! By removing the other exercises and focusing only on the barbell squat, I can perfect my form, focus and truly stimulate my legs. Don't skip leg day—make a dedicated squat day!

You'll have two rest days for every six training days with this eight-day split, so take full advantage of them! If you are lifting with a lot of intensity and quite a bit of volume, you're going to need ample time to recover. Leverage rest days to stretch and work on mobility. Try to get some blood flow and movement on those days, but don't kill yourself in the gym. Give your body time to recover and get enough sleep so you can hit it hard on the next training day.

DAY 1: SQUAT DAY

Warm-up with 3 sets of 10 reps super setting bodyweight squats and walking lunges.

- Continual pyramid in barbell squats from starting weight up to heaviest manageable weight
- Increase in increments of 10-25 lb on each side of bar until the heaviest set is reached
- 6-10 reps per set

DAY 2: HEAVY DELTS | HYPERTROPHY BACK

Warm-up with resistance bands and mobility work.

- Dumbbell Shrug (4 sets of 8 reps)
- Dumbbell Shoulder Press (4 sets of 8 reps)
- Barbell Military Press (continual pyramid set as outlined in the squat form above)

- Cable Upright Row (4 sets of 8 reps)
- Pull-ups with variation grips (4 sets of 5-15 reps)
- Cable Row (4 sets of 15 reps)
- Barbell Row (4 sets of 15 reps)

DAY 3: HEAVY TRICEPS | HYPERTROPHY CHEST

Warm-up with resistance bands and pushups.

- Single-arm Cable Extension (4 sets of 8 reps)
- Close Grip Bench Press (continual pyramid set as outlined above)
- Cable Kickbacks (4 sets of 8 reps)
- Dumbbell Skull Crusher (4 sets of 8 reps)
- Bodyweight Dips (5-15 reps)
- Cable Flat Chest Fly (4 sets of 15 reps)
- Dumbbell Bench Press (4 sets of 15 reps)
- Incline Machine Press (4 sets of 15 reps)
- Pushups (to failure)

DAY 4: REST DAY

DAY 5: HEAVY BACK | HYPERTROPHY BICEPS

Warm-up with resistance bands and mobility work.

- Pull-ups with variation grip (4 sets of 5-15 reps)
- Dumbbell Row (4 sets of 8 reps)
- Barbell Deadlift (continual pyramid set as outlined above)
- Rack Pull (4 sets of 8 reps)
- Incline Dumbbell Curls (4 sets of 15 reps)
- Heavy Hammer Curls (4 sets of 8 reps)

- Barbell Curls (4 sets of 15 reps)
- Drag Curls (4 sets of 15 reps)

DAY 6: HIGH VOLUME LEGS

Warm-up with bodyweight squats and walking lunges.

- Dumbbell Stiff-leg Deadlift (4 sets of 15 reps)
- Sumo Deadlift (4 sets of 6-8 reps *or* implement pyramid set as outlined above)
- Front Squat (4 sets of 15 reps)
- Barbell Hip Thrust (4-5 sets of 15 reps)
- Quad Extension superset with Hamstring Curls (4 sets of 15 reps)

DAY 7: HEAVY CHEST | HYPERTROPHY DELTS

Warm-up with resistance bands and mobility work.

- Cable Chest Fly (4 sets of 8 reps)
- Barbell Bench Press (continual pyramid set as outlined above)
- Dumbbell Bench Press (4 sets of 8 reps)
- Decline Dumbbell Press (4 sets of 8 reps)
- Cable Lateral Raise (4 sets of 15 reps)
- Plate Raise above head (4 sets of 15 reps)
- Reverse Dumbbell Fly (4 sets of 15 reps)

DAY 8: REST DAY

ADDITIONAL WORK

- Superset calves or abdominal work throughout the

different exercises
- These muscles typically respond better to a higher rep count between 15 and 20 reps

SAMPLE CARDIO PROGRESSION PLAN

With cardio, we can increase the time, frequency and intensity. An example of a sustainable increase in cardio using the Stairmaster machine would look something like this:

- Baseline: 10-minute session @ level 10 2x/week
- Week 2: 12-minute session @ level 10 2x/week
- Week 3: 12-minute session @ level 12 2x/week
- Week 4: 12-minute session @ level 12 3x/week
- Week 5: 14-minute session @ level 12 3x/week
- Week 6: 14-minute session @ level 14 3x/week
- Week 7: 14-minute session @ level 14 4x/week
- Week 8: 16-minute session @ level 14 4x/week
- Week 9: 16-minute session @ level 16 4x/week
- Week 10: 16-minute session @ level 16 5x/week
- Week 11: 18-minute session @ level 16 5x/week
- Week 12: 18-minute session @ level 18 5x/week
- Week 13: 18-minute session @ level 18 6x/week
- Week 14: 20-minute session @ level 18 6x/week
- Week 15: 20-minute session @ level 20 6x/week
- Week 16: 20-minute session @ level 20 7x/week
- Week 17: 22-minute session @ level 20 7x/week

If you'll notice, none of these three levers are pulled at the same time in the same week. Instead, gradually increase one of the three metrics every single week to allow your body to acclimate to the increase in duration, intensity or frequency in a sustainable manner.

The exact breakdown of your cardio duration, intensity and frequency could look a bit different from this depending on your fitness and preferred form of cardio, but this is an excellent example of what it could look like. Notice that the time spent doing cardio in this example is relatively short—10-30 minutes per cardio session should be sufficient for most individuals.

If you're spending hours and hours each day doing cardio, then you likely didn't give yourself enough time for a prep or start at a healthy composition. It also means you probably aren't implementing an effective resistance training protocol, or aren't correctly manipulating your macronutrients. Cardio is a tool to be used throughout this prep, but it isn't your primary weapon. It is a "side arm" to help you achieve the composition you're looking for.

[4]
SUPPLEMENTS APPENDIX

OVERVIEW

Supplements are one of those things that get all the press time but rarely deserve it. Supplements should be just that: supplemental. If you're following a well-formulated ketogenic diet, you're likely covering most of your body's needs, and your supplementation should be very minimal.

The need for supplements goes beyond the high-level view of macros alone. This is why I'm not a huge fan of diets that only place a significance on the macros and don't dive into the underlying quality of the foods and their micronutrients. This phenomenon isn't specific to any diet; instead, it's about how people manage their nutrition. The IIFYM community is notorious for only focusing on the macros, but that isn't necessarily indicative of the IIFYM diet.

In all, I feel that the ketogenic community places a relatively high value on the sourcing of their foods and the quality of the ingredients. Unfortunately, that hasn't stopped the rise in popularity of "dirty keto," which is a lazy way of only considering macros and ensuring total carbs are low. Any dietary protocol can and should highlight the importance of micronutrients and food sourcing and allow quality to take precedence.

The goal should be to come as close to covering all your macronutrient, micronutrient and mineral needs from the foods you consume rather than from pills, powders and potions. Once you've accomplished that, you can strategically add in any supplements as needed.

My supplement regiment is incredibly minimal. I don't like taking a bunch of pills and powders because I honestly don't see a benefit from most of them, and I also hate the inconvenience. My nutrition is on point, and I feel like a million bucks daily—no need to fix what isn't broken. All the same, I'm certainly not against supplements if they are warranted.

There are a handful of supplements I take regularly that have shown significant benefit. If your nutrition is optimized, the following list of supplements should provide you the most bang for your buck. Feel free to add or subtract from this list as you see fit; we are all unique individuals, and our needs may differ.

ELECTROLYTES

We dove pretty deep into electrolytes and how they impact our body and performance throughout the book. In short, we need them to improve muscular contraction, power our brain synapses, manage our fluid levels and so much more. Rather than hash out all the benefits of electrolytes, I want to use this section to say what I use to supplement them.

SODIUM

Sodium is an essential mineral for every animal on this planet, so don't be afraid of it! I typically consume between 5-10 g a day, depending on my goals. You can titrate your supplemental sodium intake up or down so long as you maintain a proper equilibrium with your fluid and potassium levels.

Most people seem to respond well to a 2:1 ratio of supplemental sodium to potassium. I salt my food quite heavily using Redmond Real Salt brand as it has a superior taste and quality. To keep my sodium levels in check, I'll often measure out my sodium intake for the day using an empty seasoning container. If I sprinkle that on my food throughout the day until it is empty, I'm easily able to measure my overall sodium consumption.

POTASSIUM

Potassium is another electrolyte critical for generating electrical charges throughout the body and activating nerve and cell functions. If you're following an animal-based, ketogenic diet, there is quite a bit of potassium in the meats you consume. For instance, one 3 oz piece of pork loin contains around 350 mg of potassium. Still, if you're physically active and demand quite a bit from your muscles and bodily functions, you'll benefit tremendously from some additional potassium.

As mentioned above, a 2:1 ratio of supplemental sodium to supplemental potassium seems to work well as a baseline for most people. Establish your sodium intake then cut it in half to determine your potassium intake. There are many forms of potassium available such as potassium gluconate, aspartate, chelate, chloride, phosphate, bicarbonate, citrate and orotate, and they all react a bit differently in the body. I typically like to get a blend of both chloride and citrate.

Most of the supplements out there contain potassium in the citrate form, so check the labels and try and supplement with potassium chloride as well. One great source for easily absorbed, pure potassium chloride is Upgraded Formulas Nano Potassium. Since the potassium in this product is nano-sized, you'll absorb it a bit better and likely won't need to supplement quite as much.

MAGNESIUM

Magnesium is another critical electrolyte. There is quite a bit of natural magnesium in nuts, dark chocolate and salmon, so you will likely get an adequate dose of magnesium if you consume plenty of those. Insufficient magnesium can lead to muscle cramping and discomfort, so I tend to supplement 300-500 mg daily to play it safe.

Like potassium, there are many different forms of magnesium. Magnesium citrate works fine and is inexpensive, but it may cause some gastric distress if you are sensitive to citric acid. A form of chelated magnesium will be bound to an amino acid, absorb a bit more readily and have less of a laxative effect, so go that route if you can. I'm a fan of magnesium glycinate and magnesium L-threonate.

CALCIUM

Calcium is involved in skeletal mineralization and the contraction of muscles. A well-formulated diet should cover all your calcium needs, especially if you consume quite a bit of dairy. If you're avoiding dairy, try consuming canned sardines or something similar that packs a hefty dose of calcium. Homemade bone broth is a fantastic source of calcium and is incredibly nutrient-dense.

ELECTROLYTE BLENDS

These electrolytes should be present in the foods you are consuming, but additional supplementation of electrolytes—especially on a ketogenic diet—will improve overall performance. Many companies have tried to capitalize on this by creating all-in-one electrolyte blend supplements. I'm all for convenience, so I try to leverage these blends whenever possible if I know the source and quality.

Redmond Re-Lyte powder and LMNT are two popular electrolyte blends on the market. I'm a fan of the 2:1 ratio of sodium to potassium present in the Re-Lyte powder and it makes tracking supplementation simple. That said, Re-Lyte uses potassium citrate. If your body doesn't tolerate that well, you may want to use LMNT, which uses potassium chloride. Both are fantastic options and taste phenomenal! I'll add a few servings of either to my water throughout the day and intra-training to cover all my electrolyte needs.

IODINE

Iodine is required for the synthesis of the growth-regulating thyroid hormones thyroxine and triiodothyronine. Both are tyrosine-based hormones primarily responsible for the regulation of our metabolism. If you consume much seafood, you are probably consuming adequate iodine from your nutrition. If that isn't the case, you may find it advantageous to supplement iodine as a way of ensuring proper thyroid levels. My go-to supplement for iodine is Grassland Nutrition's organic bull kelp flakes. Kelp is a fantastic source of natural iodine, and the texture of these flakes adds a nice bit of crunch and seasoning to whatever meal I'm eating.

VITAMIN D AND K2

Vitamin D has been in the media lately as a "cure-all" for every ailment. It supposedly makes your bones stronger, improves your immune system, improves hormone function, aids in muscle growth and increases life span.

I'm not sure I buy all those claims, but I think there is a benefit to supplementing it daily. Sun exposure is a great way to get more vitamin D, but that often isn't feasible in the colder months. Research shows that most of us are incredibly deficient in vitamin D. As a simple way to hedge my bets, I supplement with 5,000 IUs of vitamin D3 daily.

Vitamin D promotes vitamin K-dependent proteins, which

require vitamin K for carboxylation to function correctly. Vitamin D increases calcium levels in the body, and vitamin K helps the body use calcium by shuttling it to your bones. Current research supports the notion that supplementing vitamins D and K together might be more effective than consuming either one alone. As such, I pair my 5,000 IU dose of vitamin D3 with a 200mcg dose of vitamin K2.

FISH OIL AND OMEGA-3 FATTY ACIDS

The ratio between omega-6 and omega-3 has become incredibly skewed over the years. Ideally, we should consume close to a 1:1 ratio between the two; unfortunately, Western diets have tipped the scales in favor of omega-6. The broad use of linoleic acid from corn, soy and sunflower oils is the most likely culprit for this significant increase in omega-6 consumption.

A substantial rise in omega-6 relative to omega-3 results in increased inflammation, so anything we can do to improve that ratio is worthwhile. Simply decreasing our omega-6 consumption and increasing omega-3 consumption is low-hanging fruit when it comes to moving the needle in the right direction. As such, strive to avoid all heavily processed seed oils and dressings. Increase your omega-3 consumption via canned sardines, mackerel and anchovies. I recommend avoiding eating larger, predatory fish too often due to their higher mercury content. If you're not a fan of fish, supplement with a quality DHA and EPA oil supplement—1-2 g per day of a combined DHA and EPA supplement should be totally sufficient.

CREATINE

Creatine facilitates the recycling of adenosine triphosphate (ATP) in the muscle and brain tissues. This "recycling" is achieved by converting adenosine diphosphate (ADP) back to ATP. If you can recall your sixth-grade biology class, the mitochondrion is the "powerhouse of the cell" responsible for the production of ATP. ATP is what fuels many of the processes within the cell.

Creatine has been studied as a performance supplement for years, and its efficacy has been proven through countless studies. It's generally not used to improve performance in endurance sports, but it truly shines in the anaerobic realm, producing more power output. It has been shown to foster greater strength and recovery between lifting sets, which is precisely what we want in bodybuilding.

It is a naturally occurring compound present in the red meats we consume, but we can also synthesize it endogenously with the amino acids glycine and arginine. We can't create enough creatine internally or consume enough through our nutrition to reach a saturation point; thus, it makes sense to supplement with creatine monohydrate.

To achieve full muscle saturation of creatine, many studies suggest a "loading phase" in which you consume 20-25 g a day for the first week. Afterward, you can drop to a daily intake of 5 g/day to maintain muscle saturation. This loading phase is likely not necessary if you are consistently consuming 5 g/day of supplemental creatine in addition to what you're getting with a well-formulated, animal-based diet. The main thing to concern yourself with as it relates to creatine supplementation is consistency. If you forget to take it for several days, your body will return to its normal baseline and your muscles will no longer be at a saturation point. I add a scoop of creatine monohydrate in with my electrolyte blend once or twice a day to ensure I don't ever miss it.

Many competitors fear excess fluid retention as it relates to creatine supplementation. Creatine does draw more water into the muscle tissue itself, but this is a good thing as this volumizes the lean tissue and creates a "fuller" look. If your electrolyte supplementation is dialed in, there is no need to avoid creatine as there will not be excess fluid in your subcutaneous layer of skin. There is no need to cut your creatine intake during peak week or anything like that. Keep your supplementation consistent.

CAFFEINE

Caffeine is the world's most widely used and abused psychoactive drug. One look at your neighborhood Starbucks as you drive to work confirms this. Truth be told, I'm guilty of abusing it as well—I rarely go without my cup of coffee in the morning and I look forward to it daily!

Caffeine has been proven to create the positive neurological impacts of increased awareness and focus. It has also been shown to improve athletic performance with increased speed, power and agility. There have even been studies suggesting that caffeine has a powerful thermogenic effect and can suppress appetite. If all of this sounds like it would be a great addition to your competition prep endeavors, you are right—but in moderation.

Too much of a good thing is a bad thing, and overconsumption of caffeine is no different. Like any drug, your body can build a tolerance to caffeine, and you'll be required to supplement more to elicit the same response. This increased dosage can adversely affect your parasympathetic nervous system, creating more anxiety and less sleep and recovery. The average cup of coffee contains about 100 mg of caffeine, and many of the popular pre-workout and energy drinks have 300 mg of caffeine. That can add up quickly if you're not careful! I recommend keeping your total caffeine consumption south of 500 mg a day if possible. Ideally, avoid consuming any caffeine in the afternoon hours as you get closer to winding down for the day.

KETO BRICKS

Again, I may be a bit biased, but I'll include a discussion on supplementing with Keto Bricks just the same. I consider the bricks to be more of a food item than a supplemental source of nutrition, but they are made with a bit of protein powder, so I suppose it makes sense to include them here in the supplement section.

Each Keto Brick contains 1,000 calories and, depending on the flavor, around 90 g of dietary fat, 30 g of dietary protein and 10-12 g of dietary carbohydrates. The protein powder used in the bricks varies between a vegetable-based protein that includes digestive enzymes and a 100% grass-fed whey protein concentrate. The protein sources we employ in the bricks are of the highest quality I could source.

Many protein powders on the market are made with low-grade fillers and binding agents that can lead to gastric distress. The bricks indeed contain protein, but they are by no means a protein bar. The beauty in the bricks comes from the high-quality fat we use as the base ingredient: 100% organic raw cacao butter.

Cacao butter is a saturated fat that boasts the greatest concentration of stearic acid, a long-chain fatty acid with an 18-carbon backbone. Stearic acid has garnered a lot of attention within the scientific community as potentially having a positive effect on cholesterol levels, metabolism and reduction in fat storage potential within fat cells themselves.

The jury is still out on many of those claims, so I won't hang my hat on any of them just yet. Still, I can confidently say that stearic acid is tolerated incredibly well from a digestive standpoint and is a great energy source in terms of fat metabolism. It also has a very high melting point relative to other fatty acids, which is why the Keto Bricks stay shelf-stable at room temperature. The bricks are a high-quality, shelf-stable, 1,000-calorie ketogenic food source, plain and simple. They make meal prep easier and remove excuses for finding quality food sources to nail the fat macros. I eat one daily and have for the past several years. You certainly don't need to supplement with them, but you can rest assured that you're not sacrificing any nutrient density if you choose to consume them.

PRE-WORKOUT DRINKS

All this talk about caffeine leads to questions about pre-workout supplementation. As mentioned, most pre-workouts contain a hefty dose of caffeine as their primary stimulant (though many companies will throw in a few other compounds to hype up their formula and charge more money).

Many pre-workouts contain a blend of vasodilators like citrulline and arginine designed to increase blood flow and improve muscle pumps. Beta-alanine is a common ingredient as well, since it is converted to carnosine within the muscle tissue. It acts as a buffer for lactic acid produced while training and helps prevent fatigue.

All these amino acids are great and have a positive impact on performance. The beauty of a heavily meat-based diet is that you consume a significant amount of amino acids in your foods alone, so your need for supplementation should be greatly diminished. This doesn't necessarily mean you shouldn't opt for fancy pre-workouts and expensive supplements—just don't expect them to have a profound effect on your performance. I'll occasionally throw in a pre-workout mix when my calories are very low and energy is in short supply. I encourage you not to lean too heavily on stimulants and prioritize quality nutrition as your primary source of amino acids.

WHEY PROTEIN, BCAAS AND EAAS

Protein shakes and amino acid drinks are likely supplemented more than anything within the bodybuilding communities and fitness circles. In my early training days, I was under the impression that a protein shake within 30 minutes of my training block was a prerequisite for growth. I wrongly assumed that if I didn't consume that trusty protein shake within my "anabolic window," all my gains would melt away and the brutal training I just endured would be for naught. Luckily, this isn't the case.

Honestly, I rarely ever consume protein shakes anymore. I'll occasionally add a scoop of protein into a serving of whole-fat yogurt as a late-night snack or make a protein pancake if I'm feeling festive. Once I switched to an animal-based, ketogenic diet, two things happened:

1. I realized I didn't need to consume 300 g of protein a day to reach my goals, so my overall protein consumption decreased.
2. The optimal protein intake I needed to consume came entirely from the animal proteins I was consuming throughout the day to hit my macronutrient targets.

Both things eliminated the need for supplemental protein powders. There are times throughout this competition prep protocol when your daily protein intake will be pretty high. During those phases, you may find it advantageous to include a protein supplement to target your macros. Still, I highly encourage you to try to hit your protein targets from animal sources rather than supplements whenever possible.

This same phenomenon holds true for BCAAs and EAAs. You'll likely be consuming all necessary amino acids from your diet alone, so there's no need to waste money on expensive supplements that include undesirable filler ingredients and boatloads of sweeteners. The one caveat I have on amino acid supplementation is that I'll often supplement with a quality EAA blend during the very tail-end of my prep. Following this protocol, the last few phases of prep involve a reduced protein intake, resulting in a corresponding decrease in amino acid consumption. During these phases, it may be advantageous to supplement amino acids as a way to hedge your bets and ensure that you are leaving nothing to chance when it comes to muscle preservation.

EXOGENOUS KETONES

Exogenous ketones have flooded the market as the ketogenic diet has gotten increasingly popular. The keto diet is often heralded as a miracle weight-loss diet that causes fat to melt off your body as long as you register blood ketones. These exogenous ketone supplements help you register higher concentrations of ketones in your blood. Some brands have gone as far as to suggest you can eat all the carbohydrates you want and simply drink exogenous ketones afterward to get you back into ketosis and return to "fat-burning mode." Ladies and gents, if it sounds too good to be true, it probably is. These brands have done more damage than good, tarnishing the ketogenic diet with their exaggerated claims.

I'm not against exogenous ketone supplementation, I'm just not a fan of people supplementing them for the wrong reasons. I would never suggest anybody supplement ketones to increase fat loss or weight loss. From a fat metabolism standpoint, it makes much more sense to focus on dietary manipulations and produce ketones endogenously rather than consume them externally.

For this reason, I don't ever supplement ketones in a cutting phase; however, some promising research suggests supplemental beta-hydroxybutyrate is great for reducing inflammation and improving recovery. As such, I'm a fan of supplementing with BHB in a building phase when I'm training with a ton of progressive overload and intensity techniques. Almost all the exogenous ketone supplements are bound to a mineral of some form. These ketone salts come with a hefty dose of sodium, potassium, magnesium or calcium. Many people experience increased energy with exogenous ketone supplementation, but I feel it's often just a result of increased electrolyte consumption.

Ketone esters are another form of exogenous ketones and are generally much more expensive than the ketone salts described earlier. They are also much less tasty and much more potent. One serving of ketone esters can easily quadruple your BHB blood levels, but I don't notice a significant difference in performance with acute ester supplementation, and I can't justify the cost of supplementing the esters daily.

More research needs to be done on the efficacy of exogenous ketone supplementation for me to confidently say it's worthwhile to include in your daily supplement routine. Supplemental BHB has been shown to positively impact cancer patients and those who have Alzheimer's, dementia and other neurological disorders, but that is well beyond the scope of this book.

FAT BURNERS AND DIURETICS

Don't even consider these. They are a waste of time and money. A well-formulated diet will result in the desired fat loss, and proper electrolyte balance will ensure you aren't retaining unnecessary fluids. Fat burners and diuretics are marketing traps designed to tug at your desire for a quick fix when you find yourself in a weak moment.

STEROIDS AND OTHER SUPER SUPPLEMENTS

You have to decide what is right for you regarding the use of steroids, growth hormones, SARMS and other performance-enhancing drugs. PEDs are obviously present in the sport of bodybuilding—after all, humans aren't designed to be 5% body fat at 300 lb. None of the elite-level bodybuilders battling out for the title of Mr. Olympia have come by their physique naturally. Those competitors decided to go the route of PEDs to reach the level they have, which is their choice to make. That most certainly does not mean that they haven't had to put in a ton of work along the way.

Contrary to popular belief, steroids are not an automatic one-way ticket to the top. For this reason, I still respect and admire all the hard work that goes into building the physiques you see on the Olympia stage. I've just decided to go in a different direction for myself.

I got into the sport of bodybuilding to improve my physique, get strong, become healthier and gain more confidence. For me, injecting myself with a hormone designed to make me grow at supraphysiological levels would massively contradict my desire to be the healthiest version of myself possible.

PEDs certainly aren't a death sentence, but they can most definitely create a cascade of adverse effects I would prefer to avoid. In addition to the potential physical implications of steroid use, I don't want to go that route for psychological reasons. I like playing the long game. I like trusting the process and chipping away at my goal, day in and day out.

I'm accepting of the fact that my physique won't change drastically from one year to the next by being a natural competitor. I don't want to juggle the physical and emotional rollercoaster of coming on and off hormonal cycles. I don't want to feel like superman one week and then be plagued with depression the next—that may not always happen with steroid use, but it most certainly can.

The human body is capable of so much more than we give it credit for. My goal as a natural athlete has been to test the limits of what we can do. Anytime I think I've reached my limit, I'm able to push a bit further. This realization has led to incredible advancements in my life physically, mentally and emotionally. Rather than sell myself short and reach for a pill or potion, I've genuinely enjoyed testing myself and exceeding my expectations. The sport of natural bodybuilding is a perfect embodiment of this belief system. Natural bodybuilding has provided me an outlet to explore the extremes and then stand onstage with others of similar interests and values.

I'm not a chemist, so I won't be your greatest resource for concocting the best and safest steroid stack. If you decide to go that route, I encourage you to be smart and be safe. Please don't do it because you feel pressured by the industry or your peers. Damn sure don't do it for a cheap plastic trophy that says you won a bodybuilding show.

Recognize that there are consequences for your actions and take responsibility to learn about those consequences for yourself. I'm not here to tell you what to do, and only you can make choices about your own health. However, if you decide to go the natural route, I commend you, and I look forward to sharing a stage with you someday!

BANNED SUBSTANCES

If you decide to go the route of natural bodybuilding, be prepared to read ingredient labels like a pro! Some of the federations are incredibly relaxed toward their regulations while others are not. I typically compete in the INBF/WNBF federation, which bans competitors from competing for 10 years (unless otherwise notated) if they are found to have any of the following prohibited substances in their system:

INBF/WNBF BANNED SUBSTANCE LIST (AS OF WRITING)

All anabolic steroids including, but not limited to:

- Anadrol
- Anavar
- Anderone
- Andropen
- 1-Androstenediol
- 1-Androstenedione
- 4-Androstenediol
- 4-Androstenedione
- 5-Androstenediol
- 5-Androstenedione
- Bolazine
- Bolandiol (19-Norandrostendiol)
- Bolasterone
- Boldebal

- Boldenone– Equipoise
- Boldione
- Calusterone
- Cardarine (PPAR)
- Chioroxomesterone (dyhdrochlormethyltesterone)
- Clenbuterol (prescribed and non-prescribed clenbuterol usage will carry a two (2) year ban timeframe for new athletes wanting to join the INBF/WNBF)
- Dilaterol
- Spiropent
- Ventipulmin
- Clomid/Clomiphene (not allowed for use by men as a form of testosterone therapy, or to simply increase testosterone production even when physician prescribed and monitored)
- Clostebol
- Danazol
- Deca-Durabolin
- Dehydrochlormethyltestosterone
- Desoxymethyltestosterone
- Dianabol
- Dymethazine (DMZ)
- 5a-Dihydrostestosterone
- Drostanolone
- Epitestosterone (masking agent)
- Equipoise
- Ethisterone
- Ethylestrenol
- Fluoxymesterone
- Formebolone
- Formestane (anti-estrogen)
- Furazabol
- Halodrol
- 4-Hydroxytestosterone

- Mebolazine
- Mestanolone
- Mesterolone
- Methandienone
- Methandriol
- Methyltestosterone
- Oxandrolone
- Primobolin
- Stanozolol
- Sustanon 250
- Winstrol
- Testosterone and related compounds
- Testosterone Cypionate
- Testosterone Enanthate

TESTOSTERONE

Testosterone in any form (including creams, gels, patches, pellets and injections) for any reason, even if physician prescribed is strictly prohibited. **No Exceptions!**

The **Testosterone/Epitestosterone (T/E) Ratio** is used to measure the presence of exogenous testosterone or illicit elevation of testosterone levels. T/E ratios in excess of **6/1 are ruled as positive, no matter what the cause.**

> Note: Should the use of any substance cause a T/E ratio above the 6/1 limit, the athlete will be ruled as positive (failure).

GROWTH HORMONES AND PEPTIDES

All HGH and peptides are banned! Substances of similar chemical structure and anabolic effect that increase muscle mass even if not expressly listed impose a 10-year ban.

- Pharmaceutical HGH, HCG, and any other related compounds, including Insulin-Like Growth Factors (IGF)
- GHS (Growth Hormone Secretagogues)
- MK-677, MK-0677 (Ibutamoren)
- IGF-1
- IGF-1 LR3
- Somatomedin C
- SomaDerm
- Somatropin
- Sulfation Factor
- Oral spray or sublingual GH compounds of pharmaceutical origin (recombinant DNA technology)
- Peptides and GHRHs (Growth Hormone Releasing Hormones)
- MOD-GRF (1-29)
- CJC 1295 DAC
- HGH Fragment 176-191
- Hexarelin
- Ipamorelin
- Mechano Growth Factor with PEG
- Sermorelin
- GHRP-2, GHRP-6

ANABOLIC AGENTS, PRO-HORMONES, PRECURSORS AND METABOLITES, DERIVATIVES AND RELATED COMPOUNDS

- SARMs (Selective Androgen Receptor Modulators)
- 5-Etioallocholen-3b,7b,17b-triol and/or substances similar in structure – As of January 1, 2020, these substances shall carry a two (2) year ban timeframe.

- Any hormone, including insulin (injectable, oral, sublingual or otherwise) used for bodybuilding purposes.

DESIGNER AND PRO STEROIDS

Designer and Pro Steroids are banned and carry a 10-year ban timeframe:

- Superdrol
- Sdrol
- Ergomax LMG
- Tren
- TrenA

HORMONAL PRECURSORS AND THEIR METABOLITES AND ISOMERS

Use of the following substances requires 90 days (3 months) of abstinence prior to competing in the INBF/WNBF or affiliate federations for the first time.

- DHEA (there shall be a three-month amnesty for new athletes wanting to join the INBF/WNBF; any person supplementing with DHEA and/or it's metabolites (listed below) are ineligible for three months prior to competing with the INBF/WNBF)
- 7 Keto DHEA (there shall be a three-month amnesty for new athletes wanting to join the INBF/WNBF; any person supplementing with 7 Keto DHEA and/or it's metabolites (listed below) are ineligible for three months prior to competing with the INBF/WNBF)
- 7-ketodehydroepiandrosterone
- 7-oxodehydroepiandrosterone
- 7α-hydroxy-DHEA
- 7β-hydroxy-DHEA

PRO-HORMONAL FAT BURNING SUPPLEMENTS

The following have been identified as pro-hormonal in nature and are banned:

- 6 OXO (through 2020, there shall be a three-month amnesty for NEW athletes wanting to join the INBF/WNBF. Any person supplementing with 6 OXO and/or related compounds is ineligible for three months prior to competing with the INBF/WNBF)
- 6 Oxandrostenetrione
- 2a,17adimethyl17B-hydroxy5aandrostan3one
- 3,17keto-etiochol-triene
- 1,4,6-Androstatriene-3, 17-dione
- 5Alpha (5a-androstane-3a, 17diol)

FAT BURNING PRO-HORMONE DERIVATIVES

The presence of any banned substance in urine (i.e. nandrolone), no matter how it arrived there is ruled as positive (urine test failure).

- 3,17dihydroxydelta5etiocholane7one (A7D)
- 3,17dihydroxydelta5etiocholane7one diethylcarbonate (A7E)
- 4-androstene-3,6,17-trione
- 4-etioallocholen-3,6,17-trione

PRESCRIPTION THYROID HORMONE MEDICATION

Prescription thyroid hormone medication, when used for bodybuilding purposes, is banned!

PRESCRIPTION DIURETICS AND MASKING AGENTS

Any and all prescription diuretics, **even when doctor prescribed,** used for bodybuilding purposes, **are banned for three months prior** to WNBF competitions.

If an athlete possesses heart-related complications, a TUE can be issued for competition.

Spironolactone prescribed for acne **may not be used for 14 days prior** to competing in any INBF/WNBF Event. No exceptions!

- Acetazolamide
- Amiloride
- Bumetanide
- Bendroflumethiazide
- Canrenone
- Chlorthalidone
- Chlorothiazide
- Clopaide
- Cyclothiazide
- Dichlorphenamide
- Ethacrynic Acid
- Furosemide
- Hydrochlorothiazide
- Hydroflumethiazide
- Spironolactone
- Triamterene
- *Glycerol*: Small amounts of glycerol found in nutritional supplements are not considered banned.

CLENBUTEROL

Prescribed and non-prescribed clenbuterol usage will carry a two (2) year ban timeframe for **new** athletes wanting to join the INBF/WNBF.

- Dilaterol
- Spiropent
- Ventipulmin

GHB

GHB is banned.

MISCELLANEOUS

Muscle implants of any kind are strictly prohibited, as are chemicals/drugs used to deceive or pass the polygraph or urine test.

OTHER ANABOLIC AGENTS, HORMONES AND METABOLIC MODULATORS

Including, but not limited to:

- 17-androdione
- Androstene TRIONE
- 5AD
- Androstenedial
- 19-norandrostenedione
- Androstenolone
- Androstenedione
- Androstanolone
- Arimistane
- Androsta-3,5-Diene-7,17-Dione

- Clomid/Clomiphene (not allowed for use by men as a form of testosterone therapy, or to simply increase testosterone production even when physician prescribed and monitored)
- Trenbolone
- Testosterone
- 1-Testosterone
- Testolactone (anti-estrogen)
- Stenbolone
- Stanozolol
- Quinbolone
- Prostanozol
- Probenecid (masking agent)
- Oxymetholone
- Oxymesterone
- Oxandrolone
- Oxabolone
- Norethandrolone
- Norclostebol
- Norbolethone
- 19-Norandroster
- Nandrolone
- Mibolerone
- Methyltestosterone
- Methylnortestosterone
- Methyl-1-testosterone
- 6-Methylandrostenedione
- Methoxygonadiene
- Methenolone
- Methasterone
- Methandrostenolone
- Cardarine (Peroxisome Proliferator-Activated Receptor δ (PPARδ) agonists, GW 1516)
- Clenbuterol (Dilaterol, Spiropent, Ventipulmin)

- Selective Androgen Receptor Modulators (SARMs)
- Andarine (GSX-007 or S-4)
- Cardarine (GW-501516)
- Ligandrol (LGD-4033)
- Ostarine (GTx-024, MK-2866)
- RAD 140 (Testolone)
- Stenabolic (SR-9009)
- Tibolone
- Zeranol
- Zilpaterol
- Other SARMs similar in structure and/or physiological effect
- ACP-10
- LGD-3303
- LG-121071
- LGD-3303
- ACP-105
- Selective Estrogen Receptor Modulators (SERMs)
- Raloxifene
- Tamoxifen
- Toremifene

EPHEDRINE, EPHEDRA AND STIMULANTS

- Ephedrine and Ephedra may not have been used for three months before joining the INBF/WNBF for the first time

DMAA AND RELATED COMPOUNDS

Due to the abundance of supplements and pre-workout products containing DMAA and/or related compounds, there shall be a 30-

day amnesty period before an athlete is eligible to compete in any INBF/WNBF event for the first time.

- DMAA
- 1,3-DimethylAmylamine
- 1,3-DimethylButylamine (4 amino-2-Methylpantane citrate)
- Dimethylpentylamine
- Geranium
- Methylhexanamine
- Phenethylamine and its derivatives

WADA BANNED STIMULANT LIST

PSYCHOMOTOR STIMULANTS

Stimulants/medications prescribed or non-prescribed used for bodybuilding and/or weight loss purposes are banned in certain timeframes. Stimulants or medications that produce similar physiological effects even if not expressly listed are prohibited for use.

- Amphetamines
- Benzphetamine
- Bupropion Hydrochloride
- Cocaine
- Diethylpropion
- Dimethylamphetamine
- Ecstasy
- Ephedrine
- Ephedra
- Liraglutide
- Lorcaserin
- Methylenedioxymethamphetamine

- Naltrexone Hydrochloride
- Orlistat
- Methamphetamines
- Phendimetrazine
- Phentermine
- Sibutramine
- Speed
- Topiramate

CANNABINOIDS & CBDS

- Prohibited for use before any INBF/WNBF polygraph examination
- At this time, the INBF/WNBF has not moved toward banning cannabis and/or CBDs in season.

[5]
MISCELLANEOUS APPENDIX

The goal of this section is to shed light on all the intricate details that have incredible importance but don't necessarily deserve their own chapter. Physique competitions are all about delivering the best version of yourself to the panel of judges. That version transcends proper diet and training. It encompasses your skin conditioning, tanning color, suit detail and much more.

By creating this section as a "catch-all" to ensure that no stone is left unturned, you can be confident that you are genuinely peaking in every aspect of your full potential. Leave nothing to chance and become your best self!

POSING SUITS AND TRUNKS

Do *not* wait until the last minute to get your posing suit! Most of these are made to order and occasionally need alterations. Don't expect Amazon two-day delivery speeds when you purchase your posing suit. Keep in mind that your measurements will change throughout your prep, so you may have to do a bit of estimating when it comes to what your measurements will likely be on show day when the suit is needed.

I must say, I'm glad I'm a guy when it comes to posing suits. Most high-end suits for the male divisions can be purchased for under $100, no problem. Women, on the other hand, need much deeper pockets.

It's not uncommon for female posing suits to start at $500 and go as high as $2000. Budget accordingly, and don't let these suit expenses sneak up on you. Many competitors sell their suits after their shows, so you may be able to snag a fantastic suit for a steep discount if you are close with any other competitors who share a similar size.

Make sure to read up on suit requirements specified by the federation you are competing with. There is nothing worse than spending money on a suit that isn't allowed or that will result in a reduction in total points. Also, recognize that you'll be covered in tanning solution during show day. I encourage you to gravitate toward colors that will camouflage any smudges and smears you will most certainly encounter. I gravitate toward darker colors for this very reason. This isn't to say you should avoid bright colors at all costs; be careful and recognize that a huge tanning streak across the front of your neon pink posing suit may not be the most flattering look.

There are many reputable companies to choose from when ordering your suit. I've had great success over the years with CJ's Elite Custom Competition Suits. They offer a variety of fabric colors and finishes and provide posing suits for every competitive division. CJ's requests a longer lead time of two to three months, so keep that in mind when ordering your competition regalia.

HAIR REMOVAL

Hair removal is one of those topics that is an essential aspect of the prep process but often doesn't get the attention it deserves. I've seen competitors marred with razor burn on show day, and I've seen competitors who looked like they were next of kin to Chewbacca; neither option is ideal.

As a general rule, I highly encourage people to remove excess body hair relatively early in the prep process. There are a few advantages of going through the prep with minimal body hair. For one, you'll be able to gauge your level of conditioning with a bit more accuracy as it won't be impeded by a ton of excess hair. For instance, I can often gauge my level of body fat based on certain vascularity marks on my calves, shoulders and back. Those markers would be much less evident if I was covered in hair and couldn't readily see them.

Also, it can take quite a bit of time to condition the skin to constant shaving. The last thing you want to do is wait until the last minute, shave everything during peak week and be covered in razor burn bumps. However, if you start early in the prep and shave regularly, your skin will toughen up to that razor blade and it won't be nearly as irritating for you. As far as peak week is concerned, you certainly don't want any body hair interfering with the tanning solution. You also don't want something as simple as proper hair removal to be the reason for not placing as high as you possibly can. The following tips will ensure that this part of the puzzle isn't overlooked.

HAIR REMOVAL TECHNIQUES

Nair: I'm honestly not a huge fan of these chemical solutions. I've used them with much success in the past, but they can irritate the skin. The active ingredients in Nair break down and dissolve hair particles. You basically rub Nair lotion all over your body, wait a few moments and then start scrubbing it off to remove all of your hair.

While it is effective and relatively quick, I don't recommend subjecting yourself to the chemicals it contains. Nair is practically a dialed-down version of Drano. Your skin is your largest and most absorbent organ. I don't recommend absorbing all those chemicals since there are safer, less irritating methods.

Electric Trimmer: This is step number one. If you have quite a bit of hair to remove, I would start with a quality electric trimmer. This initial trim may take a while and can be a bit tedious, but you'll only have to do it once. Some competitors only use electric trimmers, but I've never come across an electric trimmer that shaves as close to the skin as an actual razor, so I recommend not using the electric trimmers as the "finishing cut."

Old-Fashioned Razor: Once most hair is removed with the electric trimmer, you're ready for the razor. If you're a gal, you're likely a pro at this already—I'm still amazed at how quickly my wife can shave her entire body in just a few minutes with nothing more than hot water and a fresh razor. All of you guys out there who aren't seasoned veterans, prepare yourself for a bit of struggle and a few nicks.

The first time I tried shaving my entire body, it took forever. I missed more spots than I got, and my skin was pretty irritated afterward. That doesn't sound appealing to most people, and the allure of smooth skin may seem a bit daunting.

Don't let the first few times shaving discourage you from keeping up with the regular shaving. After a week or two, you'll get the hang of it and will be zipping through the body shave process in no time. Your skin will acclimate, and you shouldn't experience as much razor burn going forward.

I recommend using a quality shaving cream and a sharp razor. If you're a yoked bodybuilder and have a hard time reaching your back, much less accurately shaving it, try and enlist the help of your spouse or some truly supportive friend to give you a helping hand. You want to ensure that no spot on your body gets left unshaved and that your skin is adequately conditioned all over before peak week. Be sure to do your final shave before applying the tanning solution.

TANNING

One topic that deserves your utmost attention to detail is tanning. We bodybuilders and figure competitors are a strange sight to see, walking around in public with a darker tan than any human should ever desire. Why then do we do it?

The stage lights are incredibly bright, and they have the power to reveal everything if your color is right; however, if you come in too light, the sheer brightness of the stage lights will wash out all your definition. Your vascularity will disappear, and the deep muscular cuts you've worked so hard for will vanish. There is nothing worse than reaching the level of conditioning necessary to be incredibly competitive and having it all gone in an instant because your color isn't dark enough.

If the judges can't see the package you've brought to the table because the lights are washing out all your definition, you simply won't place well. The "trick" is to get incredibly dark—darker than you would ever think necessary.

There are several different tanning techniques and solutions available to competitors. What follows is a list of the ones I've used myself and my recommendations. One more thing: this section on tanning is essential regardless of your skin color. If you have an incredibly dark complexion, you'll still want to get a layer of bronzer on so that everything is uniform.

TANNING BEDS AND SUN EXPOSURE

You'll never be able to reach a complexion dark enough to maximize your look onstage tanning exclusively with the sun and tanning beds; however, I highly encourage you to spend a few months before the competition day establishing a solid base tan with this light exposure.

Having a quality base tan will improve the overall look on show day. I've seen competitors as white as ghosts do incredibly well on show day with a proper spray tan or rub, but there is a significant benefit to having a base tan beneath the artificial tan.

For one, the artificial tan will blend with your skin color much better. If any of your fake color rubs off while waiting backstage or posing onstage, it will be much less noticeable if you already have a great underlying tan. Also, the darker you are in the months leading up to your show, the more accurately you'll be able to gauge your level of conditioning.

Just as the bright stage lights wash out all your definition on show day if you come in too light, the lights at your own home and gym will mask much of your definition if your skin is too light. Having a great tan will improve the visibility of your definition when gauging the effectiveness of the refeed macros in the final phases of the prep.

Being able to compare pictures that more accurately reflect your conditioning is a great asset to have. I certainly don't recommend fooling with an artificial tan in the months before stepping onstage, as that would be an incredible inconvenience and mess. I do believe there is great benefit in having a solid natural base tan to gauge your progress and improve the look of your final package on show day in tandem with the artificial tan.

SPRAY TAN

Spray tans are the most common technique for creating an incredibly dark complexion for competitors. Recognize that a spray tan for bodybuilders is not the same as a simple spray tan at your local tanning booth. The spray tans designed for physique competitors will use a much darker solution and generally require more coats.

Many of the show promoters will leverage a sponsored tanning company or have a preferred tanning partner. If this is the case, the tanning company will often have booths set up at the show venue for spraying the competitors and touchups. Most competitions will take place on a Saturday, and the initial spray tan coat will be applied on the Friday prior. An additional coat and touchups will be applied on Saturday morning and throughout the day as needed before competing.

When using the show's partnered tanning company, know that they will be swamped! They will be attending to several competitors, and you likely won't have a ton of time to get all the attention and the world's greatest tan. As such, anything you can do to condition your skin and prepare it for a good tan is time and effort well spent.

Many competitors get a poor spray tan and then totally ruin it onstage as the heat from the lights and the rigors of mandatory poses cause them to sweat profusely. This is not a good look for the judges. Fortunately, you can incorporate a few "tricks" to properly condition your skin and ensure that you fully absorb the color.

Before getting your initial spray tan, take a shower and ensure that you are clean shaven. Avoid using any shower moisturizers or cleansers that contain an oil base. I recommend using a simple bar soap and making sure everything is thoroughly rinsed off. Then, use a salt scrub and rub that all over your body—plain-old table salt will work. Rinse off thoroughly after you've scrubbed your whole body.

This salt dries out your skin and ensures that the tanning solution absorbs. When you go to get your spray tan, make sure you are warm. You don't want to be sweating at all, but you do want to be warm so that your skin's pores are open and more receptive to absorbing the tanning solution. After you get your first coat of spray tan, stand in front of a box fan for a few minutes if one is available. This ensures that the tanning solution dries before you put on clothes and risk smearing it.

The following day, you should be able to receive a second coat and any necessary touchups. What do you do if your spray tan starts to streak and run while posing onstage? Honestly, there isn't much you can do at that moment. If your show is set up to include a prejudging and a night show, you have a bit more time to correct the issue.

If your tan slips during prejudging, you can rinse in the shower, but don't scrub or use any soaps. After rinsing, use a towel to pat dry, but don't rub the towel on your skin. This improves the base coat and gives you a better foundation for additional coats and touchups before the night show. If your show uses a running format in which you only step onstage once, you likely won't have time to fix any significant tanning issues.

DREAM TAN

Dream Tan is my preferred tanning solution. It comes in two colors, Gold Brown #1 and Red Bronze #2. I've heard rumors of a third color called Brown Bronze #3, but I have never seen it in action. Dream Tan can best be described as a boot polish for your skin. It comes in a container that looks like the polish I use on my cowboy boots, and the cream itself seems to be about as dark as well.

In my opinion, Dream Tan provides the best coverage and most consistent color. The only drawback is that it's incredibly messy, and many venues don't allow it. Double-check in advance to see if your federation, show promoter or venue has any special requirements on tanning solutions and if they accept Dream Tan. If they do, I highly encourage you to go with this option for your tanning color.

I've used both the Gold Brown and the Red Bronze colors. For professional backstage photos, Gold Brown is your best bet. For stage shots and optimizing your look in front of a panel of judges, I recommend Red Bronze.

You're going to need a helping hand when it comes to applying this boot polish. Unlike the spray tan, there is no need to use a coat of this the night prior. It can take 30-45 minutes or more to apply appropriately, so make sure you wake up early enough on show day to fit this into your schedule.

Like the spray tan prep, I recommend taking a shower with a salt exfoliant and avoiding lotions or oils. Once you've dried off, enlist the help of a friend or spouse to throw on some rubber gloves and start coloring you. Don't rub this dream tan solution into your skin, as that will create a smeared look and wash out your definition. Instead, cover your rubber gloves and "slap" it onto your skin.

Using your palms, gently slap the color all over your body, overlapping as you go so there aren't any handprints or bare spots. Be sure to put a light coat on your face and the tops of your feet as well—having a perfectly tan physique and a face as white as a ghost isn't a great look. Apply a thick base coat, allow that to dry and then touch up any necessary spots that need it.

Be careful once you've applied the Dream Tan solution. It will dry slightly, but it is still subject to smears. You'll want to avoid any tight-fitting waistbands or clothes that will rub it off. Bring the container with you backstage so that you can easily touch up any areas that might rub off throughout the day. After the show is over, you'll be able to scrub off most of the Dream Tan in a hot shower with a rag. It will take a few days to disappear completely, so I recommend wearing clothes you don't mind getting stained. Be sure to use old bedsheets you can discard afterward as well.

PROTAN AND JAN TANA

Both Pro Tan and Jan Tana are popular tanning solutions. I've never competed with them, but I have helped apply them to competitors. These are both D.I.Y. tanners like Dream Tan, but I find that both of these solutions offer sub-par tans by comparison.

They are much thinner and generally require several more coats. As such, they are a bit harder to apply evenly and often don't look as consistent. I suppose these are a viable option if you don't want to use the spray tan and your venue doesn't allow Dream Tan. If you have the opportunity, though, I suggest using a different tanning solution.

HAIR AND MAKEUP

I'm honestly not your best resource for hair and makeup, as I've never had to tackle this myself. I do know that many of the competitions host a sponsored hair and makeup team similar to a sponsored tanning crew. There will likely be a section at the venue with a booth set up to provide these services if this is the case.

These services are often itemized and give the option for only doing your hair or makeup or lashes versus a complete package. The prices range anywhere from $50-$300, so plan accordingly. Make sure to schedule your appointment in advance and be on time, as they likely won't have time gaps to get you dolled up outside of your scheduled time.

Many competitors choose to either do their makeup themselves or hire a third-party provider. Either option is fine, but be proactive and ensure that everything is done in time so that you aren't rushed in getting to the venue.

TRAVEL

If your competition doesn't offer a host hotel, consider staying as close to the venue as possible. I'm a huge fan of renting a nearby Airbnb rather than a hotel for several reasons. For one, they have much more personality than drab hotel rooms, which adds to the experience. Also, they are generally more equipped for cooking and meal prep. Airbnb houses provide much more space to spread out and organize and are usually much quieter than hotels.

The more quickly you can relax and acclimate to your new surroundings, the better. Regardless of where you stay, bring a spare set of sheets to sleep in. Either bring an old pair from home or purchase a cheap pair at a local store upon your arrival. Swap out the hotel or Airbnb sheets with your sheets so that your tanning rub doesn't ruin any linens, resulting in a damage fee.

If you are driving a significant distance to compete, take advantage of every opportunity you have to stand up and stretch. Sitting in a car for hours wreaks havoc on your body's blood flow and nutrient delivery. If your electrolyte equilibrium is off, you run the risk of retaining a ton of extracellular water in your lower extremities. Ensure that you are hydrated and try to elevate your feet when possible.

Arrive in time to swing by a gym and do a light circuit training session to stimulate muscles and circulate your blood. The same concept holds if you are flying to your competition location. While the flight will undoubtedly cut down on your overall transit time, being scrunched in a tiny airplane seat certainly isn't conducive to proper blood flow and muscle stimulation.

Airplane cabins have very low humidity levels, which can result in increased dehydration. Be sure to bring some extra water. Changes in pressure experienced while flying can contribute to increased stress, GI bloat and discomfort. If you are driving a long distance or flying, try to arrive several days in advance so your body has ample time to equalize.

I've included a detailed travel checklist that you can use before your departure to ensure you have everything you may need. Feel free to add to this list or subtract from it:

- Posing suit/trunks
- Tanning touchup
- Salt for exfoliation
- Sharp razor and plenty of shaving cream
- Rubber gloves for applying the tan
- Spare bedsheets
- Any necessary makeup or jewelry
- Dark, loose-fitting clothes for after you apply the tan
- Warm blanket for backstage
- Small space heater for backstage
- All your regular supplements
- Prepped meals in Tupperware or the ingredients necessary to prepare your meals upon arrival
- Large water bottle
- Salt for seasoning/electrolytes
- Can of anchovies (if you are using them for the fathead pizza refeed)
- Keto Bricks or another convenient fat source you can take with you backstage
- Posing music and a backup just in case
- Competition federation membership card (many shows allow you to purchase this upon arrival)

- Books or music to listen to backstage
- Earbuds to listen to the above music
- Journal, camera or phone to get a few clips and document this journey
- Towels
- Pump up gear like resistance bands and a few dumbbells
- Grooming gear like trimmer, razor, comb and hair product
- Sandals
- Hygiene products like toothpaste and toothbrush
- Face wipes or hand wipes
- Small fan for improved sleep while traveling
- Eating utensils
- Umbrella to protect tan if raining

COMPETITION MUSIC

If you compete in a division that allows for an individual stage routine such as the bodybuilding division, you'll need to provide your music. Clarify with the show promoter what style and length of music are allowed. Usually, competitors are granted 60 seconds of stage time to perform their routine. The show promoter will often request that your piece be delivered in advance or that you bring a copy to the competitor check-in meeting.

Some shows allow this to be delivered in an MP3 format, whereas others still prefer this in a CD format. Regardless of format, be sure to have your music cut and mastered and have a backup copy or two. Most shows will not allow for any vulgar lyrics, so be sure to keep that in mind when selecting your music.

COMPETITOR CHECK-IN

The competitor check-in usually takes place the night before the event or the morning of. The main point is to ensure that all the competitors are onsite and accounted for. This is also when many federations allow competitors to purchase their membership card, accept their competitor number, weigh-in, provide their posing music and get instructed on the overall breakdown of events and expectations when the show starts.

Many shows will also give the competitors a "goodie bag" at these check-ins. These bags often include a branded T-shirt representing the show, some protein bars and other snacks. Most of these snacks are the furthest thing from ketogenic, so I typically give my bag away to another competitor. The check-ins are a great time to meet and greet other competitors and the show promoters. Take this time to learn who's who and have fun with it.

COMPETITOR WEIGH-IN

In physique sports, there are different divisions to showcase different poses and body compositions. These divisions range from bikini to bodybuilding. Within the divisions, competitors are broken down by different height and weight classes.

Some federations only focus on weight rather than including height. The number of weight classes is mainly dependent on the size of the show. For instance, larger shows with more competitors typically require more weight classes. Below is an example of a five-class and three-class system for the open bodybuilding division within the WNBF federation.

WEIGHT CLASSES (5) - MEN'S AMATEUR BODYBUILDING

BANTAMWEIGHT

- Under 150 lb (under 68 kg)

LIGHTWEIGHT

- 150–165 lb (68.03-74.84)

MIDDLEWEIGHT

- 165.25–176 lb (74.95-79.83 kg)

LIGHT HEAVYWEIGHT

- 176.25–190 lb (79.94-86.18 kg)

HEAVYWEIGHT

- Over 190 lb (over 86.18 kg)

WEIGHT CLASSES (3) – MEN'S AMATEUR BODYBUILDING

LIGHTWEIGHT

- Under 165 lb (under 74.84 kg)

MIDDLEWEIGHT

- 165.25–189 lb (174.85–85.73 kg)

HEAVYWEIGHT

- Over 190 lb (Over 85.73 kg)

Don't think of the weigh-in in bodybuilding the same way you would a boxing match or MMA fight. In those events, fighters cut as much weight as possible and then gorge themselves to increase their weight tremendously to provide an advantage in the fight. Not only is that incredibly unhealthy, but it will also most certainly backfire on you within the context of a bodybuilding competition.

The best advice I can give you for dealing with the weight classes within the sport of bodybuilding is simple: bring your best physique on show day and be at peace with whatever weight that winds up being. Don't overthink the weight classes with this sport. Sure, if you are shredded and on the upper weight limit for a particular class, you'll likely have an advantage within the class simply because it means you are carrying as much muscle as possible. If you win your class, you'll be battling it out for the overall title anyways, so you'll have to prepare yourself for competing against others of different weights.

I'm only 5' 7", and I typically compete in the lightweight category. I can bring a level of conditioning to the stage with my short frame that is super impressive, but it requires me to get down to a much lighter weight. I usually compete at a weight of about 157-165 lb. Sure, it would be nice to have that same level of conditioning at 190 lb, but I'm simply not there yet. Rather than come to the table with a heavier frame but much less definition, I prioritize conditioning—within the sport of natural bodybuilding, better conditioning is almost always favored over sheer size.

DRUG TESTING

If you compete in a natural federation, you will likely face a preliminary polygraph test and possibly a urinalysis test. Most natural federations structure their organization so that the purchase of their federation membership card doubles as consent to drug testing. Some federations, such as the WNBF, require a 10-year span in which the athletes have not used any of the drugs listed on the banned substance list.

Failure to comply with those standards results in the athlete's immediate disqualification and stripping of all their titles. Usually, natural federations will require all competitors to complete a polygraph test the night before the competition. This test is often scheduled in advance around the same time frame as the initial competitor weigh-in and check-in.

A polygraph test, more commonly known as a "lie detector" test, measures and records several physiological factors such as your pulse rate, blood pressure, respiration and skin conductivity. These stats are all recorded as the proctor asks you a series of questions. If you are lying, there is likely an increase in your physiological stress response, and you may fail the test.

The whole process sounds a bit nerve-racking and many competitors, myself included, worry about failing simply due to the awkwardness of the environment. Don't let the anxiety of doing something as strange as a polygraph test cause you any undue stress. If you honestly haven't taken any outlawed substances, you shouldn't have anything to worry about. The proctor will likely ask you some preliminary questions such as your name and where you are from to generate a baseline scan on the biometrics. If you have nothing to hide, you'll breeze through the polygraph test with no hiccups.

The urinalysis test is a bit more expensive and harder to scale for many athletes. Many federations choose to only perform a urinalysis test on the winners of each class and those receiving a pro card. If this is the case and you place highly, expect one of the staff members to chase you down with a urinalysis cup soon after you step off the stage. Again, if you have abided by all federation regulations and avoided any banned substances, you shouldn't have anything to worry about.

Some natural federations go as far as to randomly test athletes in the off-season. This randomized testing may seem a bit invasive, but I am in full support of it! There are ways to deceive a polygraph test and there are workarounds for urinalysis exams. Anything to create a more level playing field and ensure honest athletes is fair game, in my opinion. By randomly drug testing in the off-season, athletes are less likely to slip under the radar and cheat the system.

RUNNING FORMAT

Many shows have adopted a "running format" as opposed to the traditional prejudging and finals layout. Competitors are judged on the fly with the running format, and there is less time between prejudging and awards.

Judges bring out the entire class for their quarter turns and mandatory poses similar to a prejudging round. Then, the whole class goes backstage and waits as competitors are called out individually to perform their posing routines. After all individual routines are completed, the entire class is called back for placements and awards. With this running format, an entire division and its corresponding classes are judged and placed before moving to the subsequent division.

This running format is generally a bit more efficient from a timing standpoint since there is no need for the intermission between prejudging and finals. As such, show day is typically finished much earlier than is often the case with a traditional format.

Another benefit of this running format is that you are only really trying to peak for one moment in time rather than two. Following a conventional layout, you need to bring your best package to prejudging but then be able to hold that conditioning for several hours as you wait for the finals. The vast majority of the judging occurs at prejudging, but the finals are often used to break ties and solidify the judges' decisions. Many competitors make the mistake of overindulging on food after their prejudging rounds and look a bit soft during the finals. This is avoided entirely with this running format as there isn't nearly as much time between when the judges first lay eyes on you and when you're awarded your placings.

The upside to this is also the downside. Suppose you know what you are doing with your nutrition and have everything dialed in. In that case, it's generally easy to look amazing for prejudging, continue filling out and look just as good or better later in the day for the finals. This is a clear competitive advantage over those who are less in tune with their bodies. However, with this running format, there is no opportunity to showcase your improved physique as the day progresses because you are only onstage once.

STAGE PRESENCE

How you carry yourself onstage is of extreme importance! You never want to come across cocky or exaggerated, but you want to exude an aura of incredible confidence.

Always hold your head high with your chin up. Never allow yourself to slouch forward or appear too relaxed. Don't make the mistake of thinking the judges' eyes are not pinned on you. Assume you are constantly judged, even if you are onstage behind the primary lineup, waiting your turn. You are always being watched!

When you're onstage, the bright lights will drown out much of the audience, and your adrenaline will make it hard to focus on anything in the crowd. I like to look toward the judges and make it known that I'm confident in myself and the conditioning I've brought to the stage. I'll look toward each judge individually to make my presence known in a cool, calm and collected manner. You want to smile and be respectful throughout your entire time onstage as well.

As you cycle through your poses, do so with poise and grace. The best way to ensure this is to practice, practice, practice...and then practice some more. Start practicing long before you ever step onstage. You should glide through all your mandatory poses as if your body were designed to perform them. You never want your poses to appear forced or awkward. Lock into the pose and hold your head high with confidence.

Posing is not easy! I've battled it out onstage for 15 minutes in the past! Fifteen minutes of extreme posing in which every single muscle fiber in your body is flexed is incredibly taxing. Judges will often draw out their prejudging rounds if a class is particularly competitive or if they are trying to test the conditioning of the athletes. Fifteen minutes in, the judges can quickly tell who is in shape and who is not. Exude confidence and grace even when every part of you is screaming for a break from the brutal posing.

Continue to showcase a respectful demeanor and confidence even when the placings are established and awards are given. I've seen competitors who were unhappy with their placing throw up their hands in disgust or lash out against those who placed higher. This is incredibly unprofessional and uncalled for.

This sport is supposed to be challenging, and there will most definitely be times where a more seasoned competitor bests you. That is okay! Show them the respect they deserve and shake their hand accordingly. Everyone who competes onstage has overcome obstacles, and the mutual respect and understanding that comes with that should outweigh any differences in placement.

BACK-TO-BACK SHOWS

I highly advise against competing multiple times throughout the year, especially if there is a significant time block between shows. As I wrote in the main body of this book, that is not optimal from a muscle-building, hormonal or metabolic standpoint. However, if you are incredibly lean and dialed in, you'll likely want to capitalize on that conditioning and make the most of your current cutting phase. As such, condensing your competitive window into as tight a frame as possible and stepping onstage more than once is an understandable course of action. With such an arrangement, you may be faced with back-to-back competitions with very little time in between.

You likely won't be able to truly "peak" for numerous shows, so I encourage you to have one primary show in which you plan to look your absolute best. Optimize for that show and do everything in your power to bring your best package on that day. While you may not be able to peak for multiple shows, you can likely look incredibly dialed in and damn-near perfect for a few consecutive weekends if you stay on top of your nutrition and training. If you're lucky, you'll have a few shows in close proximity to each other. If this is the case, I highly encourage you to compete in both and make the most of your competition-level conditioning.

If you do compete in two or more consecutive shows, follow the peak week protocol as outlined in the book. The only difference is you'll want to refrain from deviating too far from the target macros after the first show is complete. Save the celebratory meals for after the entire competitive season. This way, you'll be able to maintain your composition without putting on any unnecessary body fat between shows.

Your training will also have to be slightly manipulated if you are going through back-to-back peak weeks. As is true with a traditional peak week, you'll still taper your training intensity to avoid any unnecessary inflammation. You'll only have a short window in which you can train heavy the Sunday after a show through the next Tuesday of the following week.

Try to target all your muscle groups in that window with some heavy lifting so you can continue stimulating your body with heavy loads and protect against any muscle wasting. After your heavy training days, cycle back into a standard peak week protocol with reduced intensity that continues to taper as the week progresses.

＊＊

I considered writing a comprehensive question-and-answers section in the appendix of this book as a resource for those who still may have some unique questions. However, I decided against it as I could provide a more valuable resource for those with lingering questions in an ever-evolving, online format.

I receive countless questions daily, which I try to answer via my

"Ask Me Anything" videos I post weekly on my YouTube channel and host on my website at www.ketosavage.com.

As such, I encourage you to use my website as a resource for any additional questions, recipes, scientific studies, podcast interviews and training tutorials as needed. I add new content every week, and unlike a printed book, it will continue to evolve as I receive further questions and learn additional concepts.

Ketogenic natural bodybuilding is my passion and life's purpose. I am committed to continual growth and improvement, and I'm excited to deliver the wisdom I gain to you in an actionable format. Feel free to draw on any of the resources I create and publish to better your health and fitness journey. Don't hesitate to reach out to me directly if there is ever anything I can do to aid you.

Your interest in this endeavor and the support you show me by consuming my content and following my brand help me stay motivated on this path. To keep up with what I'm doing, follow me on Instagram at @ketosavage, subscribe to Live Savage on YouTube or at KetoSavage.com. You are my oxygen, and I owe you my everything!

ACKNOWLEDGMENTS

To the natural bodybuilders out there, I owe you so much. In a world filled with quick fixes, drugs and shortcuts, it has been truly empowering to witness the rising success of so many natural athletes committed to staying true to their health and playing the long game within the sport of bodybuilding. As a natural athlete myself, I have been fortunate to stand on the shoulders of giants. Seemingly everyone within the natural bodybuilding sphere is willing and wanting to share the knowledge they've gained through years of self-experimentation and trial and error. Many of the principles developed by natural athletes before me have formed some of the bedrock concepts I apply in my coaching to this day. We are all competitive, but we all realize that a rising tide raises all ships and that an open mind and ever-flowing distribution of knowledge is mutually beneficial to all. I'm proud to call myself a natural athlete, and I'm pleased to share the company of so many others who share my love for the sport of bodybuilding. May we all continue to grow and learn together.

To all scientists and medical professionals on the cutting edge of ketogenic research, I salute you. You are changing lives in ways you don't even realize. The ketogenic diet has been used to treat children with epileptic seizures for over 100 years, but that is just the tip of the iceberg. A significant body of evidence shows the efficacy of the ketogenic diet towards mitigating the devastating effects of cancer, autoimmune issues, diabetes, neurodegenerative diseases and so much more. Witnessing this research unfold and seeing it implemented to help alleviate those suffering from these illnesses is genuinely remarkable. In a society where pharmacological, reactive remedies are often the primary narrative, it's inspiring to see the momentum gained from a more holistic, proactive intervention found in the ketogenic diet and lifestyle.

To the "haters" and those of you who have doubted me over the years, I thank you dearly. To those who said I would never compete, never get lean, never be successful without carbohydrates and never be a voice in the fitness realm, I appreciate you more than you realize. To those who doubted my ambitions towards business and entrepreneurship, I thank you as well. To those who mocked me when I quit my corporate job and pursued my passion, thank you! You have all worked to stoke the embers of the fire that now burns hotter and brighter than ever.

To my clients who have believed in me and trusted in me over the years, I honestly can't thank you enough. Working with every single one of you has been an absolute pleasure. It has taught me so much and provided me with the tools necessary to develop the principles contained in this book. Your continual feedback, biometrics and personal responses to the dietary manipulations we have made have been enlightening. Beyond the macros, the muscles and the body fat lost, I appreciate the relationships I have formed with each of you. I'm proud to call you all my friends now, more so than my clients. Our initial client/coaching relationship was the gateway that led to a much deeper bond. Life is all about relationships. I'm forever grateful for the fantastic relationships that have come from working with all of you!

To the ketogenic community, I owe you my everything! You were so gracious to give me your attention and grant me a platform from which to add value. The momentum I have gained within this community has given my life a purpose. The support you've shown me by listening to my podcast, watching my YouTube videos, interacting with me on social media and supporting our business endeavors with the Keto Bricks has truly been a remarkable experience. You are my oxygen, and I'll never take it for granted. I've dedicated my life to paying it forward and continually striving to add value to this community that has shown me so much love over the years.

To my family, I love you with all my heart. I'm proud of where I come from and the way I was raised. I'm proud to have great relationships with my mother, father, brother and extended family. I'm proud to call myself a Sikes. Many of my family members don't understand what I do for a living and can't possibly comprehend how I made a career out of it. I was raised very "old school" and was expected to go to college, get a degree and work for a company for 30-40 years to make ends meet. That is a far cry from my reality. When I left home and became my own person, things had changed. Social media, the internet, open-source education and digital entrepreneurship drastically altered the landscape of how one could find success in the modern era. I fear that the disconnect between past and present may cause tension at times, but I genuinely hope to look past that. Any success I experience in life is a direct result and byproduct of the values learned in my upbringing. My folks instilled a level of discipline and work ethic that is second to none. They taught me the importance of honesty and integrity. In short, they taught me how to be a good person, self-sufficient and independent in life. I would be nothing if it weren't for my parents, Robert Smith Sikes Jr. and Penny Lee Sikes. I would be lonely if it weren't for the companionship of my brother, Tyler Austin Sikes. I likely wouldn't be nearly as business-minded and passionate about creating the products and services if it weren't for my uncle, Mark Wayne Sikes. I wouldn't be half the person I am today if it weren't for my entire family. I love you all dearly!

To my wife Crystal, my love, you are my lifeblood. You give my life purpose and make waking up each morning exciting. From the moment I first laid eyes on you until the moment I close mine forever, I'll love you with all of my heart. No paragraph blurb in a book's acknowledgment page could do you justice. Since the beginning, you have been my partner through all my endeavors, and I would be nothing if it weren't for your love and support. You've been by my side when it wasn't easy to do so. You have been there every step of the way as we've built our business, our family and our empire. You come from a very different upbringing than I, yet you truly do complete me in every way. I am continually amazed by your passion and selfless nature. You make me want to be a better person, and I am so incredibly blessed to be able to go through life with you by my side.

To my future child, Robert Rigel Sikes, my namesake, at the time of this writing, you are brewing in Crystal's belly. It's been 17 weeks since your inception, and you've created a whirlwind of emotions for me, my future and life as I know it. At this time, I can't possibly know your interests. I don't know if you'll be keen to learn more about health and wellness and how to improve your overall well-being. I certainly hope that is the case. If you ever find yourself reading this book, know that I love you. Know that I want nothing but the best for you. Know that I support you in your endeavors and encourage you to pursue your passions. Know that I want you to become an independent individual, capable of rising to the challenges that life will most certainly throw your way. Know that I believe in you and that I'm excited to see you grow. Know that I love you with all my heart, and I'm proud of the person you'll become. Believe in yourself and become whatever it is you desire. Never sacrifice your integrity, and always strive to be better tomorrow than you were today.

ABOUT THE AUTHOR

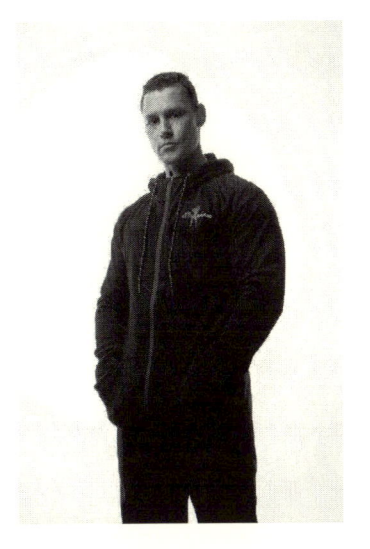

Robert Sikes is a natural ketogenic bodybuilder, author, entrepreneur, CEO and founder of Keto Savage, a health and fitness company offering coaching, training and nutrition for athletes and bodybuilders. He is also CEO and founder of Keto Brick, a company that produces ketogenic meal replacement bars for efficient nutrition with the highest quality ingredients. Sikes holds first-in-class titles from his bodybuilding competitions within the OCB and WNBF federations. Sikes lives in Northwest Arkansas with his wife Crystal. *Ketogenic Bodybuilding* is the culmination of all he has learned through his bodybuilding endeavors and client coaching practice.